AF439912

Monographs in Clinical Cytology

Vol. 23

Series Editor

Philippe Vielh Dudelange, Luxembourg

Pio Zeppa Salerno

Immacolata Cozzolino Naples

Lymph Node FNC

Cytopathology of Lymph Nodes and Extranodal Lymphoproliferative Processes

106 figures, 105 in color, and 8 tables, 2018

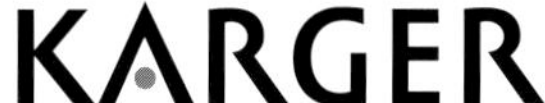

KARGER Basel · Freiburg · Paris · London · New York · Chennai · New Delhi · Bangkok · Beijing · Shanghai · Tokyo · Kuala Lumpur · Singapore · Sydney

Monographs in Clinical Cytology
Founded 1965 by Georg L. Wied, Chicago, IL

Prof. Dr. Pio Zeppa
Scuola Medica Salernitana
Pathology and Cytopathology Unit
University of Salerno
IT–84100 Salerno (Italy)

Dr. Immacolata Cozzolino
Department of Mental and Physical Health
and Preventive Medicine, Pathology Unit
Università degli Studi della Campania "Luigi Vanvitelli"
IT–80131 Naples (Italy)

Library of Congress Cataloging-in-Publication Data

Names: Zeppa, Pio, author. | Cozzolino, Immacolata, author.
Title: Lymph node FNC : lymph node cytopathology and extranodal
  lymphoproliferative processes / Pio Zeppa, Immacolata Cozzolino.
Other titles: Lymph node fine-needle cytology | Monographs in clinical
  cytology ; v. 23. 0077-0809
Description: Basel ; New York : Karger, [2018] | Series: Monographs in
  clinical cytology, ISSN 0077-0809 ; vol. 23 | Includes bibliographical
  references and index.
Identifiers: LCCN 2017036928| ISBN 9783318061147 (hard cover : alk. paper) |
  ISBN 9783318061154 (electronic version)
Subjects: | MESH: Lymphoproliferative Disorders--diagnosis | Lymph
  Nodes--cytology | Lymph Nodes--pathology | Biopsy, Fine-Needle--methods
Classification: LCC RC646 | NLM WH 700 | DDC 616.4/2075--dc23 LC record available at https://lccn.loc.gov/2017036928

Bibliographic Indices. This publication is listed in bibliographic services, including Current Contents®.

© Copyright 2018 by S. Karger AG, P.O. Box, CH-4009 Basel (Switzerland)
www.karger.com
Printed on acid-free and non-aging paper (ISO 9706)
ISSN 0077–0809
ISBN 978–3–318–06114–7
e-ISBN 978–3–318–06115–4

Contents

Preface

Whereas fine-needle cytology (FNC) is a well-established diagnostic procedure, lymph node (LN) and lymphoproliferative processes remain the most controversial application of FNC. In times that may seem very distant to the new generations of pathologists, when "nodular" or "diffuse" were the diagnostic pillars of a lymphoma and "basal membrane or capsular invasion" the almost only affordable biological markers, distrust and scepticism towards LN-FNC were almost consequential. Nonetheless, since the dawn of cytology, LN-FNC has always been requested by clinicians and mainly performed by cytopathologists who have always depended on excellent articles and books that explored and explained, in cytological terms, different and often complex lymphoproliferative processes.

In the last 50 years, pathology in general, and LN pathology overall, has undergone radical transformations, and diagnostic criteria have become less histological and more cytological, phenotypical, cytogenetical, and molecular. In the meantime, cytopathology has changed and cytopathologists have learned to apply the same ancillary techniques and procedures used in histopathology on FNC samples, including LN-FNC. Consequently, clinicians and patients have gradually grown in confidence regarding LN-FNC. Nonetheless, LN-FNC is still something different – or something more than histopathology. Ancillary techniques are indispens-able, but not sufficient for the ambitious task of producing diagnostic, prognostic, and predictive information, both affordable and clinically suitable, from cells obtained easily, quickly, and inexpensively, as is the case with FNC. For this purpose, a cytopathologist devoted to LN-FNC should be acquainted with pathology and specifically haematopathology, including its clinical aspects, should have a basic knowledge of imaging techniques and good dexterity for performing FNC and smearing and material management. He or she should also be able to execute rapid on-site evaluation (ROSE) and choose the most effective ancillary technique case by case. The cytopathologist has to thoroughly evaluate clinical data, cytological features, and the evidence from ancillary techniques to produce a timely and effective diagnostic report. Above all, the cytopathologist should realize the limits of LN-FNC and refrain from pushing the procedure beyond its own possibilities. Finally, cytopathologists should be aware that a FNC diagnosis fully confirmed by any ancillary technique but too much delayed may be useless.

Volume 18 in the *Monographs in Clinical Cytology* series (*FNA Cytology in the Diagnosis of Lymphoma* by L. Skoog and E. Tani, 2009) is a sparkling example of the transformation of LN-FNC over time; starting from the solid foundation of clinical cytology, the authors applied immunocytochemistry and other ancillary techniques to cytological samples for clonality

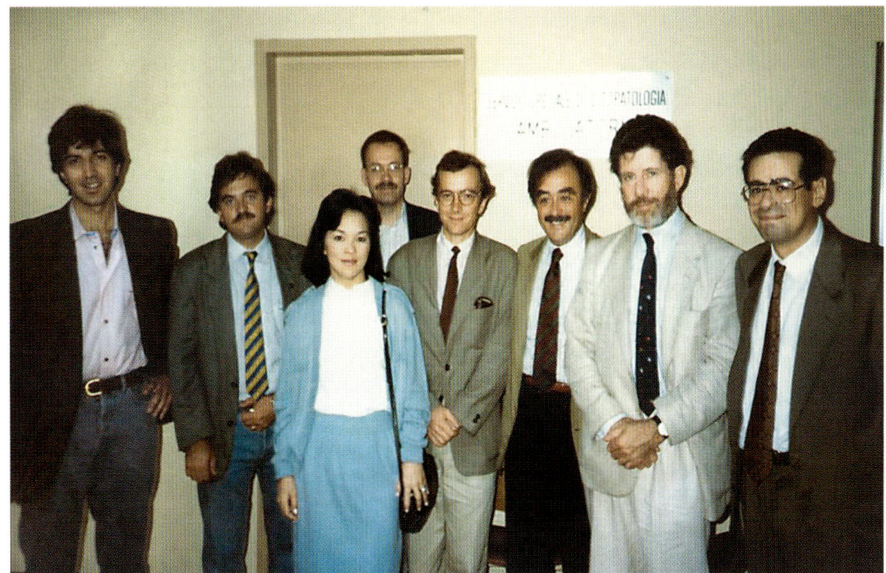

Fig. 1. The commemorative photo, taken outside the outpatients office of the FNC service on the occasion of the 8th Course on Lymph Node Cytopathology, which was held in Naples in September 1990. From left to right: Giancarlo Troncone, Giuseppe Di Benedetto, Edneia Tani, Lambert Skoog, Pio Zeppa, Lucio Palombini, David Mason, and Franco Fulciniti.

assessment and, more generally, for an accurate diagnosis and classification of different lymphoproliferative processes. Consequently, the gap between LN pathology and LN-FNC has been reduced, but the process of LN-FNC upgrading is far from complete. Recent decades have also seen the "molecular revolution" of pathology; molecular biology is going to redefine and reclassify traditional pathological entities, providing predictive information other than diagnostic and prognostic data by the application of extremely sophisticated procedures to the smallest samples. Cytopathology is involved in this new stimulating challenge and this edition of the book aims to update LN-FNC and provide basic support to cytopathologists along this uneasy and complex transformation.

In addition to the authors, different people, events, factors, and causalities contributed to the making of this monograph. Like the "dots" of Steve Jobs' life reported in his "commencement address" (2005), they were hardly connectable looking forwards but we can connect the "dots" now, looking backwards, and we will

briefly summarize them here. In 1977, Lucio Palombini spent a 6-month fellowship at the Cytopathology Service of the Karolinska Hospital, Stockholm, Sweden, where he studied FNC in that formidable school with Josef Zajicek, Torsten Lowagen, PierLuigi Esposti, and Sixten Franzén. Once back in Naples, he founded the Cytopathology Service at the Department of Pathology of the "Federico II" University of Naples. Over time, Antonio Vetrani, Franco Fulciniti, myself, Giancarlo Troncone, and Immacolata Cozzolino joined the team. In 1990, during our annual Cytopathology Course, Lambert Skoog and Edneia Tani, again from the Karolinska Hospital, and the authors of volume 18 of the *Monographs in Clinical Cytology* series on lymph nodes, as well as David Mason from Oxford University, were all invited to hold a course on LN-FNC (Fig. 1). At that time, my knowledge of the subject was very sparse and I was not particularly interested in LN cytopathology. Yet, I was fascinated by Mason's sparkling approach to haematopathology and by the disarming simplicity and effectiveness of

Skoog's and Tani's approach to LN-FNC. Since then, I, and afterwards Immacolata, have been more and more involved in LN-FNC. When Philippe Vielh asked us to prepare the new edition of the monograph, the proposal was flattering and at the same time intimidating, but on starting the job and looking backwards, these "dots" of our professional experience began to connect.

This monograph is for all cytopathologists devoted to LN-FNC. It is intended to provide them with some help in this difficult, little rewarding, and stressful, but also intriguing, challenging, and beautiful task.

Acknowledgments

This book is the result not only of our work and efforts but also of all the people mentioned above, who deserve considerable thanks. We are also grateful to the unforgotten Bruno Rotoli, and to Amalia De Renzo, Marco Picardi, Carmine Selleri, and Fabrizio Pane (haematologists), Giancarlo Villani (cytofluorimetric analyst), Rita Genesio (geneticist), Annalucia Peluso (molecular biologist), Gaetano De Rosa, Guido Pettinato, Carlo Baldi, Renato Franco (pathologists), and Ruth Katz from MD Anderson Cancer Center, Houston. Special thanks are extended to Michela Renna (interpreter and translator), and to Philippe Vielh, Thomas Nold, and Rebecca Ganz from Karger Publishers.

Pio Zeppa, Salerno
Immacolata Cozzolino, Naples

Zeppa P, Cozzolino I: Lymph Node FNC. Cytopathology of Lymph Nodes and Extranodal Lymphoproliferative Processes.
Monogr Clin Cytol. Basel, Karger, 2018, vol 23, pp 1–3 (DOI: 10.1159/000478876)

Historical Background, Clinical Applications, Controversies

Historical Background

The use of needles for diagnostic and therapeutic purposes dates back a long time [1], but the first true fine-needle cytology (FNC) was probably performed in 1904 by Greig and Gray [2], Marine officers who identified trypanosomes in lymph node (LN) smears. In 1912, Hirschfeld [3], a German haematologist, diagnosed cutaneous lymphomas and other tumours by FNC. Subsequently, in 1914, a "lymphoblastoma" was diagnosed by FNC on Romanowsky-stained smears [4]. Systematic studies on LN-FNC were then performed at John Hopkins Hospital in Baltimore [5] using 21-G needles and air-dried Romanowsky-stained smears, but Dudgeon and Patrick [6] were probably the first to define the FNC technique. In the 1920s, 2 research groups [7, 8] from the Memorial Sloan Kettering Cancer Center (MSKCC) in New York worked independently on large FNC series from different organs, with LNs significantly represented. The study carried out by Martin and Ellis [8] also documents the initial distrust towards the diagnostic potentialities of FNC; in fact, James Ewing, chief of the Pathology Department of the MSKCC, disapproved the study because he believed the procedure increased the risk of spreading cancer cells, and prevented pathologists at his Department from participating in the study that was finally published by Martin, a surgeon, and Ellis, a technician [8]. Some years later, Stewart [9], who was the successor of Ewing, published the results of another FNC study performed on a large cohort of organs, including LNs. Other sporadic studies appeared in the literature over time, but FNC was "officially" accepted as a diagnostic tool only in the 1960s at the Karolinska Hospital in Stockholm, Sweden, where a group of talented and dedicated cytopathologists established an FNC cytopathology service (Fig. 1). These cytopathologists explored all the fields of FNC, in-

cluding LNs. During the same period, other pioneers of cytopathology contributed to the development of LN-FNC, including Söderström [10], Lopes-Cardozo [11], Zajicek [12] (Fig. 2), and Linsk and Franzen [13]. Since then, FNC has spread all over the world and nowadays it is routinely used in the diagnosis of different organs. As for LN-FNC, several distinguished cytopathologists have worked on this technique, leading to significant advances. For instance, Skoog and Tani [14] from Karolinska Hospital assessed the application of immunocytochemistry on cytospins prepared from cell suspensions of LN-FNC to diagnose and classify non-Hodgkin lymphoma. Katz et al. [15], from the MD Anderson Cancer Center in Houston, applied flow cytometry on LN-FNC. In the wake of their experiences, as well as those of other leading cytopathologists, LN-FNC has been thoroughly investigated, highlighting the advantages and limitations of the technique. Nowadays, despite some criticism and distrust, LN-FNC is a generally accepted procedure in the first diagnosis of LN enlargement (LNe). Over time, cytopathologists have applied different ancillary techniques to LN-FNC, enhancing its potentialities. Finally, the exponential use of molecular techniques has involved every field of diagnostic pathology, including FNC. Numerous studies have demonstrated that vital cells obtained by FNC are excellent samples for any molecular study, opening new and challenging applications of LN-FNC.

Clinical Applications

LNe and its clinical evaluation can be an uncomfortable task for clinicians. In most cases, in a clear clinical context, the diagnosis of reactive enlargement is quite straightforward, as well as the identification of related therapeutic proce-

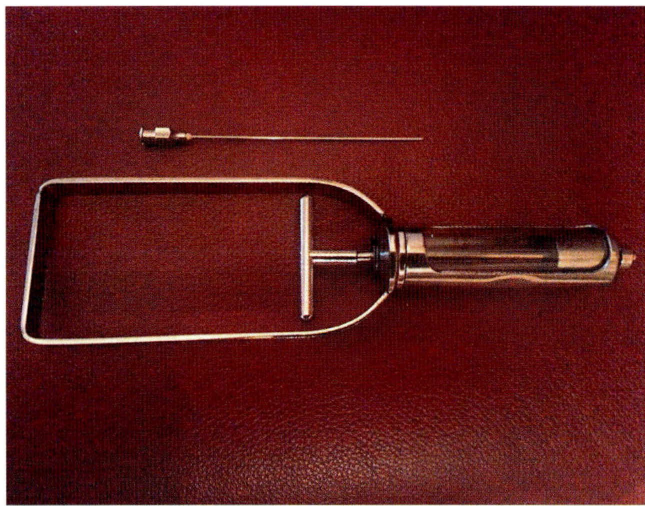

Fig. 1. A crafted aspiration biopsy syringe gun, based on an idea of Sixten Franzén, before the industrial production of similar instruments. The equipment was donated to Lucio Palombini by Torsten Lowagen in Naples during the 6th Course of Cytopathology in 1988. (Courtesy of Lucio Palombini, Professor emeritus, University of Naples "Federico II").

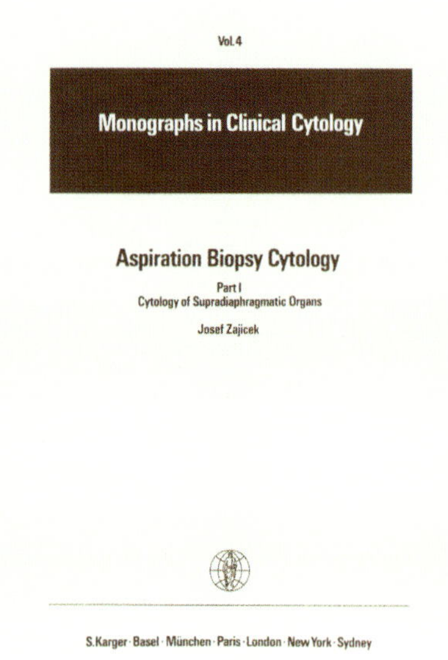

Fig. 2. *Monographs in Clinical Cytology: Aspiration Biopsy Cytology. Part I. Cytology of Supradiaphragmatic Organs* by Dr. Josef Zajicek [12] from the Karolinska Institute (Sweden). An excellent chapter of the book dealt with lymph node cytopathology.

dures. This fortunate occurrence may not always be present, because the site, the number, the size, the consistency, and the responsiveness to the therapy of involved LNs may be extremely variable. Moreover, LNe may have different clinical meanings, depending on the age and clinical history of the patient. Therefore, when the clinical presentation is less clear and serological data do not explain or do not match the clinical context, instrumental evaluations are usually required. Ultrasound evaluation, computed tomography, and other non-invasive procedures are usually helpful to obtain information that can suggest the nature of the lymphadenopathy. Unfortunately, these non-invasive procedures rarely lead to a definitive diagnosis and, if LNe persists, surgical excision and histological evaluation are the next steps. However, surgical excision is a demanding procedure for the patient and the physician, as well as for the health care system; it may require hospitalization, a complete surgical procedure, and it is not completely free from complications. The following histological examination requires additional time and costs, but is the basis for therapy and prognostic evaluations, mainly in lymphoma cases. However, the same histological examination might identify benign reactive hyperplasia or, in the worst cases, a metastasis from a known or unknown primary tumour. In these specific cases, surgical biopsy might be "too much" or "too little." FNC is an accurate, quick, and cost-effective procedure that can be used in the diagnosis of LNes. With reference to LN-FNC, in the absence of widely accepted guidelines or consensus conferences on technical procedures and diagnostic criteria, the value of FNC diagnoses varies among countries and institutions. As a consequence, the clinical relevance of LN-FNC diagnoses is lower in comparison to FNC of the thyroid, lung, or other anatomical areas in which definite FNC diagnoses are utilized for therapeutic decisions, without the need for a subsequent histological examination. The authors believe that LN-FNC diagnoses do not require histological confirmation in cases of benign reactive hyperplasia, lymphoma relapses, and metastases in which LN-FNC, provided with ancillary techniques, match clinical, instrumental, and serological data.

The histological confirmation is necessary in the case of an LN-FNC diagnosis of primary Hodgkin and non-Hodgkin lymphoma, with the exception of specific clinical situations in which biopsies cannot be performed. A histological control is also necessary when the FNC diagnosis does not match clinical, instrumental, and serological data.

Controversies

Despite its long tradition, LN-FNC is far from being a universally accepted diagnostic tool. As previously mentioned, the lack of consensus or accepted guidelines is one of the main limitations of this procedure. Moreover, its low reproducibility, its operator dependency, and the shortage of trained cytopathologists in this specific field has often generated distrust among clinicians and histopathologists. Even the efficacy of FNC on metastatic LNs has been questioned because of the possible occurrence of missing micrometastases. The main controversial field of LN-FNC is haematopathology, and specifically the lymphoma diagnosis. The zenith of distrust and criticism towards the lymphoma diagnosis by means of FNC was reached in an article published in a leading journal [16] where, on the basis of a questionable analysis of an heterogeneous series of LN-FNC diagnosed with or without the usage of ancillary techniques, the authors concluded that "FNC for lymphoma diagnosis is not helpful, not cost-effective and in addition may misguide treatment." Katz [17] countered this pointless criticism and confirmed the usefulness of LN-FNC. Distrust and criticisms rely on the fact that haematopathology is probably the most complex field of pathology, in which diagnoses and prognostic evaluations are increasingly complex, requiring ancillary techniques and highly specific knowledge. These factors led clinical haematologists and haematopathologists to circumscribe professional knowledge and tools, and this attitude restricted the access of cytopathologists and general pathologists to the field. Despite these artificial boundaries, lymphoid pathologies may involve non-lymphoid organs. Conversely, non-haematological pathologies may arise or involve lymphoid organs, leading to inextricable connections. Therefore, cytopathologists may face complex or rare "haematological" pathologies in LN and extranodal organs. Hence, they are required to have specific knowledge and professional skills in haematopathology [18]. Evaluating LN samples may be a challenging task. In the case of extranodal lymphoid pathologies, such as body cavity effusions, cerebrospinal fluid, or other organs and tissues, the task may be even more challenging. However, cytopathology may depend on well-defined diagnostic criteria that are not necessarily the same as histopathology. Moreover, haematopathology has become less "histological" and increasingly phenotypical and molecular; in the meantime cytopathologists have learned to apply the same ancillary techniques on FNC samples that are used on tissues. As a result, despite the distrust and criticism, FNC is successfully used to diagnose and subclassify lymphoproliferative processes, both in general hospitals and prestigious institutions all over the world.

References

1 Sharif K: Al-Zahwrawi Albucasis – a light in the dark Middle Ages in Europe. J Int Soc History Islamic Med 2003;1:37–38.
2 Greig E, Gray A: Note on the lymphatic glands in sleeping sickness. Proc R Soc London 1904;1:455–456.
3 Hirschfeld H: Über isolierte aleukämische Lymphadenose der Haut. Z Krebsforsch 1912;11:397–407.
4 Ward GR: Bedside Haematology: An Introduction to the Clinical Study of the So-Called Blood Diseases and of Allied Disorders. Philadelphia, WB Saunders, 1914.
5 Guthrie C: Gland puncture as a diagnostic measure. Bull Johns Hopkins Hosp 1921;32:266–269.
6 Dudgeon LS, Patrick SV: A new method for the rapid microscopical diagnosis of tumors: with an account of 200 cases examined. Br J Surg 1927;15:250–261.
7 Coley BL, Sharp GS, Ellis EB: Diagnosis of bone tumors by aspiration. Am J Surg 1931;13:215–224.
8 Martin H, Ellis EB: Biopsy by needle puncture and aspiration. Ann Surg 1930;92:169–181.
9 Stewart FW: The diagnosis of tumors by aspiration. Am J Pathol 1933;9:801–808.
10 Söderström N: Fine Needle Aspiration Biopsy. Stockholm, Almgvist and Wiksell/Gebers, 1966.
11 Lopes-Cardozo P: Atlas of Clinical Cytology. Leiden, Targa Hertogenbosch, 1975.
12 Zajicek J: Aspiration Biopsy Cytology. Part I: Cytology of Supradiaphragmatic Organs. Basel, Karger, 1974, vol 4.
13 Linsk J, Franzen S: Clinical Aspiration Cytology. Philadelphia, Lippincott, Williams & Wilkins, 1989.
14 Skoog L, Tani E: FNA Cytology in the Diagnosis of Lymphoma. Monogr Clin Cytol. Basel, Karger, 2009.
15 Katz RL, Gritsman A, Cabanillas F, Fanning CV, Dekmezian R, Ordonez NG, Barlogie B, Butler JJ: Fine-needle aspiration cytology of peripheral T-cell lymphoma: a cytologic, immunologic, and cytometric study. Am J Clin Pathol 1989;91:120–131.
16 Hehn ST, Grogan TM, Miller TP: Utility of fine-needle aspiration as a diagnostic technique in lymphoma. J Clin Oncol 2004;22:3046–3052.
17 Katz RL: Modern approach to lymphoma diagnosis by fine-needle aspiration: restoring respect to a valuable procedure. Cancer 2005;105:429–431.
18 Zeppa P: Haematocytopathology: why? Cytopathology 2012;23:73–75.

Chapter 1

Zeppa P, Cozzolino I: Lymph Node FNC. Cytopathology of Lymph Nodes and Extranodal Lymphoproliferative Processes.
Monogr Clin Cytol. Basel, Karger, 2018, vol 23, pp 4–13 (DOI: 10.1159/000478877)

Fine-Needle Cytology: Technical Procedures and Ancillary Techniques

Preliminary Aspects

Despite the efforts towards automated diagnostic procedures, fine-needle cytology (FNC), with or without aspiration, smearing, rapid on-site evaluation (ROSE), and material management remain operator-dependent procedures that require manual and professional skills. Much of the efficacy of the method and of ancillary techniques depends on the correctness of the initial procedures. Conversely, FNC non-effectiveness and many diagnostic mistakes are caused by inadequate or inaccurate FNC. Therefore, perfect sampling, smearing, staining, ROSE, and a proper management of the diagnostic material are key points to achieve an adequate and effective lymph node (LN)-FNC. In some institutions, FNC is performed by clinicians, while cytopathologists are required to evaluate and diagnose smears. However, the authors believe that LN-FNC should be performed by the cytopathologists themselves in order to optimize the procedures, as is described below. A preliminary evaluation of clinical, serological, and imaging data is required, possibly in the presence of patients. Routine laboratory data including prothrombin time, partial thromboplastin time, and platelet count should be checked before FNC, with severe coagulation disorders representing contraindications.

Steroid treatment should be interrupted before FNC because it may reduce the LN size and affect the pathological patterns. During this phase, the patient should be informed about FNC and its purposes, diagnostic possibilities, and limitations, including possible risks (pain, micro-haemorrhages, vagal stimulation). Finally, the patient should sign an informed consent form, including the permission to use residual material and obtained data for scientific purposes. This preliminary approach is useful for the diagnosis, as well as to put the patient at ease – the calmer the patient, the easier the FNC.

FNC Procedure

Perfect FNC and accurate management of the diagnostic material are crucial in diagnostic cytology, and even more so in LN-FNC, where perfect smears and ROSE are the first steps for a correct and accurate FNC. FNC requires slides, a mechanical syringe holder, 10- or 20-mL syringes that provide a sufficient negative pressure for aspiration, 22/25-G needles with different lengths, a disinfectant, cotton wool, and adhesive plasters. During FNC, the needle can be guided by palpation, by means of ultrasound (US), computed tomography (CT), or transoesophageal-transbronchial endoscopic US (EUS-EBUS). The "finger-guided" mode is generally used for palpable, superficial, and bulky LNs and/or in specific anatomical sites, such as axillary LNs, where FNC can be performed by immobilizing the LN with 2 fingers on the thoracic wall. US provides information on the nature of the target LN, its size, shape, cortex, hilum, echogenicity, vascular pattern, anatomical relations with other structures, and distance from the skin (Fig. 1). US-guided FNC is required in the case of impalpable and deeply located LNs, and it is also useful in the case of palpable LNs because it may guide the "needle tip" in specific areas of the LN (e.g., the cortex, abnormally vascular areas rather than the medulla). US-guided FNC is performed by inserting the needle in the adapter guide and following the needle track. US-assisted FNC is performed by inserting the needle tangentially to the probe, without any adaptor, with different inclinations of the needle and an angle ranging from 0° in the deeply located LN to 90° in the most superficial LN (Fig. 1). In both cases, the blunt end of the needle should be oriented towards the probe to increase US reflectivity. Therefore, if the LN is located deeply, the needle should be less inclined or almost parallel to the probe. On the contrary, the needle should be progressively inclined up to being perpendicular to the probe in a case of subcutaneous LN (Fig. 1). US-guided FNC allows an accurate hit of the target, but limits needle excursions. US-assisted FNC is less straightforward, but it allows radial excursions of the needle. Neither of the 2 options is better than the other; the selection depends on the specific context and on the operator's preference. CT-assisted FNC is generally used in thoracic, abdominal, and pelvic LNs that are not visible or attainable by US. CT assistance may also be used when US is not suitable, as in the case of obese patients, because of the attenuation of the ultrasonic beam caused by fat tissue. CT assistance allows an exact 3-dimensional localization of the target LN, even in patients with surgical wounds, bandages, and cutaneous anastomosis. In addition, CT enables an accurate choice of the access point with different angles to minimize the risk of crossing vascular structures, intestinal loops, and nonpathological tissues. Deep-located thoracic and retroperitoneal LNs can be sampled by EBUS and EUS, respectively. In these procedures, sampling is performed by endoscopists and the role of cytopathologists is limited to smearing, ROSE, and the management of diagnostic material. However, in many Institutions, ROSE is not included in the official tasks of cytopathologists and is assigned instead to cytotechnologists. As an alternative,

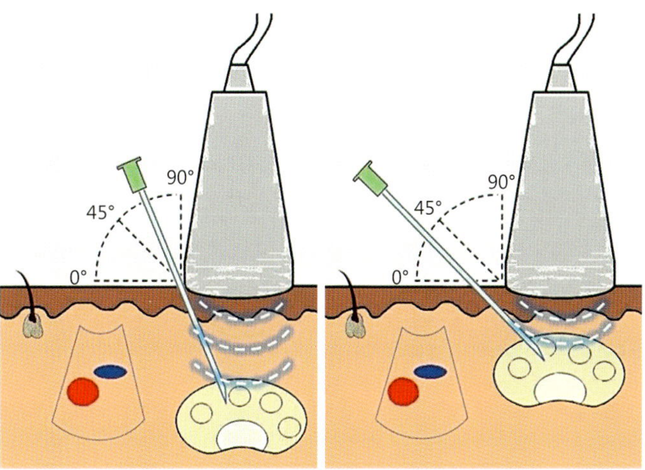

Fig. 1. "US-assisted" LN-FNC. US provides information about LN features and the power Doppler about its vascular pattern and perinodal vessels. US guidance directs the needle towards the most significant LN areas. The needle is inserted tangentially to the probe with different inclinations and an angle ranging from 0° for deeply located LNs to 90° for superficial LNs. The blunt end of the needle is oriented towards the probe to increase US reflectivity.

FNC is processed by means of liquid-based cytology (LBC). LN-FNC, with or without aspiration, is generally performed using 22/25-G needles of different lengths, on the basis of the distance of the LN from the skin and the technical approach. In the case of long needles with stylets, attention should be paid to keeping the stylets completely inserted into the needle until the LN is reached, in order to avoid the collection of cells and tissue fragments along the needle track. The needle generally finds different resistances in its path; when it passes through the LN capsule, the resistance perceived informs whether the LN is soft, hard, fibrous, or crushing; this information is also useful during smear preparation. During the aspiration, the needle should be moved gently up and down, with possible radial excursions, depending on the size of the LN. The aspiration should be interrupted when material or blood appears in the hub of the needle because it may move diagnostic material out of the needle cone into the syringe. This event can spoil the smear and cause a microhaemorrhage that could compromise a second pass. An FNC performed for more than 20 seconds should be avoided, except for "fibrous" cases, because it can be useless and cause microhaemorrhages. Attention should also be paid to the cleanliness of the slides, as dust or little glass shards may spoil the smears. Aspirated or non-aspirated material should be flushed very gently so that it can be divided into small drops to prepare

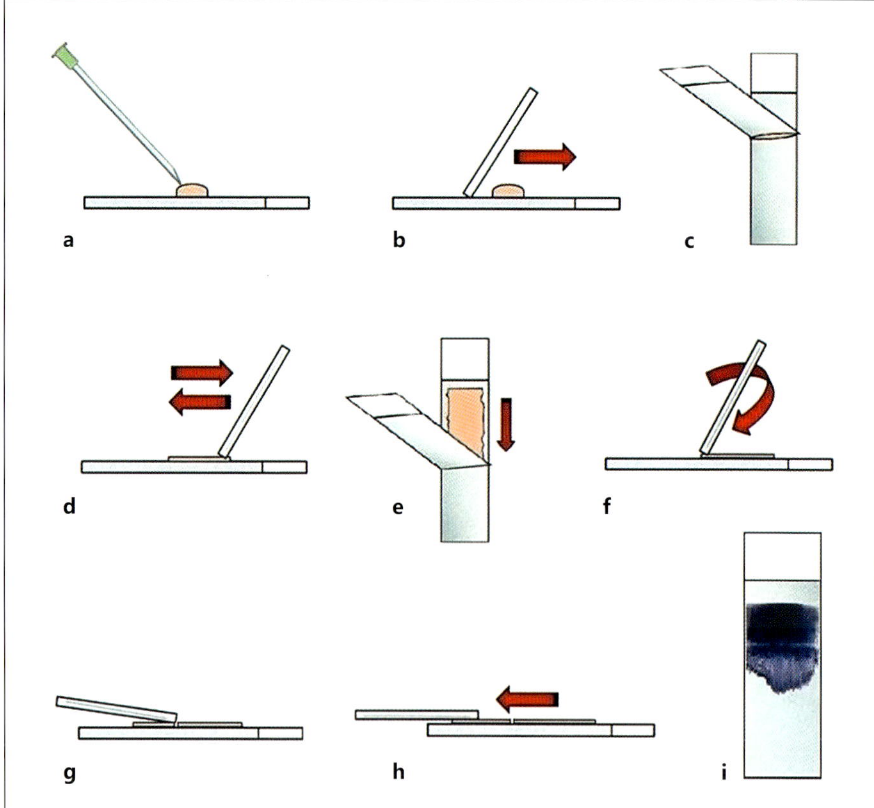

Fig. 2. Haematological smearing of fluid material. A drop of fluid is applied to the first slide (**a**); the end of the second slide is placed upright on the material of the first slide. In this way, the material is properly distributed along the width of the first slide and the end of the second slide. Then, the second slide is quickly moved forwards and backwards on the first slide (**b–e**). The second slide is then turned and juxtaposed to the distal part of the material and moved forward with a single movement and uniform pressure (**f–h**). In this way, the fluid is distributed to the proximal part of the first slide and the cells stay on its distal part (**i**). The homogeneous distribution of staining and uniform "tails" at the distal edge of the smear are key features to assess the correct execution of smearing.

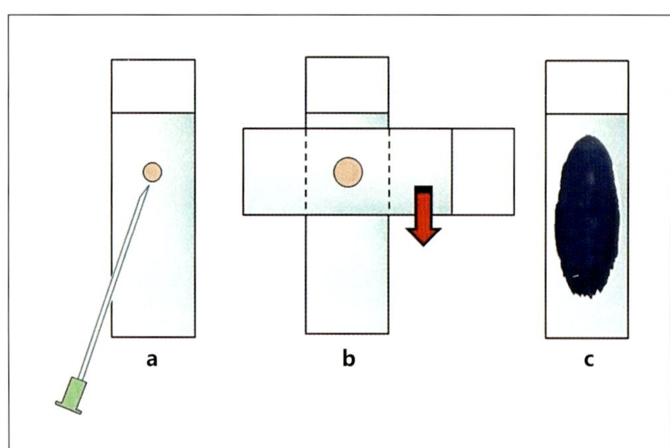

Fig. 3. Direct smearing of dense material. **a** One or more drops of dense material are gently placed on 1 or more slides, respectively. **b** A second slide is juxtaposed on the drop and moved forwards with a single movement and uniform pressure. **c** The homogeneous distribution of staining and the uniform "tails" at the distal edge of the smear are key features to assess the correct execution of smearing.

multiple conventional smears or used for ancillary techniques. The number of prepared slides depends on the quantity of material, the diagnostic needs, and the clinical data; flushing the whole material on a single slide is useless and might also hamper the smearing. The smearing technique should be chosen on the basis of the quality of the material: a haematological technique (smearing with the edge of another slide) is used in cases of fluid material (Fig. 2), while the direct smear (smearing between 2 slides) is advisable in cases of dense material (Fig. 3). Slides preparation should be rapid to prevent coagulation and cells from drying. The pressure exerted on the slides should be gentle but firm and uniform in order to avoid mechanical trauma and to preserve the morphology of the lymphoid cells that are fragile and easily crushed with pressure. In this way, it is possible to obtain thin and uniform smears along the whole glass surface (Fig. 2, 3). Two conventional smears, 1 air dried and 1 immediately alcohol fixed, Diff-Quik, and Papanicolaou stained, respectively, are the basic diagnostic tools. Residual material and additional passes should be managed according to the clinical data and ROSE.

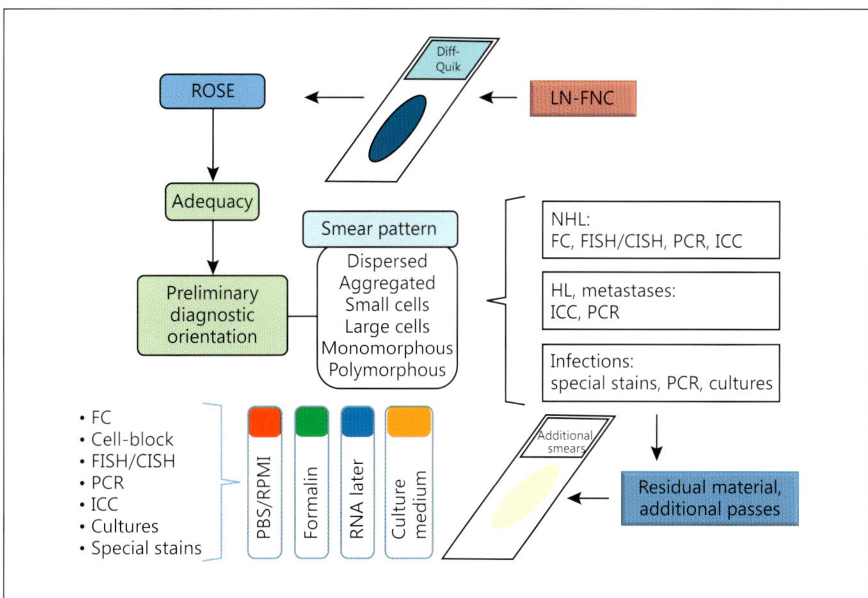

Fig. 4. ROSE allows an immediate adequacy assessment, a preliminary diagnostic orientation, and the management of residual material and additional passes. Ancillary techniques and corresponding technical supports are chosen accordingly.

LN-FNC rarely leads to complications; haematoma is the most common, occurring in less than 1% of cases [1]. Haematoma may be prevented by applying a pressure on the targeted LN using disinfectant with cotton wool. In cases of patients with mild coagulopathy and a deep-located LN, haematoma can be prevented by using appropriate blood products [1]. Pneumothorax is an extremely rare complication that may occur following deep axillary or supraclavicular LN-FNC [1]. LN damage caused by the needle track may also occur as focal haemorrhages, and segmental or total infarction. These changes are extremely rare and rarely preclude the subsequent histological assessment [2, 3].

Smear Management and ROSE

ROSE on Diff-Quik-stained smears permits an immediate adequacy evaluation, indicates the managing of residual material if any (Fig. 4), and suggests additional passes if necessary. Adequacy should be evaluated on the basis of clinical data, LN size and anatomical site, the used FNC technique (US-guided, CT-assisted, EUS-EBUS), and the ROSE evaluation. There are no "adequacy minimum criteria" for LN-FNC; adequacy should be determined case-by-case, also taking into account the nature of the location of the target LN, the difficulties in performing FNC, and the patient's compliance. Smear adequacy is also related to the smearing procedure, fixation, and staining. Air-dried Diff-Quik and 95° al-

cohol-fixed Papanicolaou or haematoxylin and eosin-stained smears are the most common used. Diff-Quik staining allows ROSE, preserves the background, and highlights fibrous cells and matrix metachromasia, as well as the orange granules of eosinophils and lymphoglandular bodies. Papanicolaou stain highlights nuclear features (chromatin texture, nucleoli, convolutions, and knobs) and cytoplasm in specific contexts (i.e., cytoplasmic orangeophilia of metastatic squamous cells). Papanicolaou stained smears may also be destained and used for immunocytochemistry (ICC).

Other Technical Supports

Residual material and additional passes (Fig. 4) may be used on different technical supports on the basis of the procedures available in each laboratory. Cell suspensions in buffer or RPMI may be divided for flow cytometry (FC) and/or cytocentrifugation and cytospin preparation. Cytospins may be used for ICC assessment and cell storage, and are the preferred method in the case of poorly cellular samples. Cell blocks (CB) of buffered-formalin or alcohol-fixed cell suspensions are another technical support, especially effective for ICC. LBC, originally conceived for cervical smears, has been extended to other cytological samples, including LN-FNC [4, 5]. As for cell storage, cytospins, CB, –80° cell suspensions, and more recently FTA cards, are suitable possibilities for any further ancillary technique [6].

Core-Needle Biopsy

Core-needle biopsy (CNB) is a more invasive diagnostic procedure in comparison to FNC [7–11]. It requires local anaesthesia, with minimum preparation of the patient. CNB and FNC share the same contraindications, and antiplatelet and/or anticoagulant therapy should be suspended before CNB. Steroid treatment should also be interrupted before CNB because it may reduce the LN size and affect the pathological patterns; CNB also requires a limited observation period of about 2–3 h [7]. CNB should be performed along the major axis on LNs larger than 20 mm. After disinfecting and circumscribing the operative area with sterile drapes, the probe with a needle holder is placed next to the point of entrance of the needle with a slight lateral inclination. The disinfected probe may be covered with a plastic biopsy bag or a sterile probe cover. Needle gauges range between 14 and 20 and each needle pass removes a tissue fragment. Automatic and semiautomatic types of biopsy gun can be used according to the experience and the needs of the operator; both systems may lead to satisfactory specimens. A CNB specimen is considered adequate when 2–3 fragments of at least 10 mm of tissue are obtained [7–11]. Fragments are fixed in buffered formalin and histologically processed. CNB complications include bleeding, haematoma and the LN necrosis [7–11].

Ancillary Techniques

Ancillary techniques include ICC, FC, fluorescence in situ hybridization (FISH), chromogenic in situ hybridization (CISH), and molecular procedures; they are useful or indispensable for an accurate LN-FNC diagnosis in most cases, especially in cases of non-Hodgkin lymphoma (NHL). Ancillary techniques are used to distinguish NHL from benign reactive hyperplasia, to classify NHL, and to identify diagnostic cells in Hodgkin lymphoma (HL) and metastasis. FNC material is usually scanty and the choice of an available specific technique is aimed at the most effective use of the material, as suggested by several algorithms [12–25].

ICC is the most commonly used technique, with high specificity and sensitivity [14]. It can be performed on different supports, such as conventional dedicated or destained smears, cytospins, Thin-Prep, and CB, with different fixations [15–17]. Both alkaline phosphatase-anti-alkaline phosphatase and immunoperoxidase can be used on cytological preparations. In the absence of official guidelines, the cytological support for ICC preferred by the authors is the CB technique. However, additional smears for ICC are preferred when only a few diagnostic cells are present on smears (i.e., CD15 and CD30 for Hodgkin and Reed-Sternberg cells). Although an unstained smear should be better than a prestained slide, the advantage of using prestained slides depends on the certainty of the quality smear and the presence of diagnostic cells. Excessive blood, background contamination, and the long-term permanence of smears in alcohol may hamper ICC and should be taken into account when selecting slides. ICC procedures have been exhaustively described [15–17]; the main advantages of ICC on CB are the number of sections available, the possibility of long-term storage, and the same antigenicity conditions of formalin-fixed CB and conventional histological sections. The main limitation of ICC on LN-FNC, on any support, is the possible need to test NHL cells for a large panel of antibodies that exceed the number of additional smears, cytospins, or CB sections available. A shortage of diagnostic material, difficulties in signals quantification (i.e., light chain expression), and the impossibility of antigen co-expression detection are other limitations of ICC on LN-FNC.

FC is the basic LN-FNC ancillary technique in the diagnosis and classification of NHL through the evaluation of B- and T-cell antigens and the clonality assessment of light chains. FC allows the assessment and simultaneous evaluation of several surface antigens, providing objective and semi-quantitative data on suspensions of vital cells. Clonality may be assessed by the kappa and lambda light chain ratio or indirectly through specific phenotypes. FC is also acquiring a role in the identification of antigens useful for prognostic evaluations [18] or potentially targeted by specific therapies. FC needs a cell suspension generally obtained by a dedicated pass and collected in a medium like PBS or RPMI-1640 solution that maintains the viability of cells; a normal buffered saline solution is also acceptable. The cell suspension should be processed as soon as possible, within 12 h, and is labelled with single or multiple fluorochrome-conjugated antibodies. After conjugation, cell degeneration may be prevented by fixation, adding a drop of buffered formalin, in this way the analysis may be postponed or repeated provided that the cell suspensions are preserved in the dark at 4°C. The analysis is then performed through flow cytometers in which cells are aligned in a laminar flow and forced to pass, one by one, through an analysis chamber. Cells are hit by laser beams that produce light in the UV and/or visible range, providing data on cell size and structural complexity. When hit by the laser beam, fluorochrome-stained cells are excited and emit fluorescent signals at a determined wavelength on the basis of the conjugated fluorochromes. Emitted fluorescent signals are measured by a photomultiplier tube and digitally converted to electronic pulses that are proportional to the emitted fluorescence of the cells. Analysed cells are reported as events on a forward scatter histogram and can be gated according to their physical parameters. FC can be performed using a large number of antibodies conjugated with different fluorochromes that may be evaluated individually or in combination to assess the expression and co-expression of the related antigens. The most commonly used fluorescent antibodies are CD3, CD5, CD7, CD2, CD4, CD8, CD19, CD20, CD10, CD23, FMC7, CD103, and Bcl2, which are generally used in predetermined combinations. The panel of antibodies is generally selected on the basis of clinical data and ROSE cytological features. An antibody is considered to be expressed when a minimum of 20% [19] of the gated cells are positive, but in specific contexts or minimal residual disease evaluation, this percentage may decrease by up to 5% [18]. With reference to clonality, kappa and lambda ratios of ≥4:1 or 1:2 are considered evidence of monoclonality, whereas even higher ratios have been reported in autoimmune or immunodepressive disease [20]. When cytological features and light chain assessment indicate an NHL, the different expressions and co-expressions of the above-reported antibodies may lead to the classification of different NHL subtypes [18, 19, 21–25]. In addition to the routinely used antibodies, others may be used in cases of specific diagnostic requests, such as CD15, CD13, and CD33, which identify myeloid and monocytic cells, and may also be aberrantly expressed in some B-cell NHL [18]. Other antibodies include CD11c and CD103, which are expressed by hairy-cell leukaemia, ZAP-70, which is normally expressed by T cells, NK cells, precursor B cells, and CD38 and CD49d that are prognostic markers of small lymphocytic lymphoma/chronic lymphocytic leukaemia. The main advantages of LN-FNC-FC are direct antigen-antibody reactions, exact quantification of antigen expression, and their possible co-expression on the same cells. The disadvantages include the absence of morphology, loss of very large cells, difficulty to identify numerically scanty cell populations (i.e., epithelial micrometastases, Hodgkin or Reed-Sternberg cells), and the difficult detection of intracellular antigens. Cell membrane integrity is the basic condition for an effective FC but may also be an obstacle for antibodies directed toward nuclear antigens. Permeation procedures may overcome this problem as in the detection of intracytoplasmic light chain in SMIG(–) NHL. Proliferative markers such as PCNA or MIB1 are less effective in FC than by ICC.

Molecular Genetic Procedures

Molecular genetic procedures are a wide, heterogeneous, and fast-growing technical field. Most of the corresponding techniques are used in specialized centres and/or for research purposes, others are routinely applied and may be conveniently used for the work-up of LN-FNC. These procedures usually focus on chromosomal abnormalities (mainly translocations and deletions), IGH, and T-cell receptor gene rearrangements and DNA amplification by polymerase chain reaction (PCR) for the sequencing and detection of specific mutations [26–60].

Fluorescence and Chromogenic in situ Hybridization

FISH is highly effective in the identification of specific NHL chromosomal abnormalities; therefore, it is used on the basis of a clear diagnostic orientation. FISH should be used after FC or ICC in LN-FNC [26–30] and has been applied to detect specific chromosomal translocations and deletions in different NHL subtypes [26–40]. FISH can be performed on different supports, such as smears, cytospins, or thin-layer slides, where the presence of intact cells allows optimal signals detection [29, 30, 33, 38]. The advantages of cytospins for FISH include a high cell concentration, probe sparing, and a short analysis time. DNA probes are labelled with a fluorochrome (e.g., Rhodamine) and hybridized with intact interphase nuclei. Commercially available probes cover almost all the variable breakpoints of chromosomal alterations. FISH is generally performed using 2 fluorescent probes that hybridize 2 regions that are close to the breakpoint of the chromosomes involved [26–39]. In case of specific translocations involving the labelled loci, 2 differently labelled probes juxtapose, providing a fusion signal; on the contrary, 2 distinct colour signals are obtained in the absence of chromosomal alterations [26–39]. Not all NHL harbour the expected translocation, such as the t(14;18)(q32;q21) translocation in follicular lymphoma (FL). Moreover, genetic abnormalities can be observed in more than 1 NHL category; for instance the t(8;14)(q24;q32) can be found in Burkitt lymphoma (BL) and, less frequently, in diffuse large B-cell lymphoma (DLBCL), FL, mantle cell lymphoma, and other subtypes. FISH may also be used to detect secondary chromosomal changes that usually occur in NHL and may have a prognostic value, such as the t(8;14)(q24;q32) translocation that characterizes BL, but may occur as a secondary aberration (double-hit) in FL (14–18t plus 8–14t) [30, 41]. CISH combines the chromogenic signal detection method of IHC techniques with in situ hybridization [32]. CISH uses bright-field microscopes rather than fluorescence microscopes used in FISH. CISH, performed after FISH, double checks data provided by the latter; in addition, the persistence of a signal beyond the decay of fluorescence allows a protracted reaction and a re-evaluation of the sample. CISH analysis on interphase nuclei is generally performed using split-signal probes, which hybridize 2 regions of the same chromosome next to a supposed breakpoint. In normal cells, the 2 hybridized regions are next to each other, generating fusion signals. Split-signal CISH, has some advantages over fusion-signal FISH, because the detection of a translocation is independent of the partner genes involved and is useful for detecting translocations involving multiple partner genes, as is the case of the IGH locus at chromosome 14q32. Another advantage of split-signal CISH is the absence of false-positive cases reported using fusion-signal FISH probes [32].

Polymerase Chain Reaction

PCR is routinely used in lymphoproliferative processes for the identification of IGH and T-cell receptor rearrangements. Other applications of PCR, not routinely used on FNC samples, are the identification and quantification of translocations by qRT-PCR strategies, the identification of IGVH somatic hypermutations by Sanger sequencing [53] and single-strand conformational polymorphisms or real-time PCR strategies. However, PCR suitability for the detection of lymphoma-associated translocations is limited when chromosomal breakpoints are spread over a large genomic region. PCR can also be used to detect specific breakpoints in NHL, such as the t(14,18)(q32;q21), involving the BCL2-IGH loci, and the t(11;14)(q13;q32), involving the BCL1-IGH loci, which occurs in 60–70% of FL and 30–40% of mantle cell lymphoma cases, respectively. Since specific NHL translocations may occur at different breakpoints in different patients, PCR might need specific primers for each possible breakpoint region. The main application of PCR on LN-FNC is IGH/TCR evaluation to assess clonality [43, 47–50]. Some authors [43] maintain that IGH/TCR PCR may replace FNC/FC be-

cause of its high efficiency and short turnaround time. However, others [42] suggest that a combined use is advisable because of a relatively high rate of monoclonality detection by PCR only. New procedures and EuroClonality/BIOMED-2 guidelines [47–49] have improved PCR specificity, reducing the risk of false negatives and positives on both tissues and FNC samples [47, 48]. TCR-PCR has been used less on FNC of T cells in comparison to B-cell NHL [49–51], whereas it is useful in the staging of T-cell NHL and cutaneous lymphoma by LN-FNC [51–52].

High-Throughput Technologies

High-throughput technologies (HTT) include different new technologies that share the capacity of multiple, parallel, and massive molecular target investigations and sample processing in a fast and reproducible manner. HTT has allowed the search for global genomic alterations responsible for the development and progression of different neoplasms, including NHL, with important clinical implications. The most used HTTs in biomedical research are gene expression profiling, comparative genomic hybridization, single-nucleotide polymorphism arrays, and next-generation sequencing (NGS) technologies [54–62].

Next-Generation Sequencing Technologies

NGS technologies are fast, relatively inexpensive, and versatile tools to analyse a wide mutational spectrum in NHL [54]. All the developed methodologies require the production of a library of extracted DNA fragments and their simultaneous sequencing in parallel that produce millions of sequenced reads for each given position of the genome, which are then aligned against the reference genome in a different database. The number of reads per stretch of DNA is called the coverage [54]. A high coverage is useful to detect tumour mutations in samples in which there is contamination of normal cells, as in NHL. At the same time, a high coverage may generate bias that can be avoided using reliable bioinformatic algorithms to interpret the sequences [55]. A number of reads above or below the mean coverage per DNA region indicates the presence of gains, amplifications, and hemizygous or homozygous deletions [54]. In addition to these large structural alterations, NGS detects translocations, single-nucleotide changes, somatic mutations, individual polymorphisms, small insertions or dele-

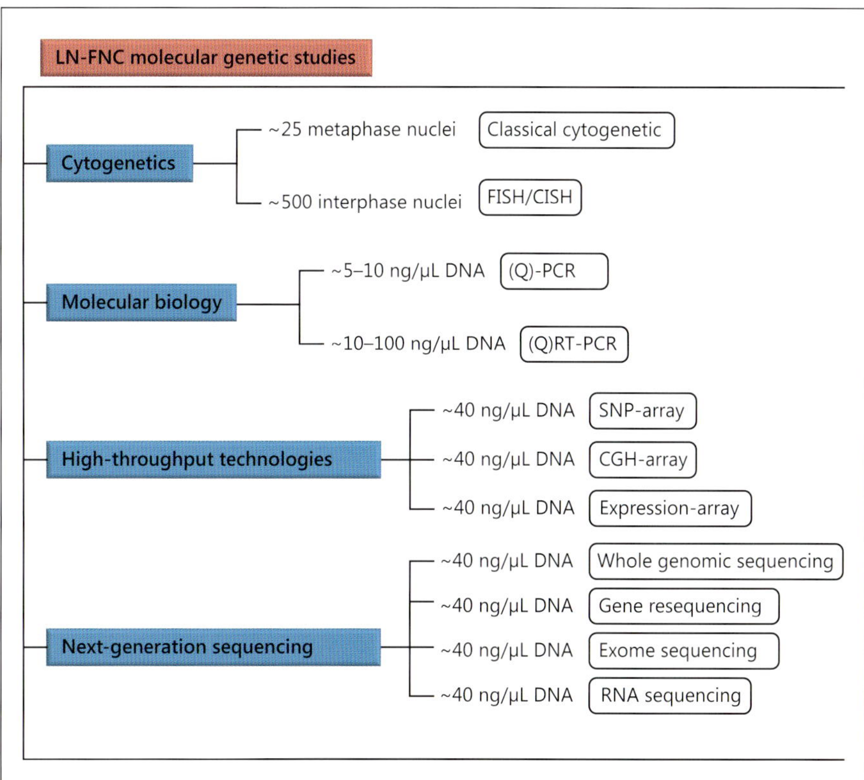

Fig. 5. The quantity of cells and nanograms of genetic material required for cytogenetic and molecular testing by each possible technique.

tions (indels). This information is obtained using whole genome, whole transcriptome, exome (specific regions of the genome including all coding exons), and specific-targeted genomic region sequencing strategies [54–57]. NGS methodologies can be performed on different platforms but obtained data need to be clinically confirmed. NGS and exome-specific targeted genomic region sequencing have been carried out in chronic lymphocytic leukaemia, hairy cell leukaemia, FL, DLBCL, and plasma cell myeloma [54–57]. NGS has highlighted new mutations in the histone methyltransferase MLL2 (in 32% of DLBCL and 89% of FL cases) [54–57], in EZH2, MLL2, CREBBP, BRAF, B2M, and EP300 (involved in the chromatin remodelling pathway) [58, 59]. NGS requires a few nanograms of DNA (about 40 ng/µL) of good-quality DNA and RNA that can be obtained by FNC of different tumours [54–60]. Therefore, NGS may enhance the LN-FNC molecular potential, providing mutational information on genes with diagnostic and predictive relevance.

LN-FNC Cell Harvesting and Preparations for Molecular Studies

The application of any molecular procedures requires a sufficient number of cells and good-quality genetic material corresponding to 10–40 ng of DNA/RNA (Fig. 5). The first issue to take into account for LN-FNC molecular testing is the number of cells obtained by FNC and its genetic content. Corresponding cell amounts are not constant, depending on the sizes of the needles, FNC technical procedures, and the nature of the lesions. It has been calculated that, using 23-G needles, a mean of 4×10^6 cells are obtained by LN-FNC, 2.5×10^6 from breast carcinoma, and 1.65×10^6 from thyroid carcinoma [61]. Considering that 40 ng of DNA/RNA may be obtained from 4×10^6 cells, a couple of additional passes from LN-FNC may be sufficient to obtain enough genetic material for any procedure (Fig. 5). Genetic material has been successfully obtained from smears, CB, or cryopreserved cells. This variability in technical supports is due to the usage of archival material or FNC performed by clinicians for routinely diagnostic purposes and only subsequently used for retrospective molecular studies.

References

1 Wieczorek TJ, Wakely PE: Lymph nodes in cytology; in Cibas ES, Ducatman BS (eds): Cytology: Diagnostic Principles and Clinical Correlates, ed 4. Philadelphia, Saunders, 2014, pp 333–374.

2 Tsang WY, Chan JK: Spectrum of morphologic changes in lymph nodes attributable to fine needle aspiration. Hum Pathol 1992;23:562–565.

3 Behm FG, O'Dowd GJ, Frable WJ: Fine needle aspiration effects on benign lymph node. Am J Clin Pathol 1985;82:195–198.

4 Zeppa P: Liquid-based cytology: a 25-year bridge between the pap smear and molecular cytopathology. Acta Cytol 2014;58:519–521.

5 Rossi ED, Martini M, Straccia P, Bizzarro T, Fadda G, Larocca LM: The potential of liquid-based cytology in lymph node cytological evaluation: the role of morphology and the aid of ancillary techniques. Cytopathology 2016;27:50–58.

6 Peluso AL, Cascone AM, Lucchese L, Cozzolino I, Ieni A, Mignogna C, Pepe S, Zeppa P: Use of FTA cards for the storage of breast carcinoma nucleic acid on fine-needle aspiration samples. Cancer Cytopathol 2015;123:582–592.

7 Amador-Ortiz C, Chen L, Hassan A, et al: Combined core needle biopsy and fine-needle aspiration with ancillary studies correlate highly with traditional techniques in the diagnosis of nodal-based lymphoma. Am J Clin Pathol 2011;135:516–524.

8 Ben-Yehuda D, Polliack A, Okon E, et al: Image-guided core-needle biopsy in malignant lymphoma: experience with 100 patients that suggests the technique is reliable. J Clin Oncol 1996;14:2431–2434.

9 Zinzani Pl, Cornelli G, Cancellieri A, et al: Core needle biopsy is effective in the initial diagnosis of mediastinal lymphoma. Haematologica 1999;84:600–603.

10 Agid R, Sklair-Levy M, Bloom Al, et al: CT-guided biopsy with cutting-edge needle for the diagnosis of malignant lymphoma: experience of 267 biopsies. Clin Radiol 2003;58:143–147.

11 Demharter J, Neukirchen S, Wagner T, et al: Do ultrasound-guided core needle biopsy of lymph nodes allow for subclassification of malignant lymphomas? Rofo 2007;179:396–400.

12 Schmitt FC: Molecular cytopathology and flow cytometry: pre-analytical procedures matter. Cytopathology 2011;22:355–357.

13 Schmitt F, Barroca H: Role of ancillary studies in fine-needle aspiration from selected tumors. Cancer Cytopathol 2012;120:145–160.

14 Schmitt F, Cochand-Priollet B, Toetsch M, Davidson B, Bondi A, Vielh P: Immunocytochemistry in Europe: results of the European Federation of Cytology Societies (EFCS) inquiry. Cytopathology 2011;22:238–242.

15 Pinheiro C, Roque R, Adriano A, Mendes P, Praça M, Reis I, Pereira T, Srebotnik Kirbis I, André S: Optimization of immunocytochemistry in cytology: comparison of two protocols for fixation and preservation on cytospin and smear preparations. Cytopathology 2015;26:38–43.

16 Tani EM, Christensson B, Porwit A, Skoog L: Immunocytochemical analysis and cytomorphologic diagnosis on fine needle aspirates of lymphoproliferative disease. Acta Cytol 1988;32:209–215.

17 Skoog L, Tani E: Immunocytochemistry: an indispensable technique in routine cytology. Cytopathology 2011;22:215–229.

18 Craig FE, Foon KA: Flow cytometric immunophenotyping for hematologic neoplasms. Blood 2008;111:3941–3967.

19 Zeppa P, Marino G, Troncone G, Fulciniti F, De Renzo A, Picardi M, Benincasa G, Rotoli B, Vetrani A, Palombini L: Fine-needle cytology and flow cytometry immunophenotyping and subclassification of non-Hodgkin lymphoma. A critical review of 307 cases with technical suggestions. Cancer 2004;102:55–65.

20 Cozzolino I, Nappa S, Picardi M, De Renzo A, Troncone G, Palombini L, Zeppa P: Clonal B-cell population in a reactive lymph node in acquired immunodeficiency syndrome. Diagn Cytopathol 2009;37:910–914.

21 Dey P: Role of ancillary techniques in diagnosing and subclassifying non-Hodgkin's lymphomas on fine needle aspiration cytology. Cytopathology 2006;17:275–287.

22 Robins DB, Katz RL, Swan F Jr, Atkinson EN, Ordonez NG, Huh YO: Immunotyping of lymphoma by fine-needle aspiration: a comparative study of cytospin preparations and flow cytometry. Am J Clin Pathol 1994;101:569–576.

23 Zardawi IM, Jain S, Bennet G: Flow-cytometric algorithm on fine-needle aspirates for the clinical workup of patients with lymphoadenopathy. Diagn Cytopathol 1998;19:274–278.

24 Bangerter M, Brudler O, Heinrich B, Griesshamnuer M: Fine needle aspiration cytology and flow cytometry in the diagnosis and subclassification of non-Hodgkin's lymphoma based on the World Health Organization classification. Acta Cytol 2007;51:390–398.

25 Zeppa P, Vigliar E, Cozzolino I, et al: Fine needle aspiration cytology and flow cytometry immunophenotyping of non-Hodgkin lymphoma: can we do better? Cytopathology 2010;21:300–310.

26 Roullet M, Bagg A: The basis and rational use of molecular genetic testing in mature B-cell lymphomas. Adv Anat Pathol 2010;17:333–358.

27 Cartagena N Jr, Katz RL, Hirsch-Ginsberg C, Childs CC, Ordonez NG, Cabanillas F: Accuracy of diagnosis of malignant lymphoma by combining fine-needle aspiration cytomorphology with immunocytochemistry and in selected cases, Southern blotting of aspirated cells: a tissue-controlled study of 86 patients. Diagn Cytopathol 1992;8:456–464.

28 Sreekantaiah C: FISH panels for hematologic malignancies. Cytogenet Genome Res 2007;118:284–296.

29 Monaco SE, Teot LA, Felgar RE, Surti U, Cai G: Fluorescence in situ hybridization studies on direct smears: an approach to enhance the fine-needle aspiration biopsy diagnosis of B-cell non-Hodgkin lymphomas. Cancer Cytopathol 2009;117:338–348.

30 da Cunha Santos G, Ko HM, Geddie WR, Boerner SL, Lai SW, Have C, Kamel-Reid S, Bailey D: Targeted use of fluorescence in situ hybridization (FISH) in cytospin preparations: results of 298 fine needle aspirates of B-cell non-Hodgkin lymphoma. Cancer Cytopathol 2010;118:250–258.

31 Zhang S, Abreo F, Lowery-Nordberg M, Veillon DM, Cotelingam JD: The role of fluorescence in situ hybridization and polymerase chain reaction in the diagnosis and classification of lymphoproliferative disorders on fine-needle aspiration. Cancer Cytopathol 2010;118:105–112.

32 Zeppa P, Sosa Fernandez LV, Cozzolino I, Ronga V, Genesio R, Salatiello M, Picardi M, Malapelle U, Troncone G, Vigliar E: Immunoglobulin heavy-chain fluorescence in situ hybridization-chromogenic in situ hybridization DNA probe split signal in the clonality assessment of lymphoproliferative processes on cytological samples. Cancer Cytopathol 2012;120:390–400.

33 Richmond J, Bryant R, Trotman W, Beatty B, Lunde J: FISH detection of t(14;18) in follicular lymphoma on Papanicolaou-stained archival cytology slides. Cancer 2006;108:198–204.

34 Kishimoto K, Kitamura T, Fujita K, Tate G, Mitsuya T: Cytologic differential diagnosis of follicular lymphoma grades 1 and 2 from reactive follicular hyperplasia: cytologic features of fine-needle aspiration smears with Pap stain and fluorescence in situ hybridization analysis to detect t(14;18)(q32;q21) chromosomal translocation. Diagn Cytopathol 2006;34:11–17.

35 Caraway NP, Gu J, Lin P, Romaguera JE, Glassman A, Katz R: The utility of interphase fluorescence in situ hybridization for the detection of the translocation t(11;14)(q13;q32) in the diagnosis of mantle cell lymphoma on fine-needle aspiration specimens. Cancer 2005;105:110–118.

36 Salaverria I, Zettl A, Bea S, et al: Specific secondary genetic alterations in mantle cell lymphoma provide prognostic information independent of the gene expression-based proliferation signature. J Clin Oncol 2007;25:1216–1222.

37 Jiang F, Lin F, Price R, Gu J, Medeiros LJ, Zhang HZ, Xie SS, Caraway NP, Katz RL: Rapid detection of IgH/BCL2 rearrangement in follicular lymphoma by interphase fluorescence in situ hybridization with bacterial artificial chromosome probes. J Mol Diagn 2002;4:144–149.

38 Bentz JS, Rowe LR, Anderson SR, Gupta PK, McGrath CM: Rapid detection of the t(11;14) translocation in mantle cell lymphoma by interphase fluorescence in situ hybridization on archival cytopathologic material. Cancer 2004;102:124–131.

39 Gong Y, Caraway N, Gu J, Zaidi T, Fernandez R, Sun X, Huh YO, Katz RL: Evaluation of interphase fluorescence in situ hybridization for the t(14;18) (q32;q21) translocation in the diagnosis of follicular lymphoma on fine-needle aspirates: a comparison with flow cytometry immunophenotyping. Cancer 2003;99:385–393.

40 Cook JR: Paraffin section interphase fluorescence in situ hybridization in the diagnosis and classification of non-Hodgkin lymphomas. Diagn Mol Pathol 2004;13:197–206.

41 Elkins CT, Wakely PE Jr: Cytopathology of "double-hit" non-Hodgkin lymphoma. Cancer Cytopathol 2011;119:263–271.

42 Shin HJ, Thorson P, Gu J, Katz RL: Detection of a subset of CD30+ anaplastic large cell lymphoma by interphase fluorescence in situ hybridization. Diagn Cytopathol 2003;29:61–66.

43 Mayall F, Johnson S: Immunoflow cytometry compared with PCR for the identification of clonality in FNAs of T-cell-rich B-cell lymphomas. Cytopathology 2007;18:117–119.

44 Davidson B, Risberg B, Berner A, Smeland EB, Torlakovic E: Evaluation of lymphoid cell populations in cytology specimens using flow cytometry and polymerase chain reaction. Diagn Mol Pathol 1999;8:183–188.

45 Aiello A, Delia D, Giardini R, Alasio L, Bartoli C, Pierotti MA, Pilotti S: PCR analysis of IgH and BCL2 gene rearrangement in the diagnosis of follicular lymphoma in lymph node fine-needle aspiration. A critical appraisal. Diagn Mol Pathol 1997;6:154–160.

46 Alkan S, Lehman C, Sarago C, Sidawy MK, Karcher DS, Garrett CT: Polymerase chain reaction detection of immunoglobulin gene rearrangement and bcl-2 translocation in archival glass slides of cytologic material. Diagn Mol Pathol 1995;4:25–31.

47 Langerak AW, Groenen PJTA, Brüggemann M, et al: EuroClonality/BIOMED-2 guidelines for interpretation and reporting of Ig/TCR clonality testing in suspected lymphoproliferations. Leukemia 2012:26:2159–2172.

48 van Dongen JJ, Langerak AW, Bruggemann M, et al: Design and standardization of PCR primers and protocols for detection of clonal immunoglobulin and T-cell receptor gene recombinations in suspect lymphoproliferations: report of the BIOMED-2 Concerted Action BMH4-CT98-3936. Leukemia 2003;17:2257–2317.

49 Van Dongen JJM, Wolvers-Tettero IL: Analysis of immunoglobulin and TCR genes. Part II. Possibilities and limitations in the diagnosis and management of lymphoproliferative diseases and related disorders. Clin Chim Acta 1991;198:93–174.

50 Dippel E, Assaf C, Hummel M, Schrag HJ, Stein H, Goerdt S, et al: Clonal T-cell receptor γ-chain gene rearrangement by PCR-based GeneScan analysis in advanced cutaneous T-cell lymphoma: a critical evaluation. J Pathol 1999;188:146–154.

51 Vigliar S, Cozzolino I, Picardi M, et al: Lymph node fine-needle cytology in the staging and follow-up of cutaneous Lymphomas. BMC Cancer 2014;14:8–18.

52 Pai RK, Mullins FM, Kim YH, Kong CS: Cytologic evaluation of lymphadenopathy associated with mycosis fungoides and Sezary syndrome: role of immunophenotypic and molecular ancillary studies. Cancer 2008;114:323–332.

53 Peková S, Baran-Marszak F, Schwarz J, Matoska V: Mutated or non-mutated? Which database to choose when determining the IgVH hypermutation status in chronic lymphocytic leukemia? Haematologica 2006;91:ELT01.

54 Migliazza A, Bosch F, Komatsu H, et al: Nucleotide sequence, transcription map, and mutation analysis of the 13q14 chromosomal region deleted in B-cell chronic lymphocytic leukemia. Blood 2001;97:2098–2104.

55 Campo E: Whole genome profiling and other high throughput technologies in lymphoid neoplasms – current contributions and future hopes. Mod Pathol 2013;26(suppl 1):S97–S110.

56 Langerak AW, Molina TJ, Lavender FL, et al: Polymerase chain reaction-based clonality testing in tissue samples with reactive lymphoproliferations: usefulness and pitfalls. A report of the BIOMED-2 Concerted Action BMH4-CT98-3936. Leukemia 2007;21:222–229.

57 Saieg MA, Geddie WR, Boerner SL, et al: The use of FTA cards for preserving unfixed cytological material for high-throughput molecular analysis. Cancer Cytopathol 2012;120:206–214.

58 Saieg MA, Geddie WR, Boerner SL, et al: EZH2 and CD97B mutational status over time in B-cell non-Hodgkin lymphomas detected by high-throughput sequencing using minimal samples. Cancer Cytopathol 2013;121:377–386.

59 da Cunha Santos G, Liu N, Tsao MS, et al: Detection of EGFR and KRAS mutations in fine-needle aspirates stored on Whatman FTA cards: is this the tool for biobanking cytological samples in the molecular era? Cancer Cytopathol 2010;118:450–456.

60 Peluso AL, Cozzolino I, Bottiglieri A, Lucchese L, Di Crescenzo RM, Langella M, Selleri C, Zeppa P: Immunoglobulin heavy and light chains and T-cell receptor beta and gamma chains PCR assessment on cytological samples: a study comparing FTA cards and cryopreserved lymph node fine-needle cytology. Cytopathology 2017;28:203–215.

61 Rajer M, Kmet M: Quantitative analysis of fine needle aspiration biopsy samples. Radiol Oncol 2005;39:269–272.

62 Roy-Chowdhuri S, Roy S, Monaco SE, Routbort MJ, Pantanowitz L: Big data from small samples: informatics of next-generation sequencing in cytopathology. Cancer 2017;125:236–244.

Zeppa P, Cozzolino I: Lymph Node FNC. Cytopathology of Lymph Nodes and Extranodal Lymphoproliferative Processes.
Monogr Clin Cytol. Basel, Karger, 2018, vol 23, pp 14–18 (DOI: 10.1159/000478878)

Lymph Nodal Structure and Cytological Patterns

Normal Histology

Lymph nodes (LN) are small, round or reniform organs located throughout the body along the lymphatic vessels. LN are more numerous in some districts and drain specific organs. Quiescent LN do not exceed 1 cm in diameter and are undetectable at a physical examination; any possible stimulus may cause their enlargement, making them clinically evident. If removed, LN are normally white-pinkish and homogenous. Any change in shape, consistency or colour of the cut surface, or a distinct nodular, haemorrhagic or necrotic change is suspicious for various pathological processes. In the quiescent state, LN show variable degrees of fatty metaplasia, especially those located in the axillary, inguinal or mesenteric regions. LN are surrounded by a fibrous capsule and are divided by septa. Beneath the capsule there is a subcapsular sinus connected to the cortical and medullary sinuses. The main role of LN is to process and present antigens that reach the cortical via the afferent lymphatic vessels to the LN immunocompetent cells.

LN are anatomically and functionally composed of 3 distinct areas: the cortex, the paracortex, and the medulla (Fig. 1a). The cortex is located underneath the capsule and is divided into follicular and diffuse regions containing primary and secondary lymphoid follicles. Lymphoid follicles contain immunocompetent cells, mainly represented by B cells and dendritic cells. There are primary follicles, which are spherical aggregates of small immature lymphocytes, and secondary follicles, which are larger and formed by a "pale" germinal centre encircled by a dark, thick border of small B lymphocytes. Secondary follicles represent the site of antigen exposure, and B cell recruitment and rearrangement (Fig. 1a). The paracortex surrounds the follicles and interposes between the cortex and the medulla. It is mainly composed of small T lymphocytes representing the zone of T cell competence (Fig. 1a). The medulla is the area below the cortex/paracortex where the lymph is conveyed towards the hilus and the efferent lymphatic ducts. The medulla is mainly structured by cords and sinuses and is immunologically a B-dependent area composed of histiocytes, plasmacytoid lymphocytes, plasma cells, and immunoblasts (Fig. 1a). Several afferent lymphatic vessels carrying lymph enter the cortical convex LN side. The lymph flows through the LN structures and reach the hilar efferent lymphatic vessels, which carry the lymph to the main lymphatic vessels. Each of these areas, far from being static, can undergo changes according to different stimuli and pathological conditions that lead to LN enlargement. This may involve corti-

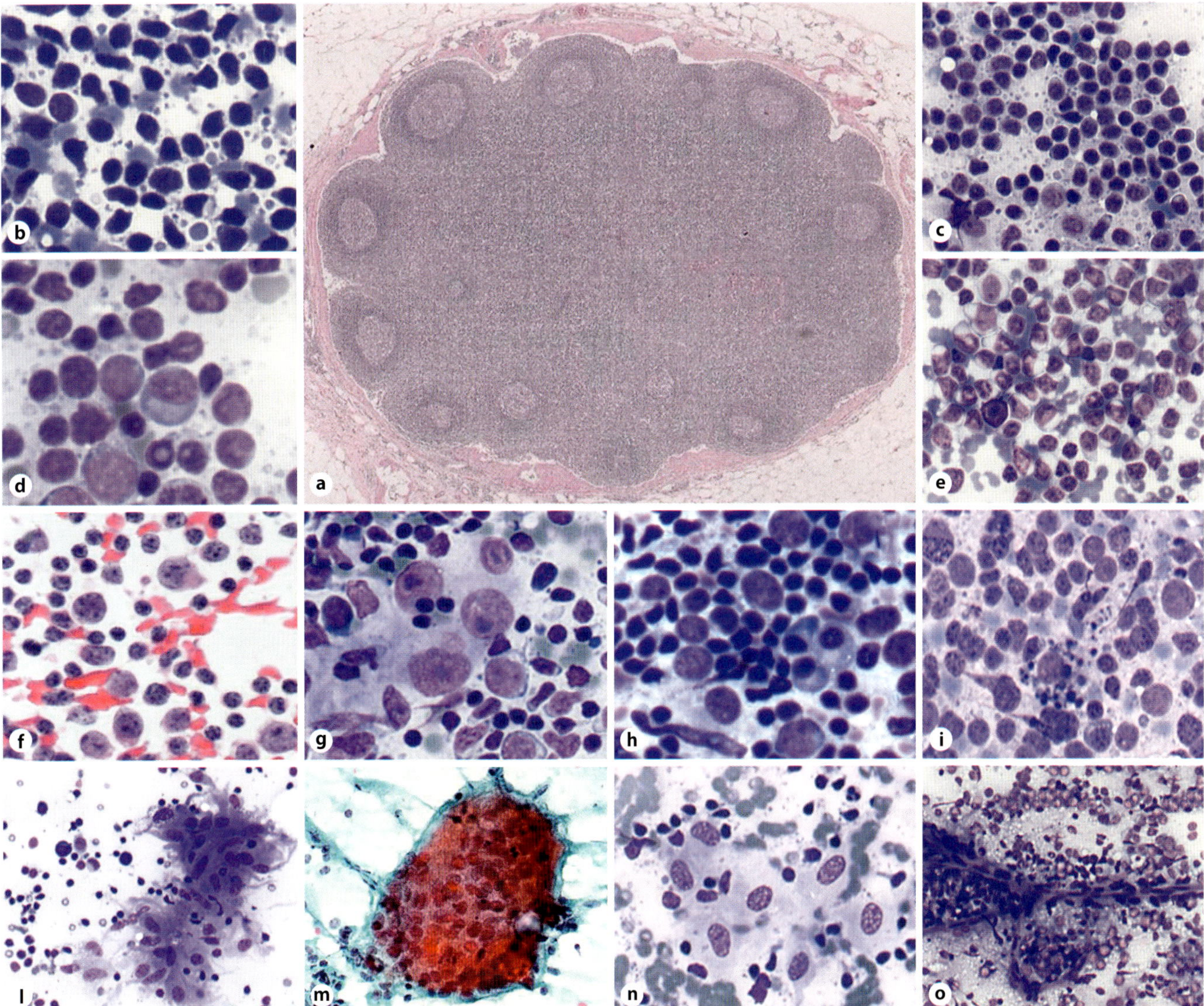

Fig. 1. Lymph node structure (**a**) and corresponding cell types. **b** "T" lymphocytes with dark and elongated nuclei. **c** Mature "B" lymphocytes with lymphoglandular bodies. **d** Plasma cells and postgerminal "B" cells with Dutcher bodies. **e** Centrocytes with slightly irregular nuclei and a scanty cytoplasm. The nuclei appear pale with dispersed chromatin and slight nuclear membrane irregularities with occasional small cleavages. **f** Follicular centre cells: centroblasts with dispersed chromatin and two or more eccentric nucleoli. **g** Immunoblasts with very large, centrally located nucleoli. **h** Plasma cells with eccentrically located nuclei with cartwheel chromatin and large, well-defined cytoplasm with a "Golgian" pale rim in the paranuclear area. **i** Macrophages with tingible bodies in the cytoplasm. **l** Epithelioid cells with 1 or 2 nuclei and a wide, dense cytoplasm that may appear pinkish in DQ stain and lymphoid cells in the background. **m** Multinucleated cell with a wide cytoplasm and numerous nuclei. **n** Dendritic cells with ovoidal, elongated, pale nuclei and an ill-defined cytoplasm. **o** Capillary structures.

cal, paracortical, and medullary expansions, either together or singularly, with different quantitative representation of the corresponding structures and cell components. Fine-needle cytology (FNC) may reflect this variability through the prevalence of the corresponding cell populations [1–6].

Normal Cytological Components on FNC Smears

LN-FNC generally reveals all the LN cell components, although not necessarily in the same quantitative proportion. Lymphoid cytoplasm fragments, also known as "lymphoglandular bodies," are considered the anatomical hallmark of lymphoid tissue and, hence, of the target LN. They appear as uniform grey-blue fragments in May-Grünwald-Giemsa (MGG) or Diff-Quik (DQ) stains. Normal cellular components are small lymphocytes, follicular centre cells (centrocytes, centroblasts, immunoblasts), and plasma cells. Other cell components are mono- or multinucleated histiocytes, with or without tingible bodies and dendritic cells. Tingible bodies in the cytoplasm of histiocytes, in a polymorphous lymphoid background, generally stand for benign reactive processes. Other than isolated cells, cohesive cell structures such as lympho-histiocytic or lympho-dendritic aggregates, capillaries, and adipose tissue fragments may also occur. Neutrophils, eosinophils, and mast cells are also present, roughly accounting for 2, 0.3, and 0.1%, respectively, in normal conditions [1–6].

- Mature lymphocytes have small, dark nuclei with dense chromatin, with or without a thin rim of cytoplasm. The B and T phenotype cannot be distinguished on the basis of its cytological features, whereas elongated nuclei and small cytoplasmic "tails" seem to be typical of T lymphocytes (Fig. 1b). As for small B lymphocytes, their cartwheel chromatin, when present, suggests a B phenotype (Fig. 1c). Postgerminal B lymphocytes may show dense intranuclear vacuoles, also known as Dutcher bodies, which represent intranuclear immunoglobulins (Fig. 1d). As expected, they occur more frequently in plasma cells and may be observed in lymphoplasmacytic non-Hodgkin lymphoma (LPCL) and plasmacytoma, but also in reactive processes.

- Centrocytes are medium-to-large sized centrofollicular cells with slightly irregular nuclei and a scanty cytoplasm (Fig. 1e). The nuclei appear paler than mature lymphocytes with dispersed chromatin and slight nuclear membrane irregularities with occasional small cleavages. One or more small nucleoli are present. Deeper nuclear cleavages are better appreciated on histological sections than in smears, where centrocytes may appear vaguely polygonal rather than roundish. Centrocytes may be numerous in any follicular expansion – whether reactive or lymphomatous.

- Centroblasts are large centrofollicular cells with pale round nuclei, dispersed chromatin, and 2 or more evident nucleoli. The latter, which are nearly adjacent to the nuclear membrane on histological sections, are often only eccentrical but not adjacent to the nuclear membrane on smears (Fig. 1f). Nucleoli are paler, larger, and more regular in shape than the chromatin clumps, whether on MGG, DQ, or Papanicolaou stains. Centroblasts may be present to a significant extent in some types of follicular hyperplasia and in high-grade follicular lymphoma (FL).

- Immunoblasts of either the B or T phenotype are the largest lymphoid cells. They appear with pale nuclei and 1 or 2 very large, centrally located nucleoli (Fig. 1g). A well-defined basophilic rim of cytoplasm is generally present. Immunoblasts may be numerous in viral, postvaccinal lymphadenitis, mononucleosis, and immunoblastic diffuse large B-cell Lymphoma (DLBCL).

- Plasma cells have eccentrically located nuclei with cartwheel chromatin and large, well-defined cytoplasm with a "Golgian" pale rim in the paranuclear area (Fig. 1d, h). Conversely to follicular centre cells, chromatin clumps should not be confused with nucleoli. Sometimes multiple cytoplasmic vacuoles (Russel bodies) may be observed. These vacuoles represent stored immunoglobulins and are defined with different terms: Grape cells, Morula cells or Mott cells. Plasma cells can be predominant in syphilis, LPCL, and plasmacytoma.

- Macrophages are large cells with variable cytological features. They generally show a wide cytoplasm, often engulfed with phagocytized cellular debris, and 1 or 2 oval eccentrically located nuclei (Fig. 1i). The latter may be round or oval, pale with "dusty" chromatin, and small or inconspicuous nucleoli. Macrophages are predominant in sinus histiocytosis, intermingled with lymphoid cells in reactive hyperplasia, and may produce a "starry sky" pattern in lymphoblastic lymphoma.

- Epithelioid cells are large cells of monocytoid origin. They have 1 or 2 nuclei and a wide, dense cytoplasm that may appear pinkish on DQ stain. Epithelioid cells may be isolated, clustered in small groups, and/or intermingled with lymphocytes (Fig. 1l). They may be found in reactive hyperplasia, mainly in toxoplasmosis, haematological diseases, and/or after chemo/radiotherapy.

- Multinucleated cells are large, sometimes enormous cells, with a wide cytoplasm and numerous (up to a dozen) nuclei (Fig. 1m). These cells may occur isolated or clustered with lymphocytes or granulomatous structures. The cytoplasm in foreign-body giant cells may contain material that betrays their origin. Multinucleated giant cells rarely show asteroid bodies, which are not necessarily expression of sarcoidosis, as was traditionally believed.

- Dendritic cells represent the LN meshwork and may occur in LN-FNC as well. These cells are generally isolated or intermingled with lymphocytes in lympho-dendritic aggregates. Dendritic cells have an oval, pale nuclei, inconspicuous nucleoli, and large ill-defined cytoplasm (Fig. 1n).

- Lympho-histiocytic or lympho-dendritic aggregates may prevalently, but not exclusively, occur in reactive LN. Sometimes they are so dense and cohesive that nuclear details may be appreciated on their edges only.
- Endothelial cells alone are not distinguishable on smears although easily recognizable capillary structures may be detected at LN-FNC. Capillaries generally appear as a bent, double-layered line of elongated endothelial cells in which erythrocytes are detectable. Capillaries may appear isolated or even organized in a meshwork (Fig. 1o). Lymphocytes, macrophages, and dendritic cells are often tightly attached to these structures. Although unspecific, capillaries often occur in LN-FNC of reactive processes.
- Adipose tissue fragments may also occur at LN-FNC, indicating partial adipose metaplasia or also contamination. Axillary and inguinal LN are those most frequently involved. LN are sometimes in almost complete adipose metaplasia, with the lymphoid tissue only present as a thin peripheral edge. In these cases, FNC may be frustratingly inadequate despite the clinical and instrumental evidence.
- LN benign non-lymphoid cell inclusions may be detected [see Chapter 9, this vol., pp 93–101].

How to Observe an LN-FNC Smear

Both pathologists inexperienced with FNC as well as expert cytopathologists should follow some basic and repetitive rules when observing LN-FNC. Smears should first be observed at low magnification to assess the cellularity, cellular pattern, and background. At this magnification, smears may be highly or poorly cellular, monomorphous or polymorphous, aggregated or dispersed. When a dispersed lymphoid cell population is observed it is important to assess its quantity and whether all the normal constituents, even in different proportions, are present, corresponding to the different stages of lymphoid differentiation. Histiocytic components, vascular structures, and small stroma fragments, if any, should also be assessed. Granulocytes and eosinophils should be identified and quantified; both may be present, even in relevant quantities, as an unspecific finding or as expression of specific pathological processes (suppurative processes, some autoimmune diseases, dermatopathic lymphadenopathies, Hodgkin lymphoma [HL]). Aggregated cells, either in small or large groups, should be scrutinized, especially those located on the edges of the smear, at high magnification, to determine whether the corresponding cells are mature or immature lymphoid cells, macrophage-lymphoid complexes, epithelioid cells, or non-lymphoid, metastatic cells. When a monomorphous cell population is observed, it should be evaluated according to its size and its more or less regular shape. Regarding cell size and shape, it is important to keep in mind that alcohol-fixed cells generally shrink by about a third compared to air-dried ones, and this mainly affects large cells, conferring a more monomorphous pattern to Papanicolaou-stained smears as compared to the MGG or DQ stains. Cell size and shape is also influenced by the smearing; in fact, cells on the distal part of the smear generally appear larger than those on the proximal part. This artefactual phenomenon should be considered when assessing cell size. For cell size assessment, it may be useful to utilize an internal control that may be represented by mature small lymphocytes, which are almost always present and scattered all over the smears. The background may also provide useful information; it may appear clean, necrotic, "dirty," mucous, and haemorrhagic. A necrotic background should be evaluated according to its own qualities. Necrosis with nuclear debris and a haemorrhagic component (dirty necrosis) may be observed in metastatic tumours, mainly from squamous cell carcinoma. Nonetheless, a "dirty" necrotic background may occur in atypical tuberculosis, in other infectious lymphadenitis, and in some autoimmune processes (i.e., lupus). Other than resulting from cellular necrosis, a dirty background may also be caused by a range of substances and microbiological agents. Silicone and other indigestible material, or specific microbiological agents like aspergillus and fungi, may be occasionally detected. "Clean" and caseous necrosis may occur in typical tuberculosis or in the rare LN infarct. The latter may occur spontaneously or in cases of damage to hilar vascular structures during FNC. A clean amorphous background may be determined by immunological amyloidosis in plasma cell tumours or autoimmune diseases, inflammatory amyloidosis in chronic inflammatory processes, or "APUD" amyloid in LN metastases from neuroendocrine tumours. Mucous-secreting tumours, such as gastric, intestinal, or ovary carcinoma, may produce large amounts of mucus either in primary sites or in metastases, hence its presence may suggest a known or unknown LN metastasis. A haemorrhagic background is a frequent FNC complication and represents a limitation to cell evaluation [1–6].

The Concept of Atypia in LN-FNC

The concept of atypia in cytology is generally related to the progressive morphological dedifferentiation of cells from their normal counterparts. This criterion is generally applied to different organs and districts but cannot be utilized outright in LN-FNC. In fact, apart from metastases and high-grade non-Hodgkin lymphoma (NHL), most low-grade NHL and reactive processes may share the same cytological atypia. For instance, centrocytes from follicular lymphoma are cytologically indistinguishable from those from a florid follicular reactive hyperplasia. Moreover, as FNC lacks architectural information on the corresponding follicles, the only, and often insufficient, cytological criteria to differentiate these 2 entities is the quantity of corresponding cells types when compared to the others present on the smear. Therefore, in most LN-FNC, lymphoid cellular atypia is more related to the monomorphism of the cell population rather than to the canonical cytological criteria, and this criterion is generally insufficient for an accurate FNC diagnosis. Conversely, some entities with even little or no "cytological atypia," such as small lymphocytic lymphoma/chronic lymphatic leukaemia, are more easily identified by FNC as malignant "clonal" processes on the basis of the sole and complete monomorphism. From a practical point of view, any reactive but not sufficiently polymorphous LN-FNC lacking follicular centre cells at different stages of maturation (centrocytes, centroblasts, immunoblasts), where macrophages with tingible bodies and vascular structures are not evident, requires proper ancillary techniques to exclude a possible low-grade NHL.

Human neoplasms generally show a significantly higher mitotic index than their normal tissues of origin. A higher mitotic index is an integrant microscopic aspect of malignancy in specific entities. In LN-FNC, with the exception of lymphoblastic lymphoma and some other high-grade NHL, mitoses may be irrelevant in the differentiation between reactive processes and NHL, and may paradoxically be more numerous in reactive hyperplasia than in low-grade NHL.

Finally, HL represents another exception to the criteria of atypia in LN-FNC. Indeed, the background of HL is not "atypical" on the basis of canonical criteria alone, but is specific enough to suggest a diagnosis of HL and the consequential microscopic research of often rare, diagnostic Hodgkin cells or Reed-Sternberg cells.

References

1 Ioachim H, Medeiros J: The normal lymph node; in: Ioachim's Lymph Node Pathology, ed 4. Philadelphia, Lippincott, Williams & Wilkins, 2009, pp 2–14.

2 Skoog L, Tani E: Lymph nodes; in Gray W, Kocjan G (eds): Diagnostic Cytopathology, ed 3. London, Churchill Livingstone, 2010, pp 409–443.

3 Sheaff MT, Singh N: Lymph nodes; in: Cytopathology: An Introduction. London, Springer, 2012, pp 179–184.

4 Caraway NP, Katz RL: Lymph Nodes; in Koss LG, Melamed MR (eds): Koss' Diagnostic Cytology and Its Histopathologic Bases. Philadelphia, Lippincott, Williams & Wilkins, 2006, pp 1186–1228.

5 Zeppa P, Cozzolino I: Normal lymph node histology and cytology. Eurocytology. http://www.eurocytology.eu/en/course/334.

6 Young NA, Al-Saleem T: Lymph nodes: cytomorphology and flow cytometry; in Bibbo M, Wilbur D (eds): Comprehensive Cytopathology, ed 4. Amsterdam, Elsevier, 2014, pp 675–708.

Chapter 3

Zeppa P, Cozzolino I: Lymph Node FNC. Cytopathology of Lymph Nodes and Extranodal Lymphoproliferative Processes.
Monogr Clin Cytol. Basel, Karger, 2018, vol 23, pp 19–33 (DOI: 10.1159/000478879)

Lymphadenitis and Lymphadenopathy

Normal lymph nodes (LN) are generally small and impalpable, and are often with adipose metaplasia. LN enlargements (LNe) are caused by different known and unknown factors, including infections, autoimmune processes, drugs, primary or metastatic neoplasms, and may also be idiopathic. The term "lymphadenitis" is generally used to indicate an LN infection caused by an agent that leads to an inflammatory reaction. The term "lymphadenopathy" refers to an LNe with a known or unknown cause, in which 1 compartment and 1 or more cell types are hyperplastic and prevail on the other(s). Lymphadenitis and lymphadenopathy patterns may overlap in LN-fine-needle cytology (FNC) and histological samples. The number, size, and the location of LNe are extremely variable, as well as their entity and duration. The severity of the process varies with the age and the individual immunological status; children may develop significant and persistent LNe in reactive processes, whereas in adults the same processes may determine a less significant LNe. Conversely, neoplastic LNe are much more frequent in adults than in children. As a consequence, LNe that are often managed by pediatricians in outpatient settings require a different clinical approach in adults because, in undefined clinical contexts, they might be suspected for different aetiologies, including lymphoproliferative processes. Other than to guide the needle during FNC, an LN ultrasound (US) evaluation is extremely useful in the identification of nodules as LN, and determining their size, number, and the anatomic relationships with other organs. US may also differentiate benign and malignant LNe, with acceptable sensitivity, through the application of standardized criteria. However, US cannot identify the aetiology of lymphadenitis or the nature of lymphadenopathy [1]. LNe may be caused by cortex, paracortex, or medullary expansion, with the ensuing shrinkage of the other compartments. The histopathology of lymphadenitis and lymphadenopathy usually reveals 5 patterns, described as follows. (1) Follicular hyperplasia with cortical expansion and increased size and number of secondary follicles. This pattern is mainly observed in infections, autoimmune disorders, lymphadenopathies, and unspecific reactions. (2) Paracortical expansion, mainly due to T lymphocytes, generally occurs in viral infections, skin diseases, drug reactions, and non-specific reactions. (3) Sinus hyperplasia with subcapsular sinuses and medullary expansion is mainly maintained by histiocytes, and it is observed in inflammatory processes, Rosai-Dorfman disease, and other pathologies. (4) Granulomatous pattern, necrotizing or non-necrotizing, is characterized by granuloma in the cortex and paracortex; it is mainly observed in tuberculosis and sarcoidosis, and may occur in other bacterial or fungal infections. (5) Suppurative pattern is characterized by a variable amount of polymorphonuclear cells intermingled in the different LN structures; this pattern is usually observed in bacterial infections. These histological patterns may also be observed on FNC, although they are less clearly identifiable.

Lymphadenitis

Lymphadenitis is an acute or chronic condition, which may show non-specific or specific features suggesting the related agent (bacteria, virus, protozoa). In most cases, morphological features are unspecific. Lymphadenitis is clinically characterized by a tender and sometimes painful swelling. Localized lymphadenitis often has an infectious aetiology and the clinical identification of an infectious focus is an indirect diagnostic aid to LN-FNC. Lymphadenitis determines the expansion of the cortex, and/or paracortex, and/or medullary, with shrinkage of the other components. FNC shows follicular centre cells, plasma cells, small lymphocytes, reticular cells, histiocytes in their different morphological presentations (macrophages with or without tingible bodies, epithelioid cells, multinucleated giant cells, granuloma), and granulocytes may be present in significant amounts. Fibroblasts and endothelial cells, generally present as "microcapillary" fragments, may also be present. LN cellular components have to be evaluated in the corresponding background (clean, necrotic, proteinaceous, suppurative). Predominant patterns and cell components in various combinations may or may not suggest the corresponding aetiology.

Acute Lymphadenitis

Acute Lymphadenitis is characterized by a rapid enlargement of the involved LNs that are generally painful and tender. Bacterial infections are the most frequent cause of acute lymphadenitis, which may produce regional suppurative lymphadenitis. Fungi may also cause suppurative lymphadenitis with similar cytological features. FNC smears are generally hypercellular and characterized by a mixed population of a variable amount of lymphocytes, neutrophils, cellular debris, and purulent material, resulting in a necrotic background (Fig. 1). Plasma cells and macrophages with tingible bodies may be observed in later stag-

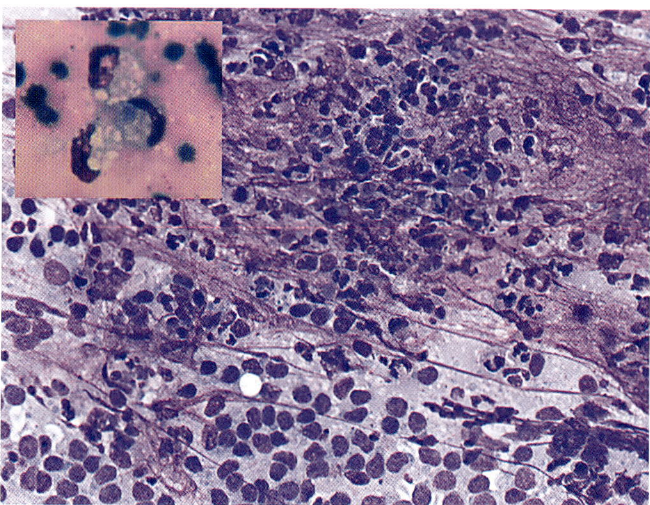

Fig. 1. Lymphoid cells at the edge of a necrotic area with nuclear debris and granulocytes. **Inset** "Kikuchi histiocytes" with eccentric, crescentic nuclei.

es. Bacteria and fungi are rarely detected in routinely stained smears, but may be identified by special stains, such as periodic acid-Schiff, mucicarmine, or Grocott methenamine silver stain. An FNC diagnosis of suppurative lymphadenitis is generally straightforward; the differential diagnosis may include necrotic metastasis, mainly squamous cell carcinoma, and rarely Hodgkin lymphoma (HL), in its "pseudo-suppurative" presentation [2]. Kikuchi-Fujimoto disease (KFD) is a self-limiting, acute, lymphadenitis mainly affecting young women. KFD generally involves cervical LNs and clinically simulates bacterial lymphadenitis. FNC, other than granulocytes, shows polymorphous lymphoid cells in a necrotic background with nuclear debris and karyorrhexis, small histiocytes that usually have an eccentrically placed round, oval, or "crescentic" nucleus ("Kikuchi histiocytes"; Fig. 1), with or without ingested nuclear debris [3]. Cytological features of KFD have been described in case reports and large series [3–7]; however, the FNC diagnosis of KFD remains descriptive in many cases because its cytological features overlap with other entities or even lymphoma [3–7].

Chronic Lymphadenitis

Chronic lymphadenitis is a persistent LNe (3–6 months or more), often caused by unknown agents. Chronic lymphadenitis may clinically simulate a neoplastic process, therefore

Table 1. Clinical and serological data of the main lymphadenitis

Agent	Symptoms and LN ultrasound	LN site prevalence	Serology [63]
Bacteria	Fever; painful, soft, sometimes necrotizing LNe; US: heterogeneous echotexture	Cervical, axillary	Throat swab with bacterial culture; RADTs, ELISA
Mononucleosis	Fever, pharyngitis; US: round, heterogeneous echotexture, possible hilum absence, indistinct margins, central vascularity	Anterior, cervical	Heterophile antibody tests, FBC and WBC, atypical lymphocytes on peripheral blood smears
CMV	Fever, malaise, night sweats; small, rubbery, mobile, tender, LNe; US: unspecific	Regional, generalized	CMV IgM and IgG antibodies, CMV PCR, CMV antigenemia test
HIV	Fever, sore throat, malaise, opportunistic infections; persistent LNe; US: variable	Axillary, cervical, occipital, inguinal	HIV antibodies (ELISA), HIV viral RNA quantitative assay, rapid HIV test, Western blot
Bartonella (Cat-scratch disease)	Fever, malaise, headache, bone and joint aches; chronic, tender LNe; US: heterogeneous echotexture	Axillary, epitrochlear, cervical, inguinal	IgM, IgG assay; PCR for *Bartonella henselae*
Chlamydia trachomatis (lymphogranuloma venereum)	Painless herpetiform, skin lesions, genital shallow ulcers (men) or cervical; persistent LNe; US: LN matting, surrounding tissue oedema	Mono/bilateral, inguinal, perianal, pelvic	Anti-chlamydia IgA, complement fixation test
Treponema (syphilis)	Macules or papules, condylomatous-like; persistent LNe; US: unspecific	Inguinal, epitrochlear	Serum VDRL, RPR, FTA-ABS tests; MHA-TP
Mycobacterium tuberculosis	Fever and myalgia; unilateral, painless, enlarged, matted LN; multiple LNs, fusion tendency, often colliquated; US: internal echoes (calcification)	Cervical, mediastinal, axillary	PCR, culture, skin tuberculin test
Mycobacterium leprae	Erythematous, skin macules, papules, plaques, nerve lesions; painless, soft rubbery LNe; US: unspecific, necrotic	Regional, generalized	AFB on Wade-Fite staining
Cryptococcus	Asymptomatic pulmonary infection (immunocompetent host); US: unspecific	Hilar, mediastinal (unusual), generalized	Serum latex agglutination test, ELISA for fungal antigens
Histoplasma	Asymptomatic pulmonary infection (immunocompetent host); US: unspecific	Mediastinal (unusual), generalized	Sputum culture
Toxoplasma	Mild, unspecific symptoms (fever and myalgia); non-tender LNe; US: unspecific	Mono/bilateral, posterior cervical	Sabin-Feldman test
Leishmania	Cutaneous and visceral lesions, persistent LNe; US: unspecific	Epitrochlear, inguinal, axillary, generalized	Serology, ELISA for *Leishmania*, PCR on tissue or serum

US, ultrasound; RADTs, rapid antigen detection tests; FBC, full blood cells exam; WBC, white blood cell; CMV, cytomegalovirus; RPR, Rapid Plasma Reagin; FTA-ABS, Fluorescent Treponemal Antibody Absorption; MHA-TP, microhaemagglutination assay; AFB, acid-fast bacilli.

direct evaluation is often required, including FNC. Some chronic lymphadenitis are caused by specific agents, such as cytomegalovirus, chlamydia, *Treponema*, fungi, HIV, and autoimmune diseases; in others the aetiology remains unknown. The anatomical site and FNC of chronic lymphadenitis contribute to identifying the aetiological agent, but usually clinical data and serological tests are needed (Table 1). When a chronic lymphadenitis does not disappear or reduce, and persists without any clear clinical explanation, FNC repetition and/or histological evaluation should be performed [8].

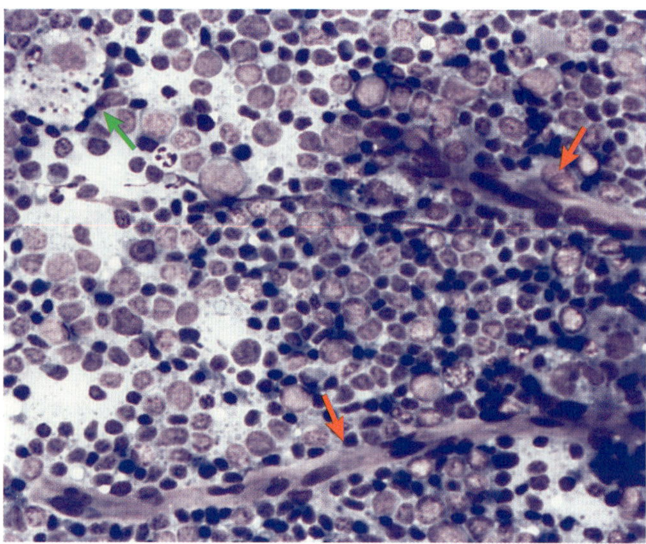

Fig. 2. Florid reactive hyperplasia showing mature lymphocytes, follicular centre cells, an immunoblast, and one macrophage (green arrow) with tingible bodies and capillary structures (red arrows).

Unspecific Reactive Hyperplasia

Many LN-FNC fall within this generic category. Smears show a variable amount of the normal constituents of LNs, including mature lymphocytes, follicular centre cells, immunoblasts, reticular cells, macrophages, with or without tingible bodies and capillary structures (Fig. 2). The presence of all the constituents and lymphoid cells in different stages of maturation generally leads to the diagnosis of reactive hyperplasia. However, in many cases the differential diagnosis with a non-Hodgkin lymphoma (NHL) is difficult or even impossible to perform on smears alone (Fig. 3). The general cytological criteria of benignity and malignancy, which are used in FNC of other organs, may be of little or no help in reactive LN. In fact, low-grade NHL usually lacks nuclear atypia and a proper phenotyping is required to assess the polyclonality of cell populations (Fig. 3b). Equally, mitoses are of little value in LN lymphoproliferative processes and may paradoxically be more numerous in reactive hyperplasia than in low-grade NHL. Scattered, and even numerous, eosinophils may occur in LN reactive hyperplasia and have been reported in Kimura disease, whereas a high number of eosinophils, HL or Langerhans cell histiocytosis (LCH) should be primarily excluded. In these cases, cytological patterns are different from reactive hyperplasia in which the presence of eosinophils usually remains cytologically unexplained.

Infectious Mononucleosis and Cytomegalovirus

Infectious mononucleosis causes cervical or generalized LNe with or without clinical symptoms and splenomegaly. FNC are relatively polymorphous and are characterized by a high number of immunoblasts with 1 or 2 large nucleoli and a rim of blue basophilic cytoplasm (Fig. 4). The background includes mature lymphocytes, plasma cells, follicular centre cells, and macrophages with tingible bodies [9, 10]. When smears appear monomorphous with a prevalence of follicular centre cells and scanty or no macrophages, a differential diagnosis with NHL is usually taken into account, and a proper immunocytochemistry (ICC) or flow cytometry (FC) phenotyping with light chain assessment is required. Binucleated cells simulating HL "mirror cells" may also be present; therefore, a differential diagnosis with HL may also be indicated. However, HL FNC generally shows a different polymorphous background with a variable amount of neutrophils and eosinophils, lacking immunoblastic proliferation, which is more evident in infectious mononucleosis [9]. Moreover, FNC of mononucleosis is generally more cellular than HL; other features favouring the diagnosis of mononucleosis on HL include the presence of mitoses and capillary structures. As for a differential diagnosis with cytomegalovirus infection, corresponding FNC findings have rarely been described [11]. FNC shows histiocytes engulfing erythrocytes, leucocytes, nuclear debris, and platelets in a background of lymphocytes, neutrophils, giant cells, and eosinophils [11]. Enlarged nuclei with typical basophilic intranuclear inclusion and peri-inclusional halo may be observed in endothelial cells [12], and are better appreciated by Papanicolaou staining [13].

HIV Lymphadenitis

HIV-related LNe may show 2 different FNC patterns, depending on the pathogenesis. In the case of bacterial and/or opportunist infections, such as mycobacteria, pneumocystis, or *Leishmania*, FNC features match with the related agents [14–17]. The second pattern is a "florid" unspecific reactive hyperplasia. This latter is caused by follicular expansion and may be due to a possible compensation of concomitant T-cell immunodeficiency. In these cases, a differential diagnosis with follicular NHL is indicated also because of the high risk of NHL in HIV patients (Fig. 5). Other viral infections and postvaccination conditions may result in LNe with non-specific patterns. In these cases, FNC shows small mature lymphocytes intermingled with centrocytes and centroblasts, plasma cells, and immunoblasts. Capillary structures, phagocytic histiocytes, and eosinophils

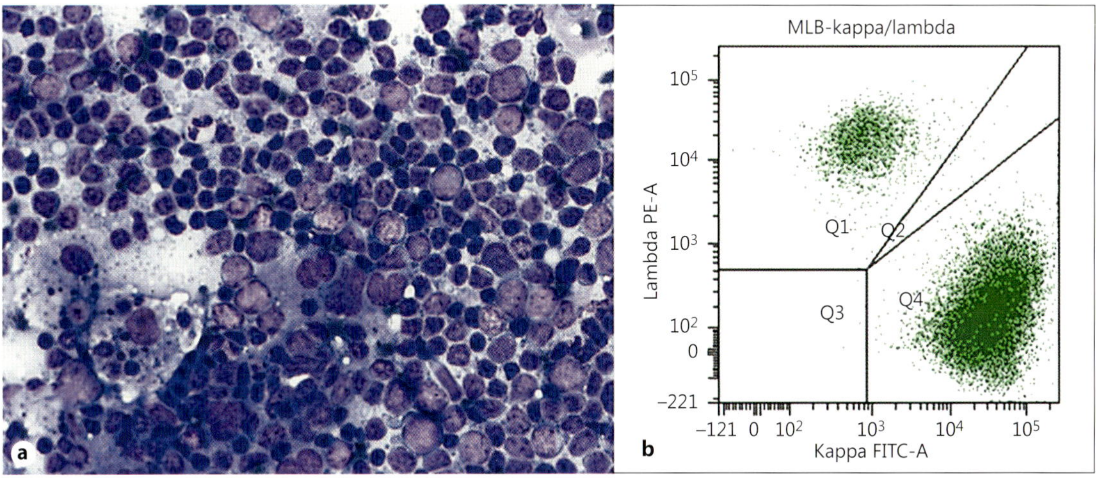

Fig. 3. a Florid unspecific reactive hyperplasia showing lymphocytes and numerous follicular centre cells. Two macrophages with cytoplasmic tingible bodies are present. **b** Flow cytometry histogram showing balanced light chain.

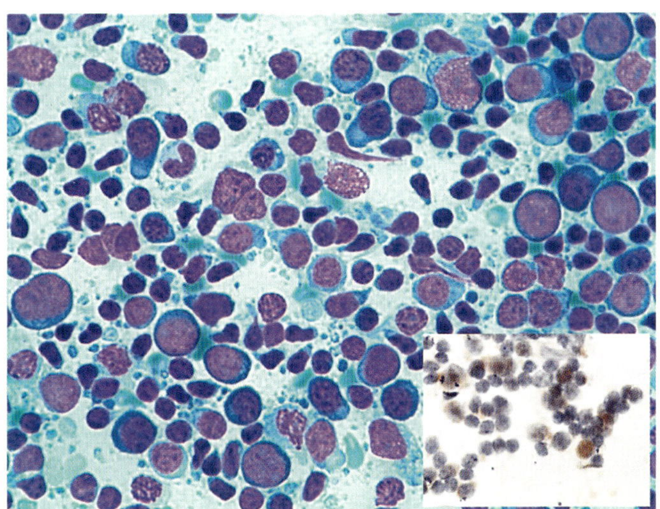

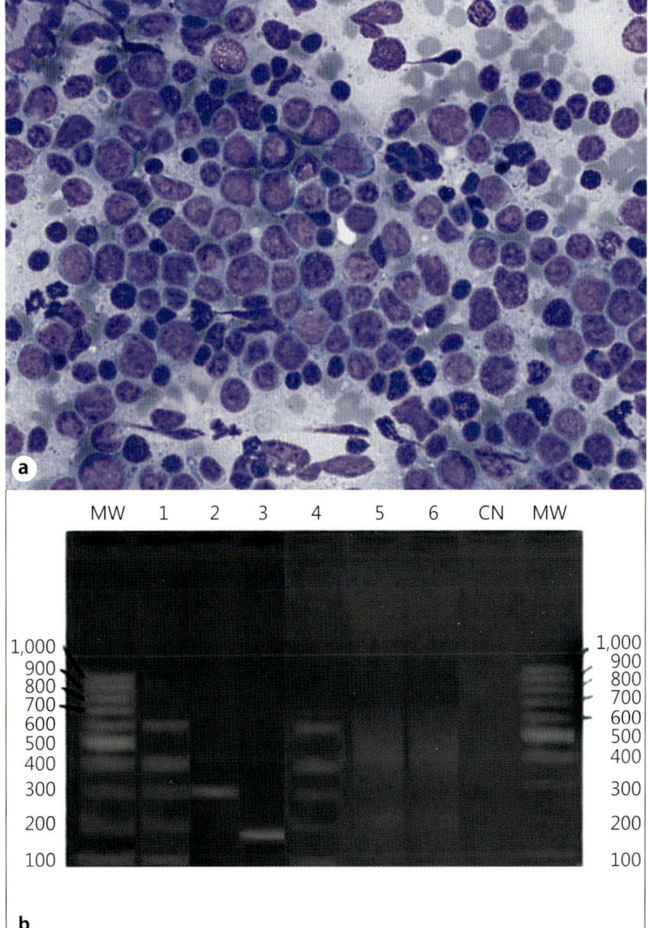

Fig. 4. Mononucleosis smear showing a polymorphous cell population. Numerous immunoblasts with large nuclei, evident nucleoli, and a rim of blue cytoplasm are scattered among lymphocytes, plasma cells, and follicular centre cells. **Inset** Focal, nuclear positivity for Epstein-Barr virus-encoded RNA in situ hybridization on an additional smear.

Fig. 5. a HIV "florid" reactive hyperplasia showing an exceeding number of follicular centre cells and scattered small lymphocytes. This pattern may be indistinguishable from follicular lymphoma on conventional smears. **b** IGHK multiplex PCR of the case: MW lane, DNA molecular weight (100 bp AA561 diluted 1:10; Nuclear Laser Medicine Srl); lanes 1–3, B-NHL control case, Gene Control Multiplex PCR (lane 1), IGH monoclonality (lane 2), IGK monoclonality (lane 3); lanes 4–6, present case, Gene Control Multiplex PCR (lane 4), IGH polyclonality (lane 5), IGK polyclonality (lane 6); CN lanes, negative controls (no DNA in PCR reactions).

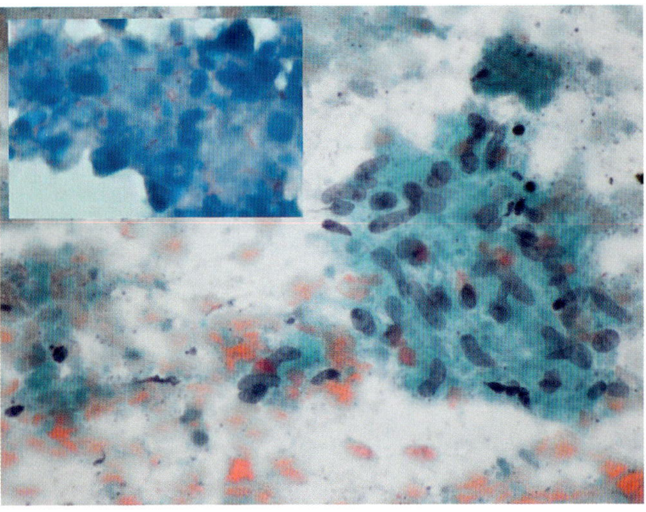 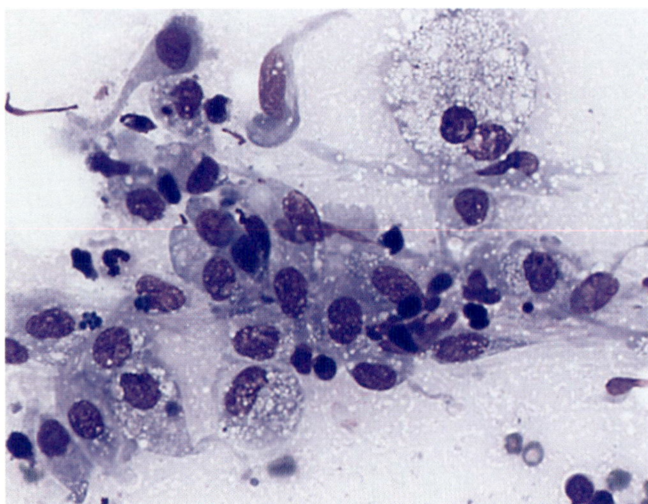

Fig. 6. Tubercular granuloma in a necrotic background. **Inset** Acid fast stain (Ziehl-Neelsen) showing mycobacteria in red.

Fig. 7. The presence of histiocytes with an abundant foamy cytoplasm in an appropriate clinical context should be considered suspicious of an atypical mycobacterial infection.

may be present. A differential diagnosis between florid follicular hyperplasia and NHL is generally indicated because of the high incidence of NHL in AIDS patients, and it mainly depends on the FC assessment of the light chain and CD19/CD10 ratio. Attention should be paid to the occurrence of small clones of B cells with light chain restriction (generally lower than 20% of the gated cells), which may cause false positive FNC diagnoses [18] and require IGHK molecular assessment. Secondary neoplasms, including LN Kaposi sarcoma, have also been reported [19] in HIV LNe.

Granulomatous Lymphadenitis
Granulomatous lymphadenitis is a chronic inflammatory reaction involving different agents and different cell types, such as T cells, macrophages, epithelioid histiocytes, and multinucleated giant cells with granulomas formation. Cytological features include epithelioid histiocytes, isolated and/or aggregated, and multinucleated cells in a variable background. Epithelioid histiocytes show ovaloid or elongated nuclei, often "boomerang" or "footprint" shaped, and dispersed granular chromatin, usually lacking nucleoli. The cytoplasm may be indistinct, showing a syncytial pattern with intermingled lymphocytes. Multinucleated giant cells may be present, both isolated or embedded in the granuloma. Multinucleated giant cells may occur in non-granulomatous lymphadenitis; therefore, aggregates of epithelioid cells only identify granulomatous lymphadenitis with

or without multinucleated giant cells. The background can be clean or dirty for the presence of necrosis and nuclear debris. In extremely necrotic patterns, Papanicolaou stain is useful to exclude atypical nuclei or orangiophilic squamous cells that might reveal squamous carcinoma with an extremely necrotic pattern. A granulomatous pattern with or without a necrotic background is observed in different infectious diseases; the identification of the related agents requires ancillary techniques (microbiological, immunohistochemical, biochemical, and special staining techniques) on different supports.

Tuberculosis
Tuberculosis (TB) is the most common cause of granulomatous lymphadenitis, caused by the "mycobacterium tuberculosis complex" and atypical mycobacteria. This latter, also known as "non-tuberculous mycobacteria," mainly causes opportunistic infections in immunocompromised patients. LN-FNC shows epithelioid histiocytes and granulomas with or without caseous necrosis (Fig. 6), lymphoid cells, Langerhans multinucleated giant cells, either isolated or embedded in the granuloma. Necrotic-suppurative inflammation with a variable number of neutrophils in a watery background, is often observed [20]. Caseous necrotic material is granular, eosinophilic, usually without nuclear debris. In atypical mycobacterial infections, cytological features may differ from the standard granulomatous pattern. Smears

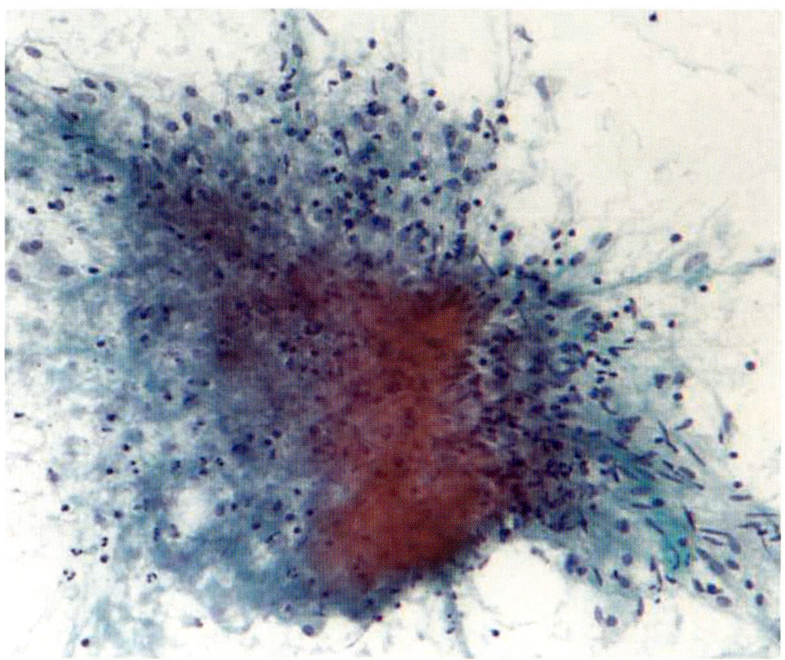

Fig. 8. Cat-scratch disease lymphadenitis. A dense fragment of epithelioid cells, lymphocytes, and neutrophils with a necrotic "core."

may show histiocytes with an abundant, pale, finely vacuolated and ill-defined cytoplasm and less granulomas than those observed in typical TB (Fig. 7). Necrosis may be absent and suppurative changes may occur. The diagnosis of TB needs to be confirmed by acid-fast bacilli (AFB) by Ziehl-Neelsen stain (Fig. 6), mycobacterial culture, or PCR [20–22]. AFB positivity is higher in samples with necrosis only, followed by those with epithelioid histiocytes and granulomas plus necrosis, and lower in samples with granuloma only. Mycobacterial culture is quite specific and sensitivity is influenced by the necrotic content. The disadvantages of mycobacterial culture are poor sensitivity and prolonged times. ICC can be used to detect TB bacilli using the anti-MBP64 antibody on aspirated material with a reported 68% sensitivity and 95% specificity [23]. The distinction between typical and atypical mycobacteria is necessary because they require different treatments and depend on molecular procedures. Recently, an automated semi-nested PCR technique (Xpert MTB/RIF) has been introduced. It is a closed system that carries less biohazard and contamination risk, and can distinguish typical from atypical mycobacteria other than assessing the Rifampicin resistance. Xpert MTB/RIF has been recommended by the WHO for the initial TB diagnosis, especially in children, immunocompromised patients, and in cases of multidrug resistance [20].

Cat-Scratch Lymphadenitis

Cat-scratch lymphadenitis is caused by *Bartonella* and generally involves cervical and axillary LN. FNC shows numerous neutrophils, B lymphocytes, epithelioid histiocytes, and Langerhans giant cells; necrosis is also present (Fig. 8). In the early stage of infection there are increased histiocytes and follicular hyperplasia with no neutrophil predominance or suppurative necrosis. A granulomatous pattern may be observed in the intermediate phase of the disease; smears show granuloma with peripheral palisading epithelioid histiocytes and centrally located neutrophils (micro-abscesses), associated with polymorphous lymphoid cells [24–27]. Like most lymphadenitis, cat-scratch FNC features are not specific and the diagnosis is based on *Bartonella* identification by indirect immunofluorescent antibody, enzyme-linked immunosorbent assay (ELISA), or PCR [24].

Toxoplasmosis

Toxoplasmosis should be considered in the case of any non-necrotizing granulomatous lymphadenitis, especially when posterior cervical LN are involved. FNC shows epithelioid histiocytes (Fig. 9), either isolated or in small clusters (microgranuloma). Isolated epithelioid histiocytes show dense and well-defined cytoplasm and eccentrically located nuclei. These are the same epithelioid histiocytes that enter the follicular centre on histological sections.

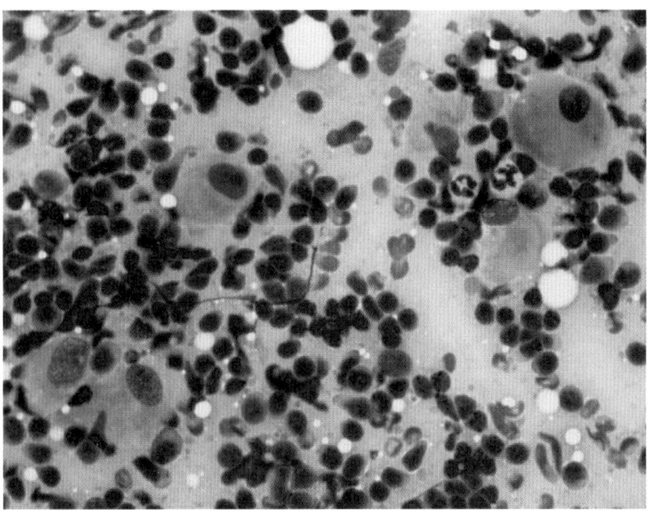

Fig. 9. Epithelioid cells with large, dense, well-defined cytoplasm and eccentric nuclei. Lymphoid cells in different maturative stages are present in the background. This pattern may suggest a serological screening for toxoplasmosis.

Lymphocytes, immunoblasts, and plasma cells may also be observed. Necrosis or suppurative changes do not usually occur [28]. The FNC pattern is unspecific and overlaps other granulomatous lymphadenitis, such as leprosy, lymphogranuloma venereum, and post-vaccine granulomatous. Therefore, the toxoplasma aetiology has to be serologically confirmed.

Lymphadenopathies

Lymphadenopathies are a heterogeneous group of LNe, not directly caused by biological agents and often related to autoimmune processes. Lymphadenopathies are characterized by the expansion of 1 LN compartment and 1 or more cell types that are hyperplastic and may be predominant. Lymphadenopathies are most frequently determined by sarcoidosis, lupus erythematous, rheumatoid arthritis, Castleman disease, angioimmunoblastic hyperplasia, drug hypersensitivity, Rosai-Dorfman disease (RDD), silicone lymphadenopathies, and dermatopathic lymphadenopathies (Table 2). Lymphadenopathies usually show unspecific cytological features whereas sarcoidosis, RDD, dermatopathic and silicone lymphadenopathies FNC are quite typical. In the case of an unspecific follicular pattern, FNC alone is usually not sufficient to provide a definite diagnosis. A

phenotypic profile of the cell population, including light chain assessment by FC, is usually necessary for a correct FNC diagnosis. When light chains are unexpressed or undetected, or when the kappa/lambda ratio is quantitatively insufficient or unclear, FNC repetition, additional molecular tests, or excision may be necessary to exclude NHL.

Sarcoidosis
FNC features of sarcoidosis have been described since the 1980s [29]. Its clinical relevance has acquired importance since the introduction of endoscopic US and endobronchial US FNC [30]. Smears show epithelioid histiocytes, mainly in cohesive groups, and lymphoid cells (Fig. 10). Multinucleated giant cells may be present and the background is generally clean. Different patterns of granuloma have been reported, but they do not distinguish sarcoidosis from TB. Asteroid and Schaumann bodies, which were emphasized as typical of sarcoidosis in the past, may be observed on FNC, but they are neither frequent nor specific [31, 32]. The distinction between sarcoidosis and other types of lymphadenitis and lymphadenopathies with a granulomatous pattern depends on the correlation of FNC with clinical, radiological, and microbiological data [33]. Attention should be paid when few atypical cells occur, because granulomatous pattern may hide a neoplasm. Moreover, HL and large-cell NHL may also have a granulomatous component, adding difficulties to the FNC diagnosis [34–36].

Silicone Lymphadenopathy
The high diffusion of breast reconstruction/augmentation has increased the incidence of silicone lymphadenopathy. Silicone globules phagocytized by macrophages may reach LN through lymphatic vessels. The FNC hallmark of silicone lymphadenopathies is the presence of numerous macrophages with a foamy cytoplasm, deformed by rigid large globules of non-birefringent material, transparent on Diff-Quik or faint yellow on PAP [37, 38] (Fig. 11). Histiocytes engulfed by non-silicone amorphous material in LN may occur in storage diseases and other pathologies, which usually do not determine clinically relevant LNe [39, 40].

Lupus Erythematosus, Rheumatoid Arthritis, Syphilis
These pathologies may cause localized or generalized LNe with cortical expansion and follicular hyperplasia. FNC is similar in these conditions, showing hypercellularity with mature lymphocytes, follicular centre cells, reticular cells, histiocytes, and immunoblasts. Plasma cells, also containing

Table 2. Clinical and cytological features of the main lymphadenopathies

Disease	LN site prevalence	Cytological features
Kimura lymphadenopathy	Head and neck, retroauricular	Eosinophilic microabscesses
Rosai-Dorfman lymphadenopathy	Bilateral cervical region	Histiocytes (SHML cells) with engulfed lymphocytes (emperipolesis)
Kikuchi lymphadenopathy	Unilateral posterior cervical triangle	Histiocytes non-phagocytic and phagocytic with crescent nuclei, nuclear debris; fibrinoid deposits, neutrophil absence
Sarcoidosis lymphadenopathy	Bilateral and symmetric, peribronchial	Epithelioid cells, scattered multinucleated giant cells, lymphocytes, collagen fibres
Lupus lymphadenopathy	Localized or generalized; cervical, axillary	Nuclear dust, "fibrinoid" necrosis, lipid-laden histiocytes, neutrophil absence
Rheumatoid lymphadenopathy	Localized or generalized; axillary, cervical, supraclavicular	Polymorphous with plasma cells and numerous tingible body histiocytes
Dermatopathic lymphadenopathy	Axillary and inguinal	Interdigitating, dendritic cells, Langerhans cells and small lymphocytes; eosinophils, melanin, hemosiderin, lipid-laden macrophages may occur
Drug-induced lymphadenopathy	Generalized or localized	Mixed cellular infiltrate of immunoblasts, eosinophils, plasma cells, necrosis
Silicone lymphadenopathy	Axillary	Extracellular empty-looking vacuoles of various sizes, histiocytes with intracellular foamy vacuoles; multinucleated giant cells
Castleman lymphadenopathy	Unicentric (cervical or mediastinal) or multicentric (immunocompromised patients)	Small lymphocytes, hyaline material (vascular variant); follicular centre cells and numerous plasma cells (plasma cell variant)
Angioimmunoblastic lymphadenopathy	Generalized	Polymorphous cellular infiltrate (lymphocytes, plasma cells, immunoblasts, scattered eosinophils), follicular dendritic cells (CD21 positive)

Russel bodies, are usually present in cases of lupus erythematosus (LE; Fig. 12) and syphilis (Fig. 13). Necrosis and karyorrhexis may be observed in the absence of granulocytes, especially when LE overlaps KFD features, to which LE has often been associated [41–43]. In most of these cases, a differential diagnosis with NHL is indicated and a proper phenotyping is required.

Castleman Disease
Castleman disease (CD), also known as angiofollicular LN hyperplasia, refers to a group of uncommon lymphadenopathies with the same morphological features that involve a single LN or occurs as a systemic process. The 2 main histological subtypes of CD are the hyaline-vascular variant that mainly occurs in single LNe, and the plasma cell variant with a main multicentre occurrence (Fig. 14). CD is characterized by lymphoid benign proliferation determined by interleukin-6 hypersecretion. Human herpes virus-8 infection may be the driver of the process. Patients show systemic inflammatory symptoms and autoimmune manifestations. FNC are generally highly cellular, showing small lymphocytes, follicular centre cells, immunoblasts, and macrophages with tingible bodies. Plasma cells, more evident in the plasma cell variant, are also present; hyaline eosinophilic material within aggregates of follicular centre cells have been described [44]. Epithelioid cells, giant cells, and necrosis are generally absent. Despite these specific cytological features, a differential diagnosis with NHL is usually taken into account and cell phenotyping by ICC or FC is necessary [38, 45–51].

Angioimmunoblastic Lymphadenopathy
Angioimmunoblastic lymphadenopathy (AILD) is a systemic disorder with unknown aetiology. Allergic, infective, neoplastic, drug induced, and immunological theories have

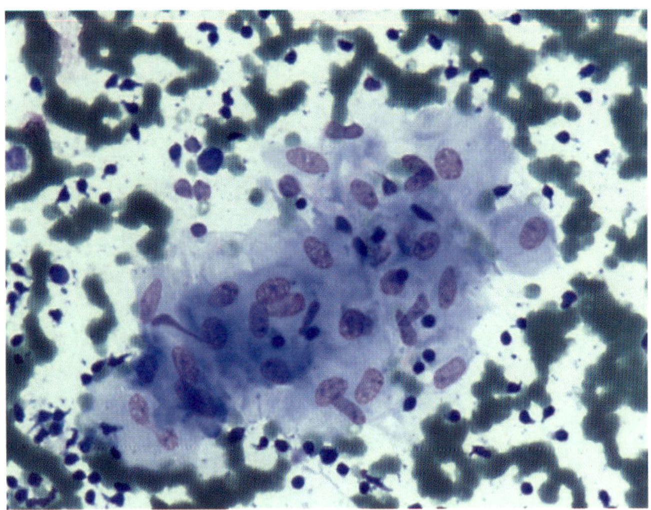

Fig. 10. Granulomatous lymphadenopathy in sarcoidosis: a cohesive granulomatous cluster of epithelioid cells with a large cytoplasm and oval, eccentric nuclei. A few small lymphocytes are intermingled or present in the background.

been considered. AILD is still considered a reactive non-lymphomatous disorder, but immunological and molecular studies demonstrated that the majority of AILD are T-cell clonal processes. AILD patients generally suffer from night sweats, weight loss, hepatosplenomegalia, fever, and skin rashes. LN-FNC and cell blocks show capillary fragments, with a polymorphous population of cells consisting of immunoblasts, plasma cells, eosinophils, and follicular dendritic cells (CD21+; Fig. 15). Follicular cells are generally absent [52]. These unspecific cytological features, in the absence of specific clinical data, do not allow a definite FNC diagnosis of AILD, and a histological assessment is necessary.

Drug Hypersensitivity

LNe may occur after vaccinations or drug assumption. The relation between LNe and phenytoin/dilantin or methotrexate is well known. In other cases, LNe is caused by individual hypersensitivity to different drugs. FNC usually shows unspecific reactive hyperplasia. Numerous eosinophils, plasma cells, and Reed-Sternberg-like cells have also been reported [38]. In most cases, LNe from drug hypersensitivity disappears after the interruption of the corresponding treatment.

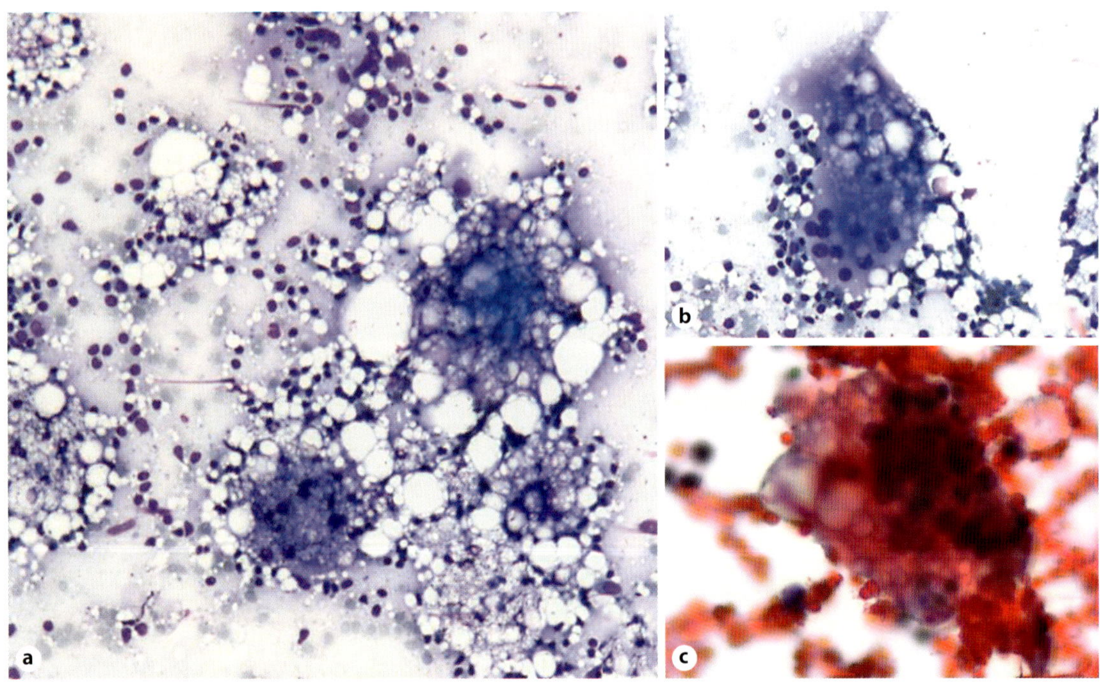

Fig. 11. Silicone lymphadenopathy. Multinucleated histiocytes with a foamy cytoplasm engulfed by roundish large globules (**a**), which are transparent on Diff-Quik (**b**) or faint yellow on Papanicolaou (**c**).

Rosai-Dorfman Disease
Rosai-Dorfman disease (RDD) or sinus histiocytosis with massive lymphadenopathy (SHML), is a rare, extremely large, self-limiting lymphadenopathy that may occur in LN and extra-LN locations. Histologically, RDD is characterized by medullary expansion due to histiocytic proliferation. FNC hallmarks are histiocytes and multinucleated giant cells with emperipolesis of lymphocytes in a background of mixed lymphoid cells (Fig. 16). RDD histiocytes are S100 positive and CD1a negative at ICC evaluation. A

differential diagnosis with Langerhans cell hystiocytosis (LCH) may be indicated. Nonetheless, LCH histiocytes show typical "coffee bean" nuclei and are CD1a positive and S100 negative. FC in RDD is generally useless [38, 53–57].

Dermatopathic Lymphadenitis
Dermatopathic lymphadenitis may occur in long-standing different cutaneous diseases. FNC are variably cellular, with macrophages containing brown melanin pigment. Histio-

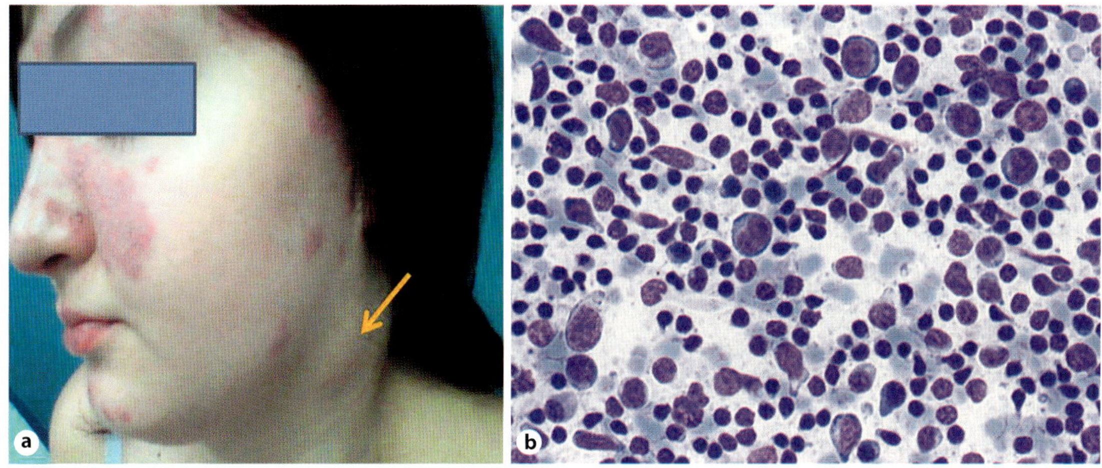

Fig. 12. Lupus erythematosus: a young girl with a butterfly erythema and left cervical, enlarged LN (arrow; **a**); LN-FNC reactive hyperplasia with follicular centre cells and plasma cells (**b**).

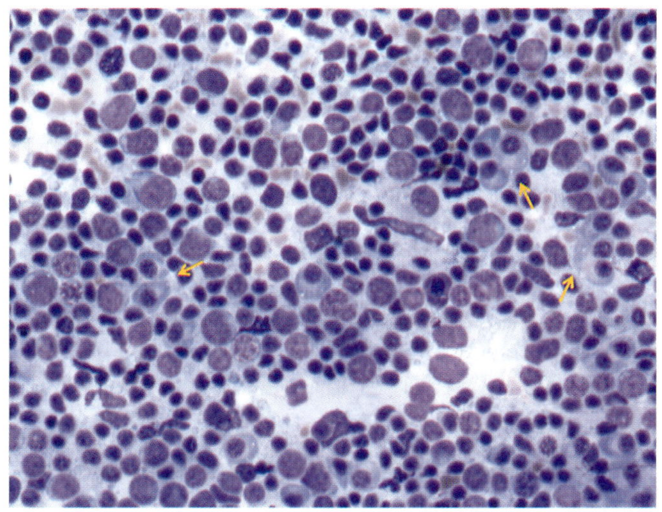

Fig. 13. Reactive polymorphous pattern showing follicular centre cells, small lymphocytes, and numerous mature plasma cells (arrows). Serological data only were indicative of syphilis.

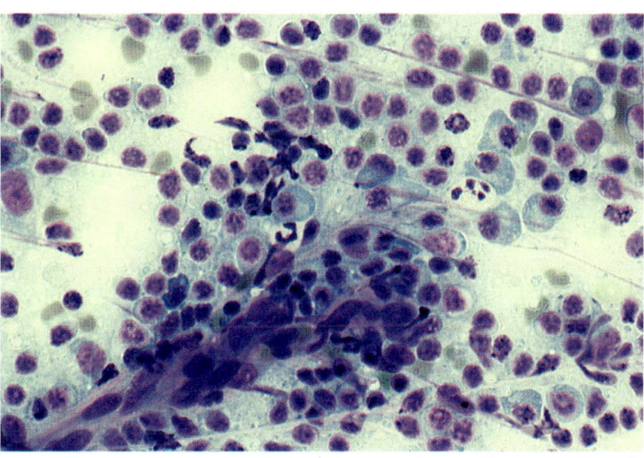

Fig. 14. LN-FNC of Castleman disease case: smear showed capillary structures, small lymphocytes, follicular centre cells, and immunoblasts. Numerous plasma cells were detected. FC showed a polyclonal pattern. The case was diagnosed as negative unspecific. A histological control revealed a Castleman disease plasma cell variant.

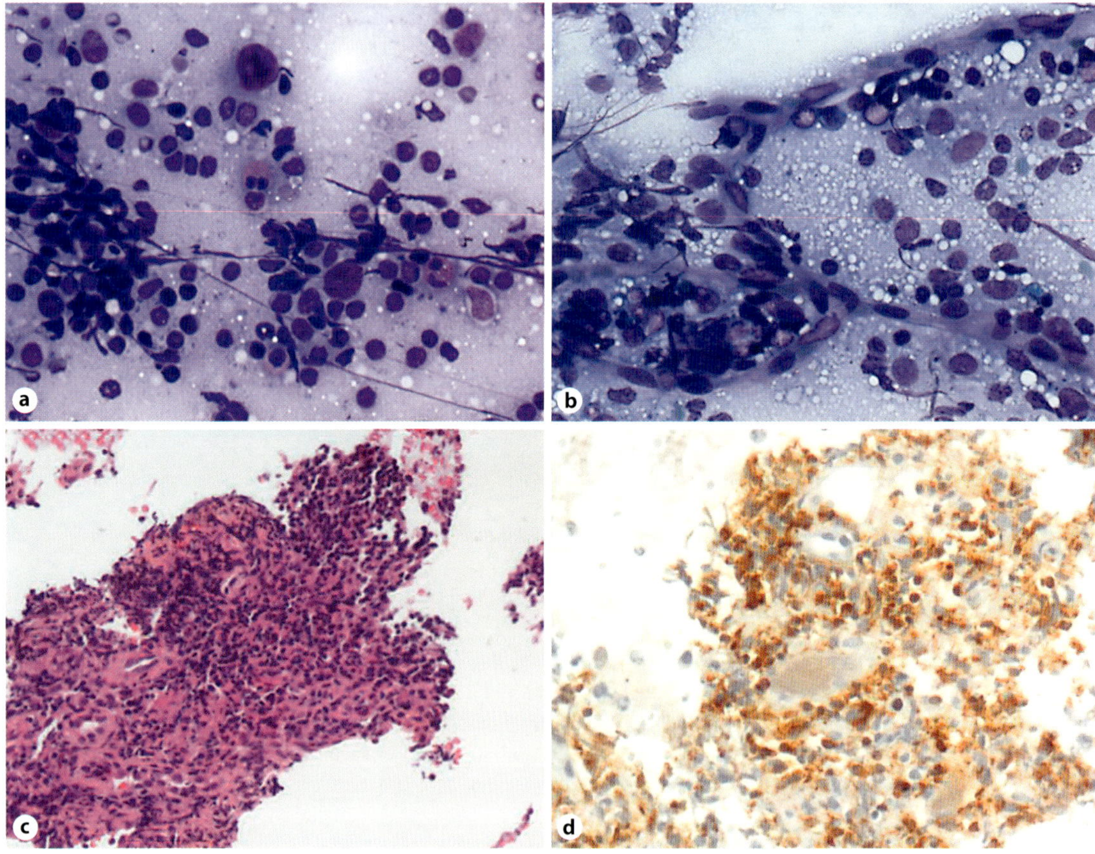

Fig. 15. a Angioimmunoblastic lymphadenopathy showing a polymorphous cell population with small lymphocytes, immunoblasts, plasma cells, and eosinophils. Follicular cells are absent. **b** Capillary structures. **c** Cell block showing a fragment of vascular stroma in the absence of follicles. **d** CD21 strong positivity of dendritic cells.

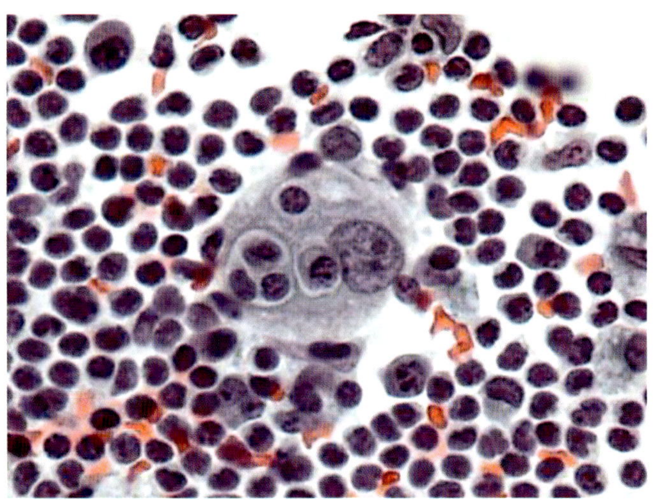

Fig. 16. Rosai-Dorfman disease lymphadenopathy: a typical histiocyte with emperipolesis of lymphocytes in a background of mixed lymphoid cells.

cytic-dendritic cells, sometimes clustered around vascular structures, may occur (Fig. 17). Histiocytes have an abundant, pale, blue cytoplasm and indistinct cytoplasmic borders. Mature lymphocytes, eosinophils, and plasma cells are present in the background. Follicular centre cells are scanty when compared to unspecific reactive hyperplasia [38, 58–63]. FNC diagnosis of dermatopathic lymphadenitis is quite straightforward in the presence of chronic dermatitis such as psoriasis, but it may be challenging in cases of cutaneous lymphoma [58].

Lymph Node Infarction
LN infarction is a coagulative necrosis usually caused by vascular thrombosis that may occur in superficial and deeply located LN [64]. As LNs are supplied by numerous anastomosing vessels, LN infarct is extremely rare and may occur in NHL or metastases in 30–40% of cases. FNC may show dense amorphous, basophilic material in which

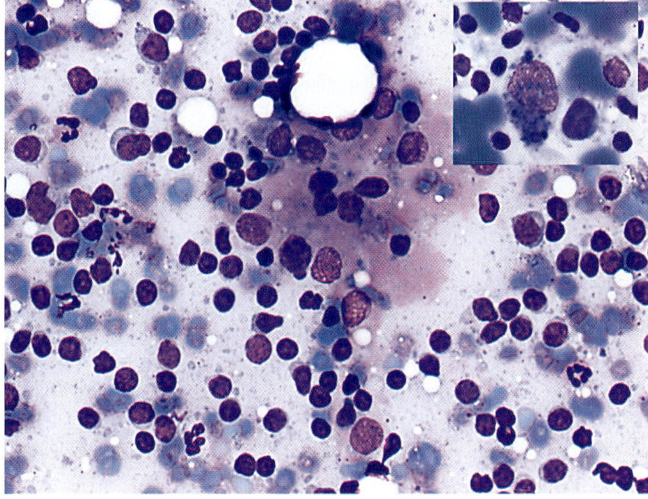

Fig. 17. Dermatopathic lymphadenitis showing histiocytic-dendritic cells in a polymorphous background. Macrophages containing brown melanin pigment (**inset**) are scattered on the smear.

Fig. 18. Lymph node infarction FNC showing dense amorphous, basophilic material. Few whole nuclei are present in the background.

whole nuclei are present on the edges only (Fig. 18). A variable number of vital cells may be observed in the background. A differential diagnosis with Kikuchi disease may be indicated, whereas this latter usually occurs in younger patients [see Chapter 6, this vol., p. 66]. ROSE may be helpful to avoid ineffective ancillary techniques, to choose another LN, if any, and its report prevents FNC to be considered responsible for the LN infarct [65].

References

1 Gupta A, Rahman K, Shahid M, Kumar A, Qaseem SM, Hassan SA, Siddiqui FA: Sonographic assessment of cervical lymphadenopathy: role of high resolution and color Doppler imaging. Head Neck 2011;33:297–302.

2 Fulciniti F, Zeppa P, Vetrani A, Troncone G, Palombini L: Hodgkin's disease mimicking suppurative lymphadenitis: a possible pitfall in fine-needle aspiration biopsy cytology. Diagn Cytopathol 1989;5:282–285.

3 Das DK, Mallik MK, Dashti HA, Sathar SA, Jaragh M, Junaid TA: Kikuchi-Fujimoto disease in fine-needle aspiration smears: a clinico-cytologic study of 76 cases of KFD and 684 cases of reactive hyperplasia of the lymph node. Diagn Cytopathol 2013;41:288–295.

4 Hong L, Wang X, Huang Z, Cheng L, Wang J: Histiocytic necrotizing lymphadenitis diagnosed by conventional cytology and liquid based cytology. Int J Clin Exp Pathol 2014;7:6186–6190.

5 Das DK, Haji BI, Al-Boijan RA, Sheikh ZA, Pathan SK, Mannan AA: Fujimoto disease in fine needle aspiration smears: a clinico-cytologic study of 18 pediatric cases and correlation with 68 adult patients. Indian J Pathol Microbiol 2012;55:333–338.

6 Sivakumar S, Ramamoorthy R: Fine needle aspiration cytology of Kikuchi-Fujimoto's disease: a report of 2 cases with emphasis on cytologic features and differential diagnosis. Acta Cytol 2012;56:457–462.

7 Tong TR, Chan OW, Lee KC: Diagnosing Kikuchi disease on fine needle aspiration biopsy: a retrospective study of 44 cases diagnosed by cytology and 8 by histopathology. Acta Cytol 2001;45:953–957.

8 Thomas JO, Adeyi D, Amanguno H: Fine-needle aspiration in the management of peripheral lymphadenopathy in a developing country. Diagn Cytopathol 1999;21:159–162.

9 Stanley MW, Steeper TA, Horwitz CA, Burton LG, Strickler JG, Borken S: Fine-needle aspiration of lymph nodes in patients with acute infectious mononucleosis. Diagn Cytopathol 1990;6:323–329.

10 Kardos TF, Kornstein MJ, Frable WJ: Cytology and immunocytology of infectious mononucleosis in fine needle aspirates of lymph nodes. Acta Cytol 1988;32:722–726.

11 Gupta A, Sen R, Batra C, Banerjee D, Gupta A, Jain M: Hemophagocytic syndrome secondary to cytomegalovirus infection in an infant. J Cytol 2011;28:36–38.

12 Zhang X, El-Sahrigy D, Elhosseiny A, Melamed MR: Simultaneous cytomegalovirus infection and Kaposi's sarcoma of the thyroid diagnosed by fine needle aspiration in an AIDS patient: a case report and first cytologic description of the two entities occurring together. Acta Cytol 2003;47:645–648.

13 Wax TD, Layfield LJ, Zaleski S, Bhargara V, Cohen M, Lyerly HK, Fisher SR: Cytomegalovirus sialadenitis in patients with the acquired immunodeficiency syndrome: a potential diagnostic pitfall with fine-needle aspiration cytology. Diagn Cytopathol 1994;10:169–174.

14 Anuradha, Sinha A: Extrapulmonary *Pneumocystis carinii* infection in an AIDS patient: a case report. Acta Cytol 2007;51:599–601.

15 Sarma PK, Chowhan AK, Agrawal V, Agarwal V: Fine needle aspiration cytology in HIV-related lymphadenopathy: experience at a single centre in north India. Cytopathology 2010;21:234–239.

16 de Faria FB, Barroca H: Fine needle aspiration of a lymph node in an HIV patient with chronic infection by *Leishmania*: a case report. Acta Cytol 2010;54(5 suppl):946–948.

17 Reddy DL, Venter WD, Pather S: Patterns of lymph node pathology; fine needle aspiration biopsy as an evaluation tool for lymphadenopathy: a retrospective descriptive study conducted at the largest hospital in Africa. PLoS One 2015;10: e0130148.

18 Cozzolino I, Nappa S, Picardi M, De Renzo A, Troncone G, Palombini L, Zeppa P: Clonal B-cell population in a reactive lymph node in acquired immunodeficiency syndrome. Diagn Cytopathol 2009;37:910–914.

19 Fulciniti F, De Chiara A, Apice G, Petrillo A, Botti G, Feroce F, Mozzillo N: Fine-needle cytology of Kaposi's sarcoma in an intramammary lymphnode: report of one case. Diagn Cytopathol 2012;40(suppl 2):E149–E152.

20 Chatterjee D, Dey P: Tuberculosis revisited: cytological perspective. Diagn Cytopathol 2014;42: 993–1001.

21 Kim DW, Jung SJ, Ha TK, Park HK: Individual and combined diagnostic accuracy of ultrasound diagnosis, ultrasound-guided fine-needle aspiration and polymerase chain reaction in identifying tuberculous lymph nodes in the neck. Ultrasound Med Biol 2013;39:2308–2314.

22 Mittal P, Handa U, Mohan H, Gupta V: Comparative evaluation of fine needle aspiration cytology, culture, and PCR in diagnosis of tuberculous lymphadenitis. Diagn Cytopathol 2011;39:822–826.

23 Purohit MR, Mustafa T, Wiker HG, Sviland L: Rapid diagnosis of tuberculosis in aspirate, effusions, and cerebrospinal fluid by immunocytochemical detection of *Mycobacterium tuberculosis* complex specific antigen MPT64. Diagn Cytopathol 2012;40:782–791.

24 Choi AH, Bolaris M, Nguyen DK, Panosyan EH, Lasky JL 3rd, Duane GB: Clinico cytopathologic correlation in atypical presentation of lymphadenopathy with review of literature. Am J Clin Pathol 2015;143:749–754.

25 Stastny JF, Wakely PE Jr, Frable WJ: Cytologic features of necrotizing granulomatous inflammation consistent with cat-scratch disease. Diagn Cytopathol 1996;15:108–115.

26 Donnelly A, Hendricks G, Martens S, Strovers C, Wiemerslage S, Thomas PA: Cytologic diagnosis of cat scratch disease (CSD) by fine-needle aspiration. Diagn Cytopathol 1995;13:103–106.

27 Silverman JF: Fine needle aspiration cytology of cat scratch disease. Acta Cytol 1985;29:542–547.

28 Viguer JM, Jiménez-Heffernan JA, López-Ferrer P, González-Peramato P, Vicandi B: Fine needle aspiration of toxoplasmic (Piringer-Kuchinka) lymphadenitis: a cytohistologic correlation study. Acta Cytol 2005;49:139–143.

29 Frable MA, Frable WJ: Fine-needle aspiration biopsy: efficacy in the diagnosis of head and neck sarcoidosis. Laryngoscope 1984;94:1281–1283.

30 Fritscher-Ravens A, Sriram PV, Topalidis T, Hauber HP, Meyer A, Soehendra N, Pforte A: Diagnosing sarcoidosis using endosonography-guided fine-needle aspiration. Chest 2000;118:928–935.

31 Jorns JM, Knoepp SM: Asteroid bodies in lymph node cytology: infrequently seen and still mysterious. Diagn Cytopathol 2011;39:35–36.

32 Das DK, Muqim AA, Sheikh ZA, Al-Kandari M, Junaid TA: Sarcoidosis diagnosed on transbronchial fine needle aspiration smears: a case report with new information on asteroid bodies. Acta Cytol 2010;54:225–228.

33 Kaur G, Dhamija A, Augustine J, Bakshi P, Verma K: Can cytomorphology of granulomas distinguish sarcoidosis from tuberculosis? Retrospective study of endobronchial ultrasound guided transbronchial needle aspirate of 49 granulomatous lymph nodes. Cytojournal 2013;10:19.

34 Paksoy N: Cervical lymph node metastasis of extramedullary plasmacytoma of the tonsil presenting with granulomatous lymphadenitis in fine needle aspiration cytology. Acta Cytol 2010;54: 733–736.

35 Koo V, Lioe TF, Spence RA: Fine needle aspiration cytology (FNAC) in the diagnosis of granulomatous lymphadenitis. Ulster Med J 2006;75:59–64.

36 Zardawi IM, Barker BJ, Simons DP: Hodgkin's disease masquerading as granulomatous lymphadenitis on fine needle aspiration cytology. Acta Cytol 2005;49:224–226.

37 Malzone MG, Campanile AC, Gioioso A, Fucito A, D'Aiuto G, Botti G, Fulciniti F: Silicone lymphadenopathy: presentation of a further case containing asteroid bodies on fine-needle cytology sample. Diagn Cytopathol 2015;43:57–59.

38 Monaco SE, Khalbuss WE, Pantanowitz L: Benign non-infectious causes of lymphadenopathy: a review of cytomorphology and differential diagnosis. Diagn Cytopathol 2012;40:925–938.

39 Cozzolino I, Picardi M, Pagliuca S, Ciancia G, Luigia L, Pettinato G, Vetrani A: B-cell non-Hodgkin lymphoma and pseudo-Gaucher cells in a lymph node fine needle aspiration. Cytopathology 2016; 27:134–136.

40 Zeppa P, Vetrani A, Ciancia G, Cuccuru A, Palombini L: Hemophagocytic histiocytosis diagnosed by fine needle aspiration cytology of the spleen: a case report. Acta Cytol 2004;48:415–419.

41 Rao GS, Vohra D, Kuruvilla M: Is Kikuchi-Fujimoto disease a manifestation of systemic lupus erythematosus? Int J Dermatol 2006;45:454–456.

42 Pai MR, Adhikari P, Coimbatore RV, Ahmed S: Fine needle aspiration cytology in systemic lupus erythematosus lymphadenopathy: a case report. Acta Cytol 2000;44:67–69.

43 Sudha A, Vivekanand N: Cytologic picture of Castleman's disease: a report of two cases. J Cytol 2010;27:152–154.

44 Tsang WY, Chan JK: Fine-needle aspiration cytologic diagnosis of Kikuchi's lymphadenitis: a report of 27 cases. Am J Clin Pathol 1994;102:454–458.

45 Naik LP, Fernandes G, Mahapatra L: Cytology of Castleman disease hyaline vascular type: a close differential diagnosis with Hodgkin's lymphoma. Acta Cytol 2010;54(5 suppl):1093–1094.

46 Nanda A, Handa U, Punia RS, Mohan H: Fine needle aspiration in retroperitoneal Castleman's disease: a case report. Acta Cytol 2009;53:316–318.

47 Deschênes M, Michel RP, Tabah R, Auger M: Fine-needle aspiration cytology of Castleman disease: case report with review of the literature. Diagn Cytopathol 2008;36:904–908.

48 Mallik MK, Kapila K, Das DK, Haji BE, Anim JT: Cytomorphology of hyaline-vascular Castleman's disease: a diagnostic challenge. Cytopathology 2007;18:168–174.

49 Taylor GB, Smeeton IW: Cytologic demonstration of "dysplastic" follicular dendritic cells in a case of hyaline-vascular Castleman's disease. Diagn Cytopathol 2000,22.230–234.

50 Meyer L, Gibbons D, Ashfaq R, Vuitch F, Saboorian MH: Fine-needle aspiration findings in Castleman's disease. Diagn Cytopathol 1999;21:57–60.

51 Dey P, Radhika S, Das A: Fine-needle aspiration biopsy of angio-immunoblastic lymphadenopathy. Diagn Cytopathol 1996;15:412–414.

52 Mallick S, Ghosh R, Iyer VK, Jain D, Mathur SR: Cytomorphological and morphometric analysis of 22 cases of Rosai-Dorfman disease: a large series from a tertiary care centre. Acta Cytol 2013;57: 625–632.

53 Majumdar K, Tyagi I, Saran RK, Kumar S, Gondal R: Multicentric extranodal Rosai Dorfman disease – a cytological diagnosis, with histological corroboration. Acta Cytol 2012;56:214–218.

54 Schein C, Kluskens L, Gattuso P: Fine-needle aspiration of primary Rosai-Dorfman disease of the bone without peripheral lymphadenopathy: a challenging diagnosis. Diagn Cytopathol 2013;41: 230–231.

55 Shi Y, Griffin AC, Zhang PJ, Palmer JN, Gupta P: Sinus histiocytosis with massive lymphadenopathy (Rosai-Dorfman disease): a case report and review of 49 cases with fine needle aspiration cytology. Cytojournal 2011;8:3.

56 Layfield LJ: Fine needle aspiration cytologic findings in a case of sinus histiocytosis with massive lymphadenopathy (Rosai-Dorfman syndrome). Acta Cytol 1990;34:767–770.

57 Vigliar E, Cozzolino I, Picardi M, Peluso AL, Fernandez LV, Vetrani A, Botti G, Pane F, Selleri C, Zeppa P: Lymph node fine needle cytology in the staging and follow-up of cutaneous lymphomas. BMC Cancer 2014;14:8.

58 Verma SK, Chowdhury N: A case of dermatopathic lymphadenitis diagnosed by fine needle aspiration. Pathology 2006;38:466–468.

59 Galed-Placed I: Fine needle aspiration cytology of dermatopathic lymphadenitis. Acta Cytol 2000;44: 931–932.

60 Galindo LM, Garcia FU, Hanau CA, Lessin SR, Jhala N, Bigler RD, Vonderheid EC: Fine-needle aspiration biopsy in the evaluation of lymphadenopathy associated with cutaneous T-cell lymphoma (mycosis fungoides/Sézary syndrome). Am J Clin Pathol 2000;113:865–871.

61 Iyer VK, Kapila K, Verma K: Fine needle aspiration cytology of dermatopathic lymphadenitis. Acta Cytol 1998;42:1347–1351.

62 Sudilovsky D, Cha I: Fine needle aspiration cytology of dermatopathic lymphadenitis. Acta Cytol 1998;42:1341–1346.

63 BMJ Best Practice: Assessment of lymphadenopathy. http://bestpractice.bmj.com/best-practice/monograph/838/diagnosis/differential-diagnosis.html.

64 Ioachim HL, Medeiros LJ: Metastatic tumors in lymph nodes; in: Ioachim's Lymph Node Pathology, ed 4. Philadelphia, Lippincott, Williams & Watkins, 2009, pp 590–598.

65 Strauchen JA, Miller LK: Lymph node infarction: an immunohistochemical study of 11 cases. Arch Pathol Lab Med 2003;127:60–63.

Chapter 4

Zeppa P, Cozzolino I: Lymph Node FNC. Cytopathology of Lymph Nodes and Extranodal Lymphoproliferative Processes.
Monogr Clin Cytol. Basel, Karger, 2018, vol 23, pp 34–51 (DOI: 10.1159/000478880)

Non-Hodgkin Lymphoma

The last WHO classification [1] still divides non-Hodgkin lymphoma (NHL) into B-cell type, which accounts for about 90% of cases, T-cell type (about 10%), and a very small number of "null-cell" type. According to morphology and cell size, NHL may be basically distinguished as small-cell NHL or medium/large-cell NHL, and this broad subdivision is reliable at fine-needle cytology (FNC) as well. According to the cell size criterion, the most common small-cell NHL are generally monomorphous entities: small lymphocytic lymphoma/chronic lymphocytic leukaemia (SLL/CLL), mantle cell lymphoma (MCL), marginal zone lymphoma (MZL), follicular lymphoma (FL) grades I and II, and lymphoplasmacytic lymphoma (LpcL). This group almost exclusively includes B-cell NHL and natural killer lymphoma. The medium-to-large group is more polymorphous and heterogeneous, and includes diffuse large B-cell lymphoma (DLBCL), FL grade III, Burkitt and Burkitt-like lymphoma (BL and BL-like), precursor B- and T-cell lymphoma (LL-T), peripheral T-cell lymphoma not otherwise specified (PTCL NOS), and anaplastic large-cell lymphoma (ALCL). Whereas cytological features may suggest a specific entity, morphology alone cannot identify the definite phenotype of each NHL, which needs to be assessed by appropriate immunocytochemistry (ICC) or flow cytometry (FC) phenotypization.

Small B-Cell Non-Hodgkin Lymphoma

On FNC smears, small-cell NHL generally shows a monomorphous, dissociated, small-size cell population, with little nuclear abnormalities. These features are shared by different entities, corresponding to different subtypes with different clinical behaviours. Therefore, an accurate classification depends only partially upon morphological features, and mainly upon phenotypic and genetic characteristics.

Small Lymphocytic Lymphoma/Chronic Lymphocytic Leukaemia

SLL/CLL are 2 different, often interchangeable, presentations of the same disease. In many patients, SLL/CLL is already in an advanced stage at clinical onset. Compromised lymph nodes (LN) are slightly enlarged or even of normal size. SLL/CLL cells are small, well-differentiated lymphocytes with a scant cytoplasm; the nuclei are roundish or slightly irregular with chromatin aggregated in coarse clumps, without evident nucleoli (Fig. 1). Mitoses, apoptotic cells or necrosis are generally absent. The typical phenotype of SLL/CLL cells is CD20+, CD19+, CD5+, CD23+, CD10–, and CD38+/– (Fig. 1). Two-thirds of SLL/CLL cells are genetically similar to hypermutated post-germinal cen-

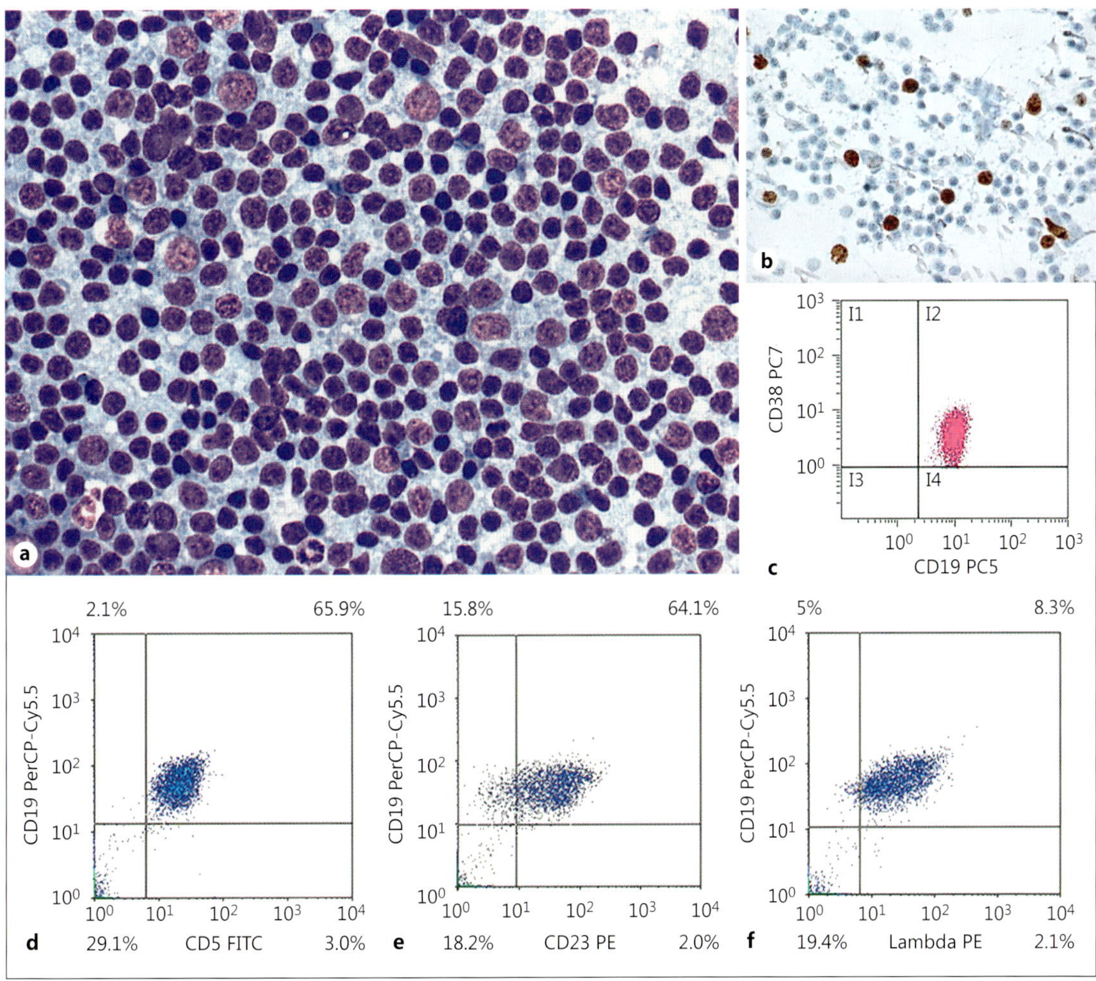

Fig. 1. Cytology and flow cytometry (FC) of small lymphocytic lymphoma/chronic lymphocytic leukemia. **a** Smear showing a monomorphous population of small lymphocytes; nuclei have granular chromatin, light membrane irregularities and occasional small nucleoli. **b** Ki67 positivity in less than 10% of the cells. FC showing: CD19/CD38 co-expression (**c**), CD5/CD19 co-expression (**d**), CD23/CD19 co-expression (**e**), and λ light chain restriction (**f**).

tre B (GCB) cells; the remaining third are similar to mature pre-GCB cells that have not yet undergone antigen selection and have a more clinically aggressive behaviour [2–8]. A phenotypical differentiation between the 2 groups is possible because the first has a hypermutated VH region and does not express ZAP-70 and CD38; conversely, the second group has wild VH regions and expresses ZAP-70 and CD38 [2–8]. SLL/CLL generally has an indolent clinical course, whereas, in a variable percentage of cases, it may progress to large B-cell NHL (Richter syndrome) or evolve towards Hodgkin lymphoma (HL) or an even more aggressive form of leukaemia (prolymphocytic or blast leukaemia). SLL/CLL relapses may occur in an "accelerated phase" (SLL/CLL-AP) showing intermediate-to-large cells with prominent nucleoli, plasmacytoid cells, and numerous mitoses (Fig. 2); Ki67 on additional smears or cell blocks may highlight this aspect (Fig. 2). Apoptotic bodies and necrosis may occur in SLL/CLL-AP. It is important to differentiate SLL-AP from Richter syndrome, which carries a different prognosis and requires different therapy [9]. Notably, SLL/CLL-AP patients are often chronic, immunosuppressed patients who may develop a second neoplasia. Therefore, possible metastases should be considered when dealing with LN-FNC in SLL/CLL patients [10].

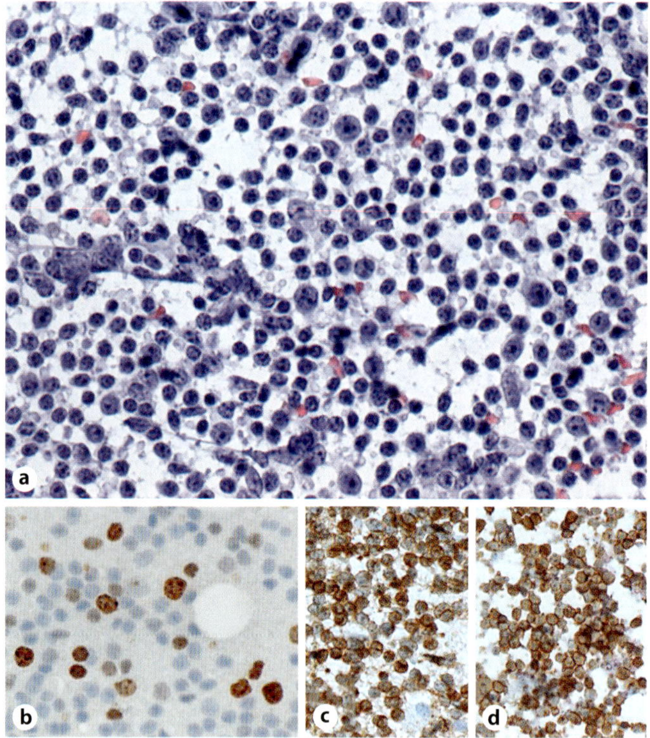

Fig. 2. a Small lymphocytic lymphoma/chronic lymphocytic leukemia in an accelerated phase showing scattered larger cells with 1 or 2 central nucleoli (paraimmunoblasts) and mitoses. **b** Ki67 is positive in an unusual exceeding number of cells. CD23 (**c**) and CD5 (**d**) positivity.

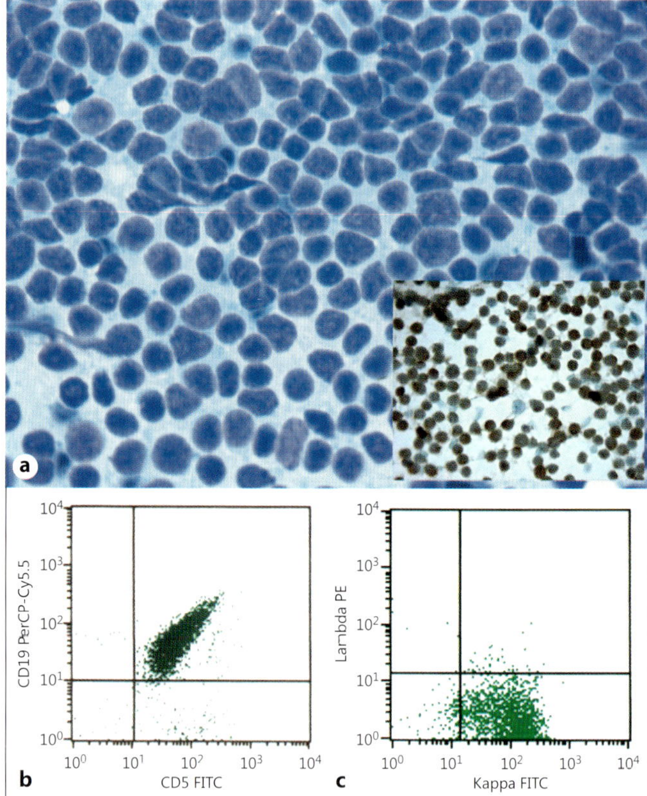

Fig. 3. Mantle cell lymphoma. **a** Dispersed small- to medium-sized cells with coarse granular chromatin and small nucleoli. Nuclei have an irregular shape and a rough "cobblestone" arrangement. **Inset** Cyclin D1 nuclear positivity. Flow cytometry showing CD19/CD5 co-expression (**b**) and κ light chain restriction (**c**).

Mantle Cell Lymphoma

MCL represents 4–10% of all NHL. In most cases it is determined by the t(11–14)(q13;q32) translocation, with the deregulation of the cyclin-D1 translocated gene on the immunoglobulin heavy-chain (IGH) locus [1]. The age at onset is approximately 60 years and it is often diagnosed in advanced stages with generalized lymphadenopathy, and the possible involvement of extranodal sites. MCL generally has a poor prognosis compared to other small-cell NHL [1]. In 20% of cases, MCL appears in the "blastoid variant" that has a more clinically aggressive behaviour. FNC of MCL shows small- to medium-sized cells with a scanty cytoplasm and irregularly shaped nuclei. The nuclear cleavages typically observed on MCL histological sections may not be evident on smears where, conversely, MCL cells may show irregular nuclear borders and a "moulding" arrangement with nuclei more polygonal than roundish in shape. The chromatin is dispersed and the nucleoli are small or irrelevant (Fig. 3). The MCL "blastoid variant" shows larger cells with higher proliferative activity and heavier nuclear atypia (Fig. 4) determined by additional genetic alterations. The typical MCL phenotype is CD19+, CD20+, CD22+, CD79a+, CD5+, CD10–, CD23– (Fig. 3). Additional cyclin D1 (Fig. 3) and more recently SOX11 are highly sensitive and specific for MCL on smears or cell blocks [11]. MCL generally responds to treatment but frequently relapses; therefore, FNC performed twice or more in the same patients over time is not unusual in LN-FNC series [12–24].

Marginal Zone Lymphoma

The WHO [1] classifies MZL into 3 types: extranodal mucosa-associated lymphoid tissue lymphoma (MALT NHL), splenic MZL, and nodal MZL. Despite their morphological and immunophenotypic similarities, molecular data suggest different pathogenic mechanisms. For instance, MZL shows the t(11,18) translocation in half of the extranodal cases and rarely in the nodal ones. MALT NHL is the most frequent presen-

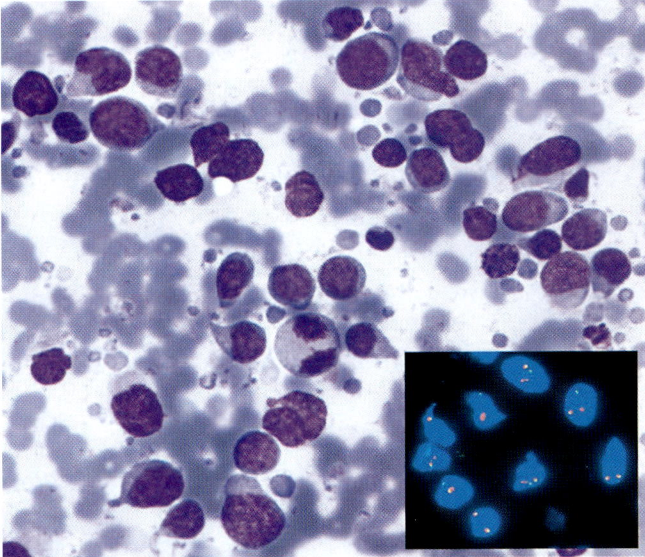

Fig. 4. Mantle cell lymphoma blastoid variant showing medium to large cells with irregular nuclei and numerous mitoses. **Inset** FISH t(11;14)(q13;q32) using CCND1 (spectrum orange) and IGH probes (spectrum green) showing single and double fusion signals.

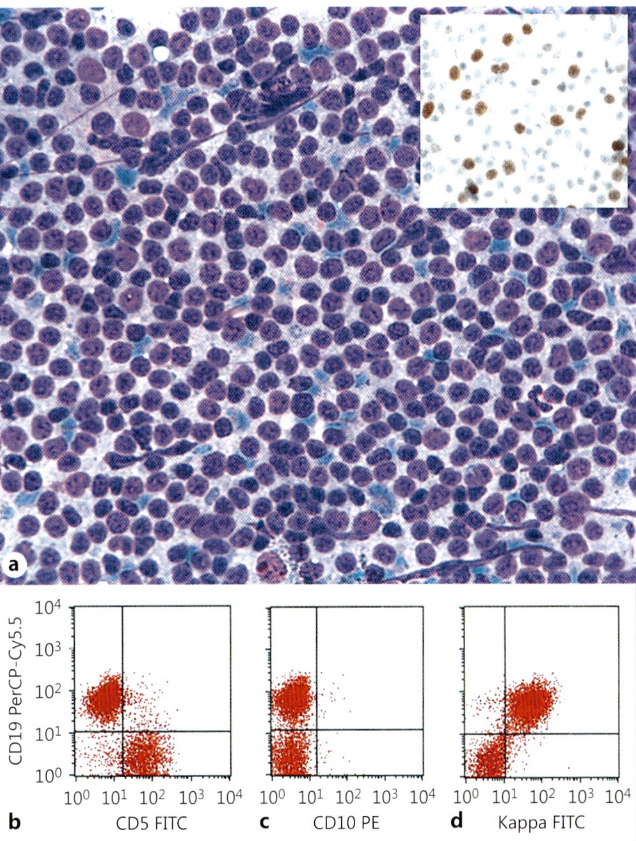

Fig. 5. Marginal zone lymphoma. **a** Monomorphous, small-sized lymphocytes with granular chromatin. **Inset** T-bet nuclear positivity. CD5– (**b**), CD10– (**c**), and κ light chain (**d**) restriction.

tation [see Chapter 9, this vol., pp. 93–101]. Nodal MZL is more aggressive than the other 2; it occurs in more advanced stages and frequently evolves into DLBCL with a generally shorter survival [1]. MZL cells are defined as centrocyte-like when they show slightly indented nuclei, or monocytoid if they have an evident, clear cytoplasm; this last aspect is more frequent in the nodal type and is not easily detectable on FNC (Fig. 5). The MZL phenotype is CD20+, CD79a+, CD23+/–, CD5–, CD10– (Fig. 5). Given the lack of specific cytological features and the CD5–/CD10– phenotype, their classification on FNC is almost impossible to date. Polymorphic and monomorphic MZL might be differentiated from other small cell NHL by T-bet (Fig. 5) and IRTA1 positivity in CD5– and CD10– small cell NHL. Their ICC expression may be detected on cell blocks or additional smears.

Follicular Lymphoma (Grades I and II)
FL represents about 20% of NHL and occurs primarily in the fifth to sixth decades of life; two-thirds of patients are in stages III-IV at diagnosis [1]. In most cases, FL is determined by the t(14;18)(q32;q21) translocation with deregulation of the translocated bcl-2 gene on the IGH locus. Additional genetic changes may involve the bcl-6 gene and in some cases MYC, determining a clinical pathological switch of the disease. FL typically arises in LNs and rarely in extra-

nodal sites. The clinical course of FL is generally indolent with a median survival of 8–10 years. On LN-FNC, the shape of FL cells ranges from small and irregular with coarse chromatin and small nucleoli, to larger and roundish with dispersed chromatin and 1 or more evident nucleoli (Fig. 6). A variable number of reactive T lymphocytes and dendritic cells are present in the background. The FL immunophenotype is CD19+, CD20+, CD22+, CD79a+, CD10+, BCL6+, BCL2+, CD23–/+, CD5– (Fig. 6). FNC grading of FL is rather difficult and may be suggested by the proliferative index on an additional smear (Fig. 6) [25]. The risk of transformation of FL in DLBCL increases with disease duration.

Lymphoplasmacytic Lymphoma
LpcL is a rare variant of SLL/CLL often associated with monoclonal gammopathies [1]. In addition to the LN, possible extranodal localizations are the spleen and bone mar-

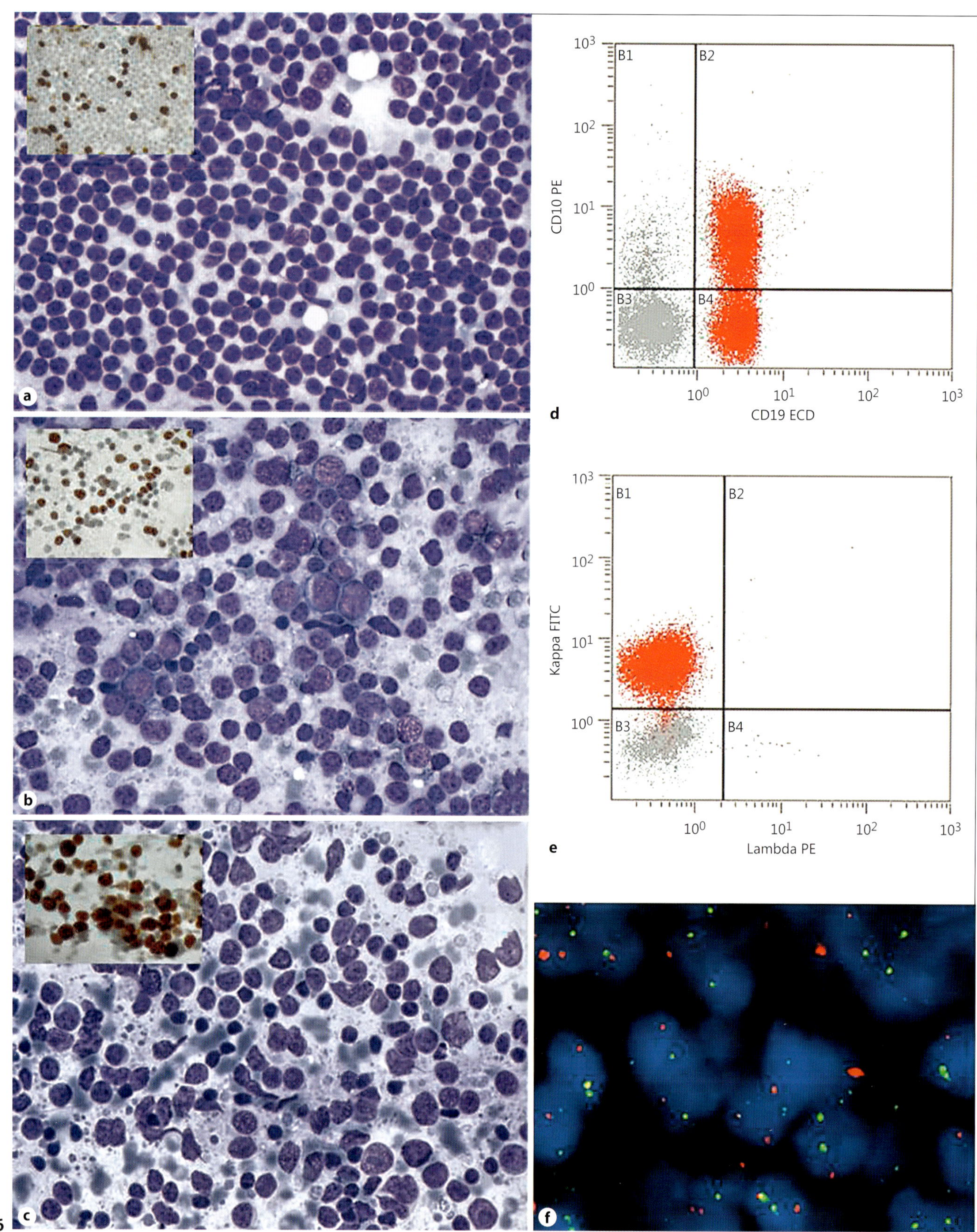

(For legend see next page.)

row. LpcL sometimes initially affects the peripheral blood and bone marrow before spreading to the spleen and LN. LpcL frequently shows the t(9;14)(p13;q32) translocation, and in some cases the 6q21 deletion as well. LpcL FNC shows a diffuse infiltration of small lymphocytes similar to those of SLL/CLL and a variable number of cells with nuclear and cytoplasmic plasmacytoid differentiation (Fig. 7). The neoplastic cells are CD20+, CD19+, CD79a+, CD38+/−, CD5−, CD10−.

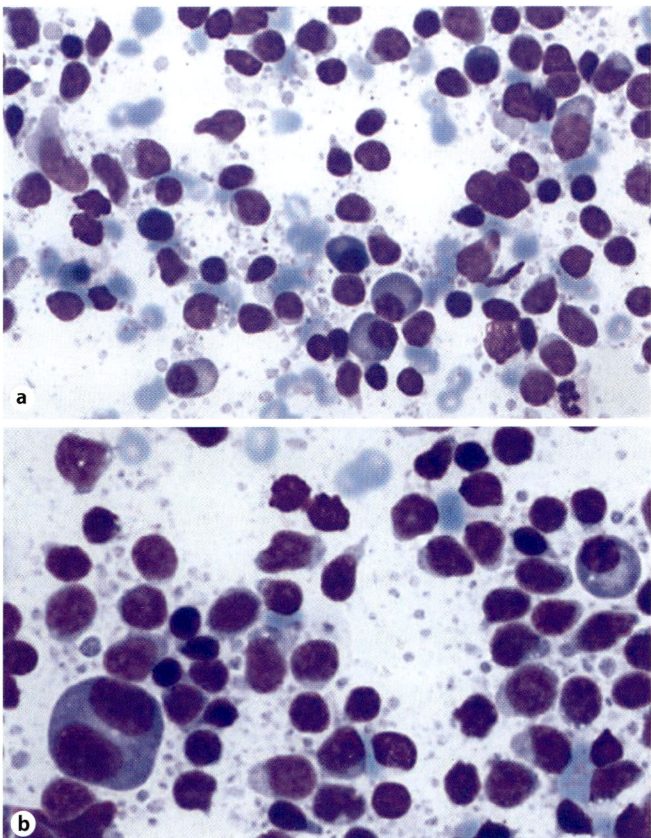

Fig. 7. a, **b** Lymphoplasmacytic lymphoma showing plasma cells-like in an SLL/CLL background with occasional large, binucleated plasmablasts.

Fig. 6. Follicular lymphoma (FL). **a** Grade I FL: monomorphous small cells with chromatin in clumps and Ki67 positivity in <10% of the cells (**inset**). **b** Grade II FL smear showing medium and occasional large cells with more dispersed chromatin and nucleoli in the large cells; the Ki67 index is positive in up to 30% of the cells (**inset**). **c** Grade III FL showing large irregular cell nuclei with dispersed chromatin and evident nucleoli; Ki67 is positive in up to 50% of the cells (**inset**). **d**, **e** FC showing CD19/CD10 co-expression and κ light chain restriction. **f** FISH t(14;18)(q32;q21) using the IGH probe (spectrum green) and BCL2 probe (spectrum orange) showing numerous fusion signals.

Natural Killer/T Lymphoma
Natural killer/T lymphoma (NK/T-L) is an aggressive and extremely rare entity that includes the extranodal NK/T-nasal type and NK/T-cell leukaemia [1]. NK/T-L frequently occurs with systemic symptoms (cytopenia, fever, hepatic enzyme increase, etc.) and may affect other extranodal sites at onset. LN-FNC shows dispersed and poorly differentiated small cells with coarse, compact chromatin and a scanty or absent cytoplasm; the mitotic index is high (Fig. 8). The NK/T-L phenotype is CD3+, CD56+, CD4−, CD8−, CD20−, CD19−, CD5−, CD10−, CD23− (Fig. 8) [26, 27]. When NK/T-L is not initially suspected at rapid on-site evaluation (ROSE), additional FNC-flow cytometry (FC) should be required to add CD56 to the panel [28, 29]. Other useful markers for NK/T-L are TIA-1, granzyme-B, and perforin, which may be tested by ICC [1].

Medium-Large B-Cell Non-Hodgkin Lymphoma

Diffuse Large B-Cell Lymphoma and FL Grade 3
DLBCL is the most frequent NHL histotype, accounting for about 40% of NHL cases. It is generally aggressive, although its course and prognosis are quite variable [1]. Different genetic abnormalities may occur, involving Bcl-2, Bcl-6, MYC, EZH2, PTEN, and other genes, conferring the varied and heterogeneous genetic profiles of DLBCL [30, 31]. Consequently, different morphological variants of DLBCL are known; the most common is the "centroblastic" variant (80%), where cells resemble centroblasts of germinal centres. Other types are the "immunoblastic" variant, accounting for 10%, and the "anaplastic" variant. In this latter, the cells show bizarre, pleomorphic nuclei, multinucleation, and an abundant cytoplasm. The rare "T-cell-rich/histiocyte-rich" variant shows a background of non-neoplastic T lymphocytes, more rarely histiocytes, and atypical large lymphoid cells that may even represent only 10% of the whole cell population. Therefore, DLBCL is considered as a "basket" containing at least 2 or 3 different biological entities. Gene expression profiling (GEP) studies have identified 3 DLBCL subtypes with prognostic and predictive differences, namely the GCB type with a better prognosis, the activated B-cell type, and unclassifiable type (non-GCB type); the latter two with a worse prognosis [30]. DLBCL FNC shows variable cellularity ranging from scanty to moderate, presenting different cytological patterns, namely immunoblastic-like with large monomorphous cells, with 1 or 2 central, large nucleoli

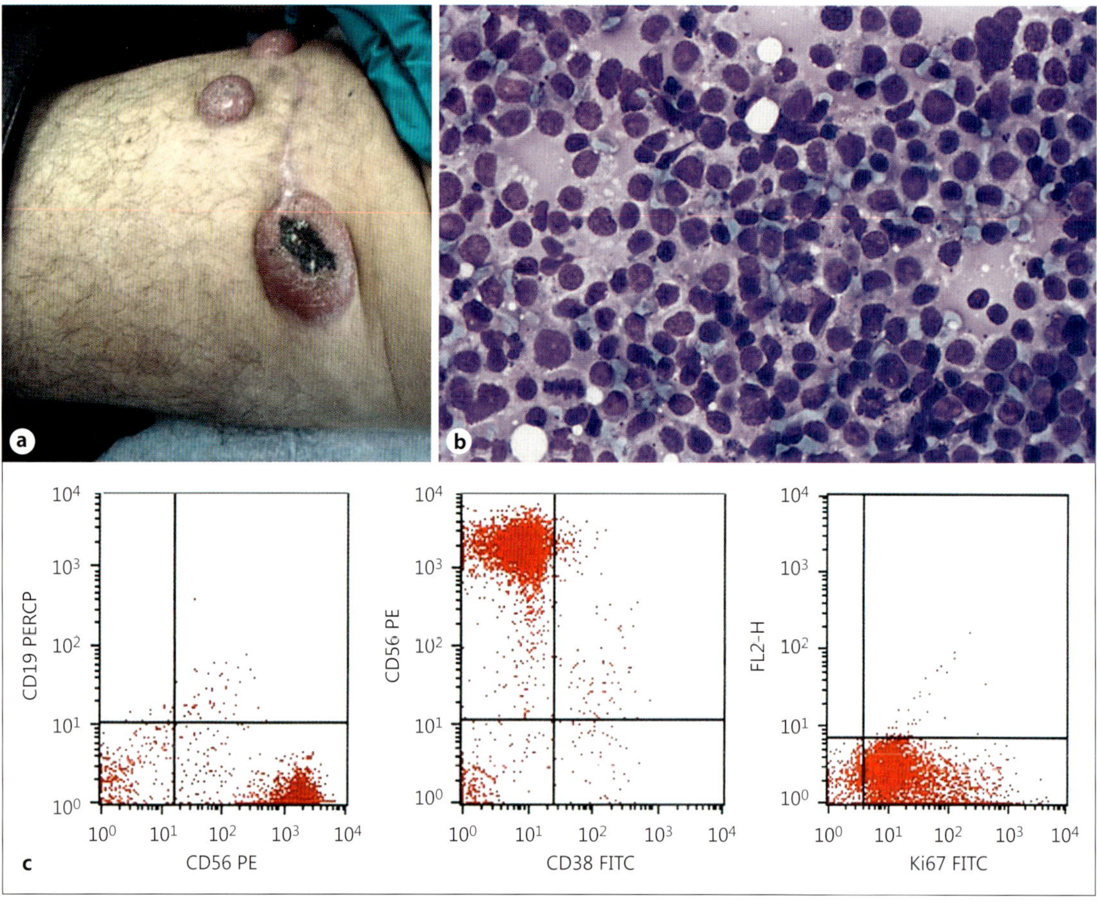

Fig. 8. a Pericicatricial nodules of natural killer/T lymphoma (NK/T-L) relapse; the primary lesion was removed just 1 month prior. **b** NK/T-L FNC showing dispersed and poorly differentiated small cells with nuclear irregularities, coarse chromatin, and a scanty or absent cytoplasm. Note the numerous mitoses. **c** Flow cytometry showed CD56 positivity, CD19 and CD38 negativity, and Ki67 positivity in almost all the gated cells.

and a polymorphous pattern with atypical cells with round or very irregular nuclei, single or multiple nucleoli, and a scanty cytoplasm, or round/irregular nuclei with a single prominent nucleolus and an evident cytoplasm. The FNC presentation of DLBCL may be also influenced by possible and variable LN fibrosis that can hamper the cells harvesting and influence the cytological features. A variable amount of non-neoplastic, reactive lymphocytes is generally present (Fig. 9). The proliferative index is high and necrosis may be occasionally observed. The DLBCL phenotype is CD19+, CD20+, CD79a+, CD5–, CD23–. The different expression of a series of antigens, such as CD10, MUM1, BCL6, FOXP1, GCET1, and LMO2, is helpful to differentiate the GCB-type from the non-GCB-type, and may be tested on cell blocks or additional smears (Fig. 10).

[30–32]. FL grade 3 FNC (Fig. 6) is generally more monomorphous than DLBCL and shows large nucleated cells, whereas the distinction is almost impossible on smears. The phenotype is similar to CD10+ DLBCL (Fig. 10).

Burkitt Lymphoma

BL is an aggressive NHL occurring more frequently in children and often involving extranodal sites [1]. BL may occur in epidemic or sporadic forms. The former more frequently involves the facial area and the sporadic form the subdiaphragmatic organs. Nodal BL arises more frequently in adults. Epstein-Barr virus infections are considered the main pathological promoter, whereas *Plasmodium falciparum*, arbovirus, and other agents have been considered possible local cofactors in the endemic form. BL is deter-

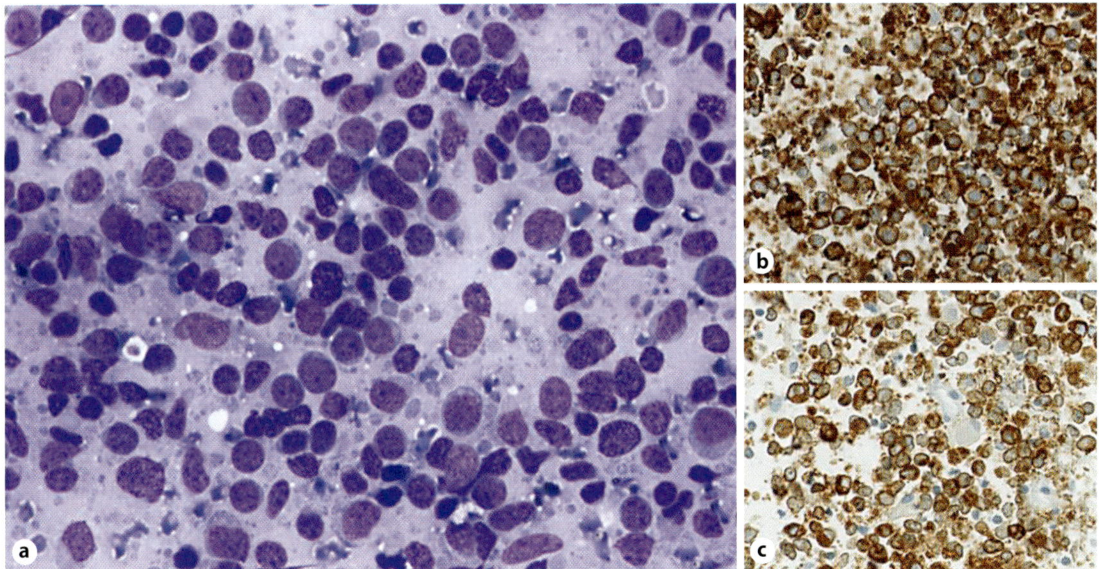

Fig. 9. Diffuse large B-cell lymphoma, GCB-type. **a** A dispersed lymphoid large cell population with an irregular, round-oval nuclei, with small but evident nucleoli. **b** CD20 ICC positivity. **c** CD10 ICC positivity.

mined by the t(8;14) translocation involving the MYC gene that represents the genetic hallmark of BL, whereas it is also detectable in a subset of DLBCL and FL, which is called double-hit B-cell NHL [33]. BL grows as a solid mass infiltrating organs and tissues, and progresses rapidly because of its high mitotic index. FNC shows medium-sized cells with round nuclei and coarse chromatin and multiple small nucleoli. A scanty blue cytoplasm (Fig. 11) with frequent small vacuoles and indistinct edges is generally observed. Macrophages with tingible bodies in a clear cytoplasm are usually intermingled with the neoplastic population producing the "starry sky pattern" also detectable on FNC (Fig. 11). Numerous mitoses and apoptotic figures are usually observed. The cells are CD19+, CD20+, CD79a+, CD10+, CD3–, CD5–, Bcl2–, TdT–. CD10 positivity of almost all of the lymphomatous cells is a relevant feature detectable by the CD10/CD19 co-expression by FC. Additional diagnostic criteria for BL are light chain restriction, Ki67 positivity of up to 90% of the neoplastic cells, nuclear c-myc positivity at ICC, and t(8;14)(q24;q32) by fluorescence in situ hybridization (FISH). The FNC diagnosis of BL has greater clinical relevance compared to other high-grade NHL because a timely and aggressive treatment is required. Such cases of BL, formerly defined as atypical BL, may show evident nuclear pleomorphism and prominent nucleoli similar to other high-grade B-cell NHL. These features represent the wide morphological spectrum recognized by the current WHO classification for BL that over-rules atypical BL. GEP recognizes a gene expression signature in BL that is distinct from DLBCL [1].

Precursor B-Cell Lymphoma/Acute B-Cell Lymphoblastic Leukaemia

This group encompasses different entities with or without specific recognized genetic abnormalities that share similar morphological and clinical features [1], some of which are not yet classified. Precursor B-cell lymphoma has a high incidence in childhood and rarely affects adults (3–5% of all NHL). FNC may be requested in advanced stages with LN and/or extranodal involvements. "Leukaemic-lymphomatous conversions" are frequent. The neoplastic cells are medium sized, the nuclei may be convoluted with finely granular chromatin and no nucleoli, and the cytoplasm is scanty. The cells are generally positive for TdT and B markers.

Precursor T-Cell Lymphoma

T-cell lymphoblastic lymphoma (T-LBL) is a blastic NHL that more frequently affects adolescents or young adults [1]. The typical presentation is a mediastinal/thymic mass with peripheral blood and bone marrow involvement. T-LBL cells are medium sized, with a scanty cytoplasm and roundish nucleus, with finely distributed chromatin and some-

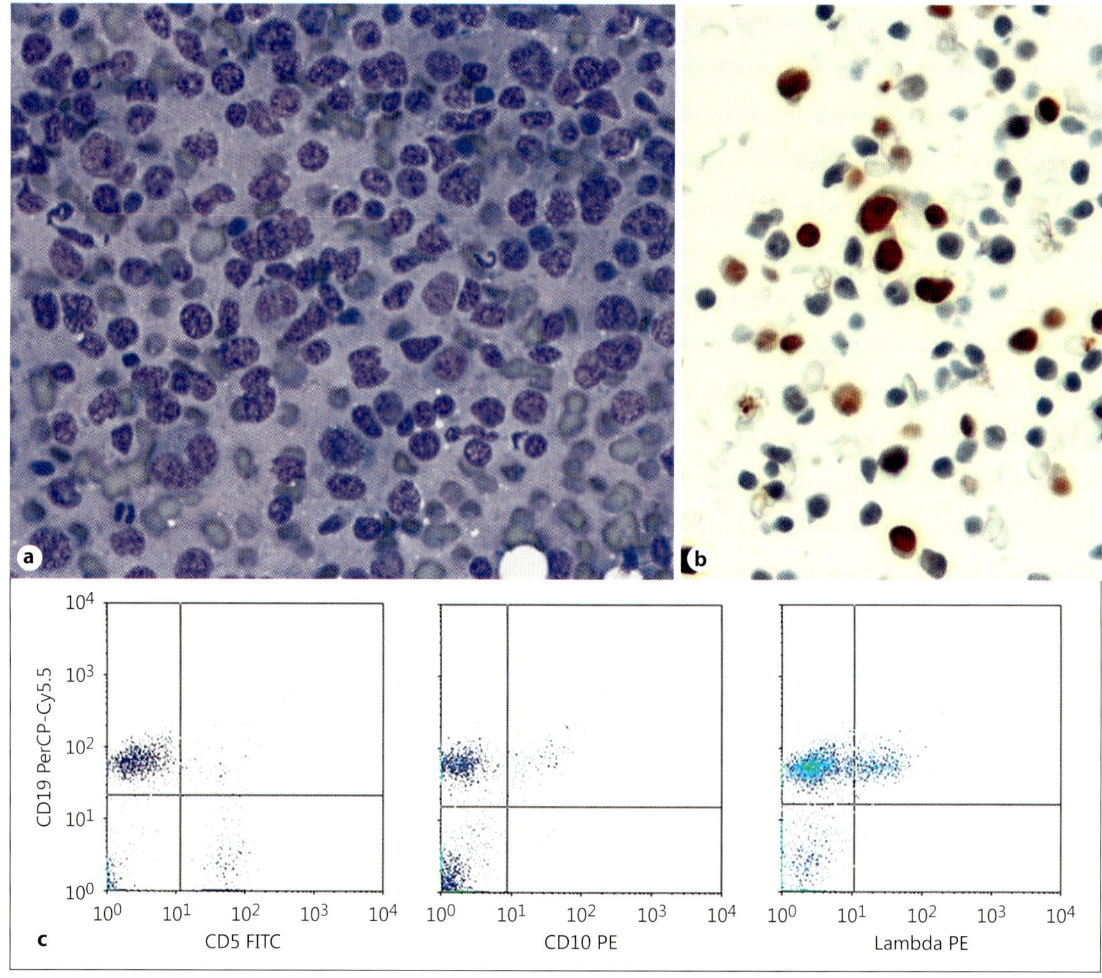

Fig. 10. Diffuse large B-cell lymphoma, non-GCB-type. **a** A dispersed lymphoid large cell population with irregular, round-oval nuclei and scattered small lymphocytes in the background. **b** Nuclear MUM1 ICC on cell block positivity. **c** Flow cytometry: a faint CD19 positivity and λ restriction with co-expression in the upper right quadrant; CD5 and CD10 negativity.

times convoluted contours (Fig. 12). Mitoses and apoptotic bodies are frequent, and a "starry sky pattern" may be observed. ICC or FC are essential to attempting an FNC diagnosis; T-LBL cells are TdT+, CD99+, CD34+, CD1a+, CD3+, CD7+, CD2+/–, CD5+/–, CD4+/–, CD8+/–, CD10+/–. The corresponding antigens are expressed in a variable manner, depending on T-grade maturation. The expression of at least 2 T-markers (more frequently CD7 and CD3) are the minimum criteria for identifying them as belonging to the T lineage.

Peripheral T-Cell Lymphoma Not Otherwise Specified
Peripheral T-cell lymphoma not otherwise specified (PTCL NOS) represents a heterogeneous group of NHL, mainly with LN localization. These share a T-cell phenotype and a generally more aggressive behaviour than their B-cell counterpart. PTCL NOS includes about half of mature T-NHL cases, with patients being mainly adults [1]. LNs are the most common site but, at the time of diagnosis, the disease often presents generalized involvement (bone marrow, liver, spleen, and skin), and sometimes peripheral blood involvement (leukaemia conversion) as well. The FNC features are quite heterogeneous; in some cases the cells are small to medium in size, while in others they are large and quite irregular. The nuclei,

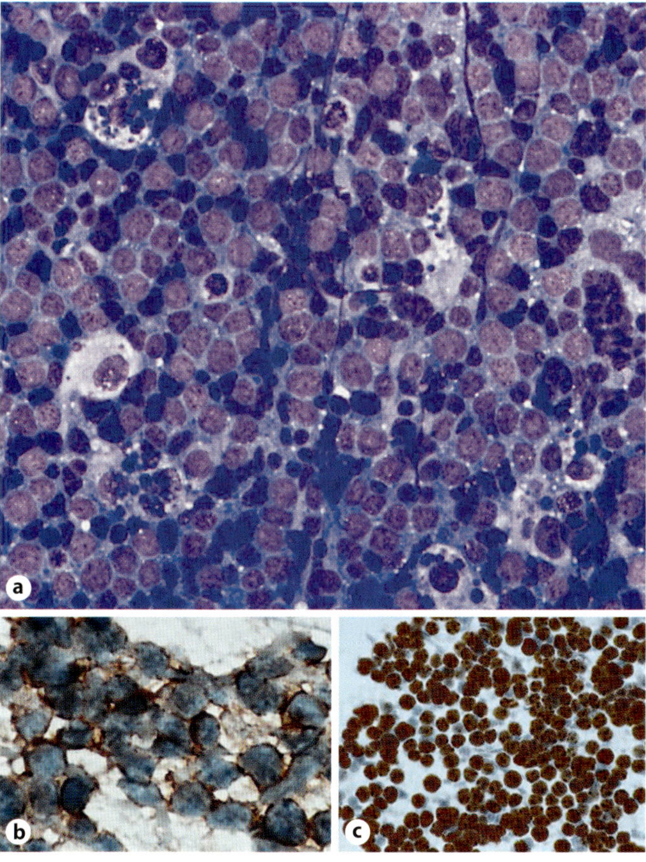

Fig. 11. a Burkitt lymphoma showing undifferentiated medium-sized cells with roundish nuclei, coarse chromatin and small nucleoli. Macrophages with tingible bodies and clear cytoplasm are present conferring a "starry sky pattern." **b** Membranous CD10 positivity. **c** Ki67 positivity in more than 90% of the cells.

in this latter case, are polymorphous, irregular, hyperchromatic or vesicular, with or without macronucleoli, and mitoses are frequent (Fig. 13). Eosinophils, plasma cells, and epithelioid histiocytes are frequently observed in the background. The distinctive high endothelium venules, found on histological samples, are not detectable on smears. PTCL cells express T-cell markers frequently characterized by the loss of some of them, particularly CD7. The most frequent phenotype is CD3+, CD2+, CD4+, CD8−, CD5−, CD7−. A CD8+ form, also expressing CD56, has been reported, mainly in extranodal sites [1, 34].

Anaplastic Large Cell Lymphoma

Anaplastic large cell lymphoma (ALCL) is a rare T-NHL (3%) occurring in childhood (30%), and mainly in males. The t(2;5)(p23;q35) translocation involving the ALK gene is the most frequent (84%) chromosomal anomaly [1]. ALCL is divided into ALK-positive and ALK-negative types. LNs are the most common localizations, while extranodal sites are frequently the skin, bones, soft tissues, lungs, and liver. ALCL is characterized by large, pleomorphic cells with an anaplastic aspect, CD30 positivity (membranous and Golgian positivity) and, in a percentage of cases, ALK positivity, mainly in young patients. Diagnostic cells are large, with a reniform, embryo-like or horseshoe nucleus, and abundant, well-represented cytoplasm (Fig. 14). ICC is CD30+/ALK+/−, EMA+/−, and shows variable positivity for T-cell markers (Fig. 14). ALK+ (generally cytoplasmic and nuclear) ALCL has distinctive molecular modifications [1]. Frequently, T-cell markers are lost and the phenotype may appear as a "null type." Therefore, it is appropriate to use T-cell markers that are less easily lost, such as CD2, CD4, rather than CD3, CD5, or CD7.

Non-Hodgkin Lymphoma and Ancillary Techniques

Ancillary techniques are fundamental in the FNC NHL diagnosis and the management of the corresponding specimen is a key step for an accurate LN diagnosis. For this purpose, ROSE is indispensable for the evaluation of adequacy, the diagnostic orientation, the choice of ancillary techniques, and the storage of the material. The most commonly used ancillary techniques for NHL diagnosis are ICC, FC, FISH, PCR-based techniques and, more recently in a few laboratories, GEP. These procedures are routinely employed in surgical pathology, and work perfectly on FNC samples provided by accurate and specific technical application. The role of ancillary techniques in LN-FNC is enhanced by the relative value of cytological atypia in LN evaluation. In fact, low-grade NHL may show mild or even absent nuclear atypia when compared to some reactive LN; conversely, in high-grade NHL, nuclear atypia may be sufficient to assess malignancy but not to identify specific subtypes or even to exclude metastases. Therefore, assessment of malignancy, differential diagnosis, and NHL classification depend on appropriate ancillary techniques, which need to be chosen according to the clinical data and ROSE results. Provided that cytological atypia are not sufficient for low-grade NHL diagnosis, clonality assessment and specific phenotypic profiles by FC are very effective and counterbalance the little contribution of the nuclear atypia. As far as high-grade NHL is concerned, ICC is highly effective compared to FC, main-

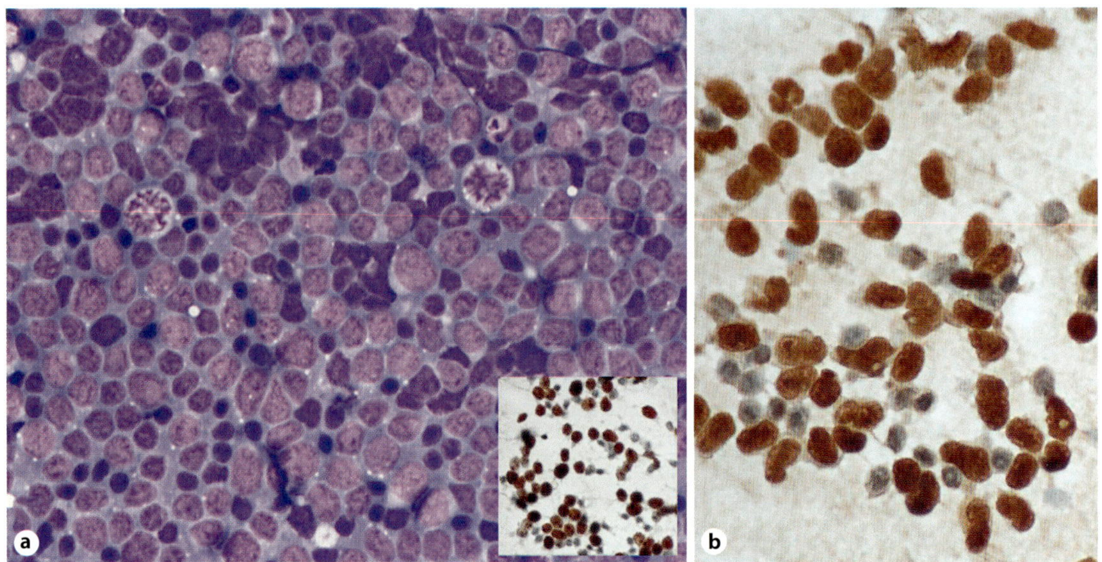

Fig. 12. T-cell lymphoblastic lymphoma. **a** Cells are medium sized, with a scanty cytoplasm and irregular, sometimes convoluted nuclei and granular chromatin. **Inset** Mitoses are frequent with a high Ki67 index. **b** Nuclear TdT positivity.

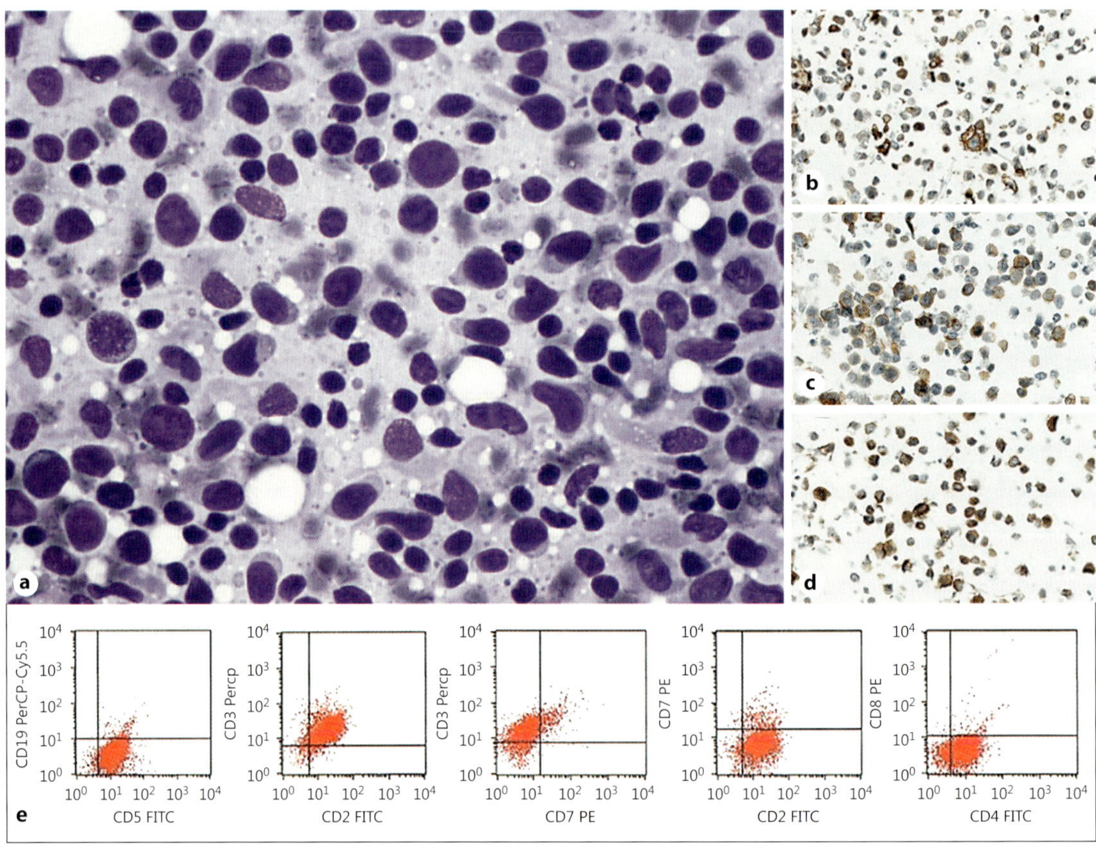

Fig. 13. Peripheral T-cell lymphoma not otherwise specified. **a** Polymorphous irregular small, medium, and large cells. CD3 (**b**) and CD30 (**c**) positivity. **d** Aberrant CD38 positivity. **e** FC: CD5/CD3/CD2 co-expression, loss of CD7, CD8–/CD4+.

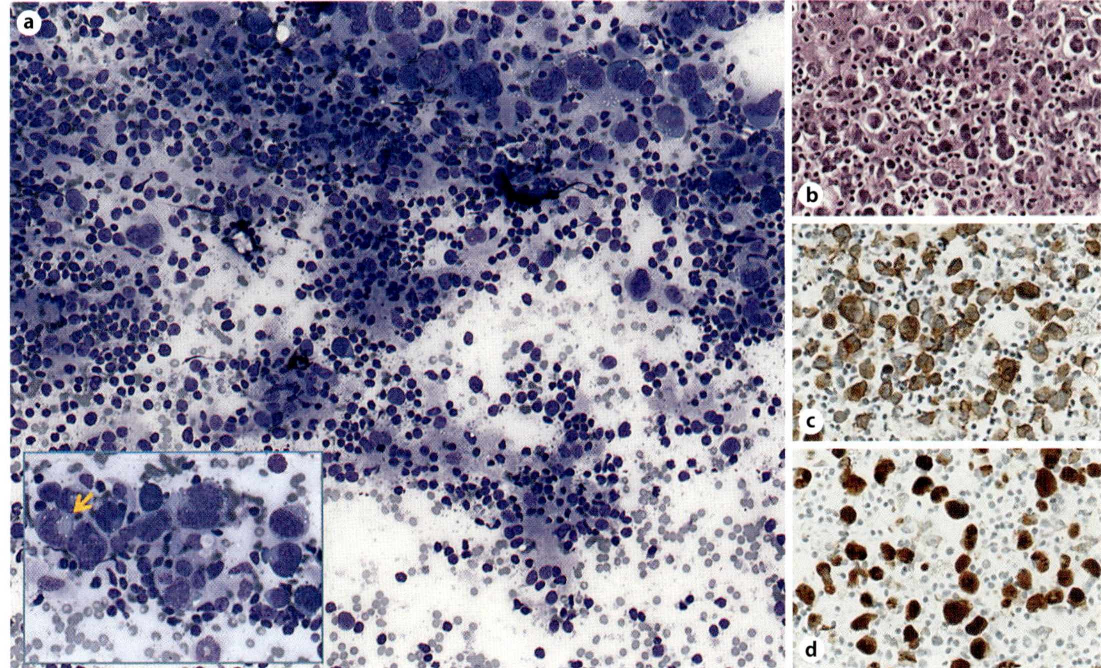

Fig. 14. Anaplastic large cell lymphoma. **a** Large, atypical, and pleomorphic cells on the top in a background of small lymphocytes and plasma cells simulating a metastasis. **Inset** Nuclear details of diagnostic mononucleated and binucleated cells and an embryo-like cell (arrow). **b** HE cell block showing a "chessboard distribution" of the neoplastic cells. **c** CD30 cytoplasmic positivity. **d** ALK1 nuclear positivity.

ly when the differential diagnosis is with non-hematopoietic, poorly differentiated malignancies. Once a basic NHL diagnosis is defined, a classification of specific entities may be attempted by FC and ICC, or FISH. FISH is particularly useful when the FNC/FC or clinical data suggest a subtype carrying a specific translocation (Fig. 4, 6) or in case of already known NHL-subtypes with insufficient material to perform ICC or FC. PCR is mainly useful when FC and ICC fail to assess clonality and/or identify the cell lineage. Moreover, PCR is highly effective in T-cell NHL where clonality assessment by FC or ICC is difficult or impossible, respectively [35, 36]. GEP uses microarray analysis to study gene expression patterns and to assess their expression in a given cell population. FNC material can be rinsed in RNA-stabilization reagent and GEP performed by hybridising RNA to gene chips. Among its potential applications, GEP contributes to identifying new drug targets and new therapeutic regimens and helps discriminate among the different prognostic subtypes in DLBCL. However, as this is a time-consuming and costly method, it is not very practical in routine laboratories so far.

NHL Diagnosis and Clonality Assessment

Clonality testing is an important procedure in the FNC diagnosis of NHL because, in the absence of histological criteria and/or significant cytological atypia, it may be the only diagnostic criteria. Cytological atypia, which is fundamental in epithelial tumours, is less relevant in NHL malignancy assessment because it can be mild or even absent in low-grade NHL.

Flow Cytometry

Clonality can be detected by the kappa/lambda (κ/λ) light chain ratio and/or specific phenotypes. As for FC κ/λ light chain assessment, a ≥4:1 or 1:2 ratio is generally considered to be an expression of monoclonality. Nonetheless, in specific clinical-pathological contexts, 3.1 or 1:1 κ:λ ratios have to be carefully evaluated as they may express clonality. Conversely, κ:λ ratios >4:1 or 1:2 may occur in non-lymphomatous LN enlargements (LNe), mainly in autoimmune processes and T-cell immunodeficiencies [39, 40]. The cut-offs suggested for clonal cell percentages of the gated cells range from 5%, in the case of NHL relapse or minimal residual

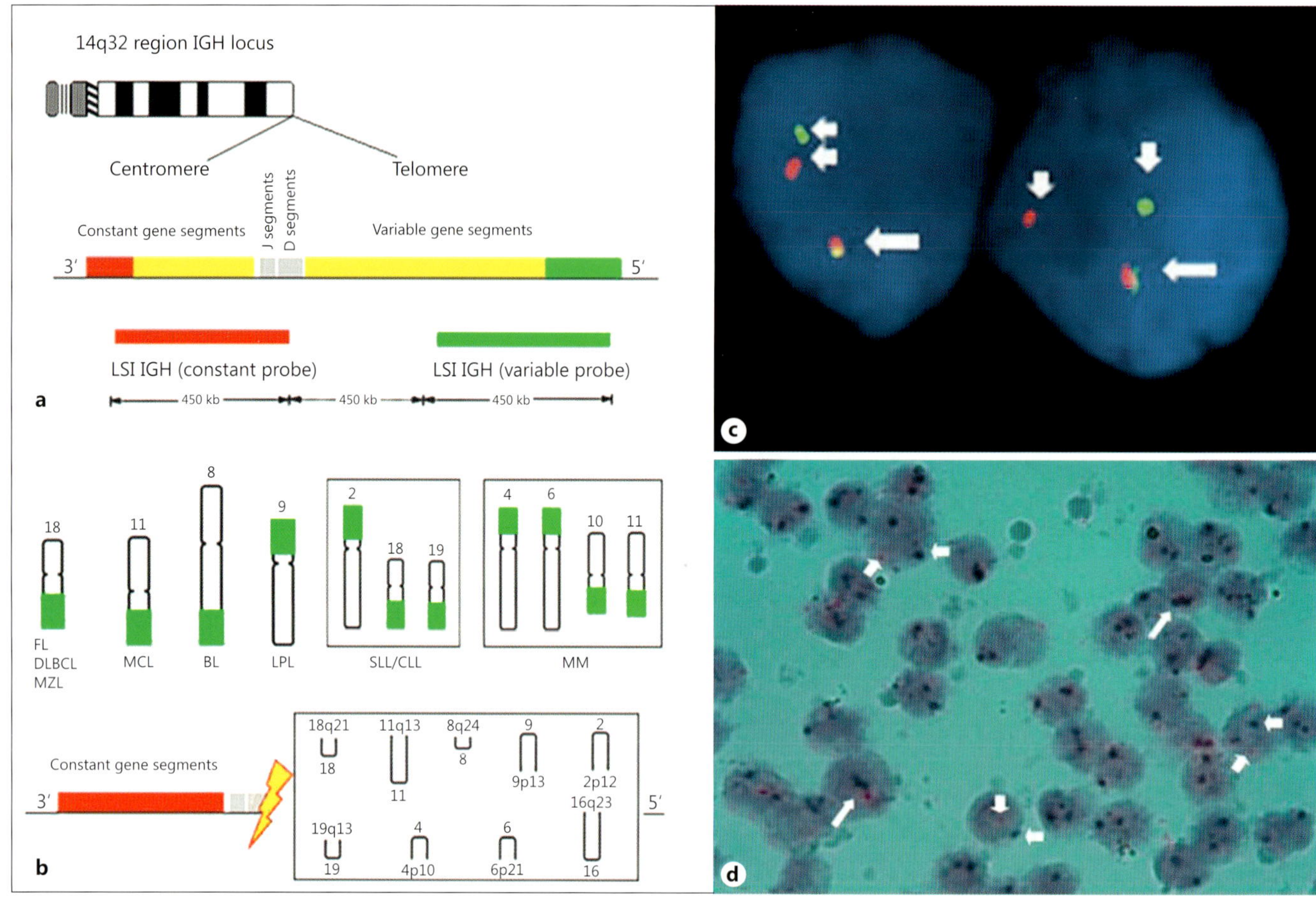

Fig. 15. a The IGH locus hybridized with the split-signal IGH-FISH DNA probe; the green-labeled DNA probe (IGH-Flu) binds the 612-kb telomeric segment and the red-labeled DNA probe (IGH-TR) binds the 460-kb centromeric segment, generating a fusion signal (yellow). **b** The IGH breakpoint with translocation of 1 segment generating split signals (red and green). The corresponding chromosomal partners (green) are shown: FL, DLBCL, MZL, MCL, BL, LpcL, SLL/CLL, and MM (multiple myeloma). **c** IGH translocation by IGH-FISH: the long arrows indicate fusion signals and the short arrows the split signals. **d** CISH of the same IGH-FISH DNA probe split signals: blue signals reveal the green-labeled DNA probe (IGH-Flu) and the red signals indicate the red-labeled DNA probe (IGH-TR). The long arrows indicate fusion signals and the short arrows the split signals.

disease [41], to as much as 20% for LN-FNC [18]. A lack of expression of surface light chain in B-cell NHL may occur [18, 23, 35, 42] with different incidence rates in different subtypes. DLBCL and MZL are the NHL types with a higher incidence of minimal or absent light chain expression (30% for both) [43]. This occurrence may be related to a low expression of surface light chain, or to a low proportion of diagnostic cells due to the admixture of reactive cells, as occurs in T-rich DLBCL and MZL, or the lack of detection of plasmacytoid cells by the CD45 gating by FC. In these cases, monoclonality should be considered in the case of a higher CD19 or CD20 rate in appropriate clinical cytological settings [13, 14, 22, 44–46]. In addition to light chain restriction, clonality may be suggested by aberrant co-expressions of CD5/CD19 or CD5/CD20 that are generally indicative of SLL/CLL and MCL, whereas CD5/CD19 co-expression may occasionally occur in a limited number of cells in peripheral blood and LNes of autoimmune diseases [41]. High values of CD10/CD19 co-expression may also be indicative of B-cell clonality (mainly FL or BL) with or without light chain restriction. Bcl-2 is expressed on different mature and immature B cells; it may indicate an FL or DLBCL, but only when CD10 is co-expressed [47]. FC clonality assessment of T-cell NHL is less effective than B-cell NHL because T-cell NHL lacks specific immunophenotypic profiles and TCR-proteins corresponding to the κ/λ light chain of the B-cell

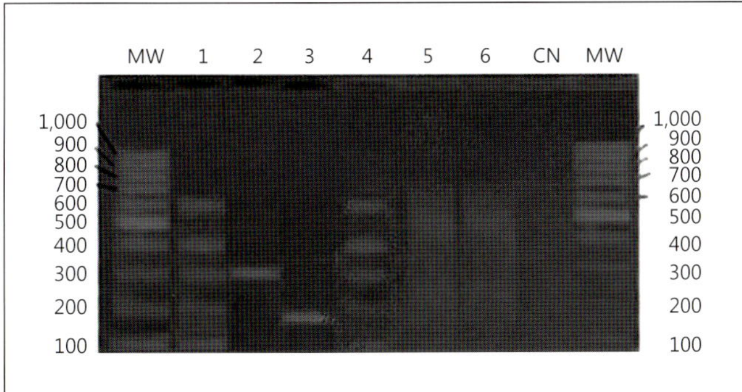

Fig. 16. Heteroduplex analysis of the IGHK multiplex PCR. MW lanes: DNA molecular weight (100 bp AA561 diluted 1:10; Nuclear Laser Medicine Srl). Lanes 1–3: B-cell NHL case No. 1, Gene Control Multiplex PCR (lane 1), IGH monoclonality (lane 2), IGK monoclonality (lane 3). Lanes 4–6: BRH case No. 2, Gene Control Multiplex PCR (lane 4), IGH polyclonality (lane 5), IGK polyclonality (lane 6). CN lane: negative controls (no DNA in PCR reactions).

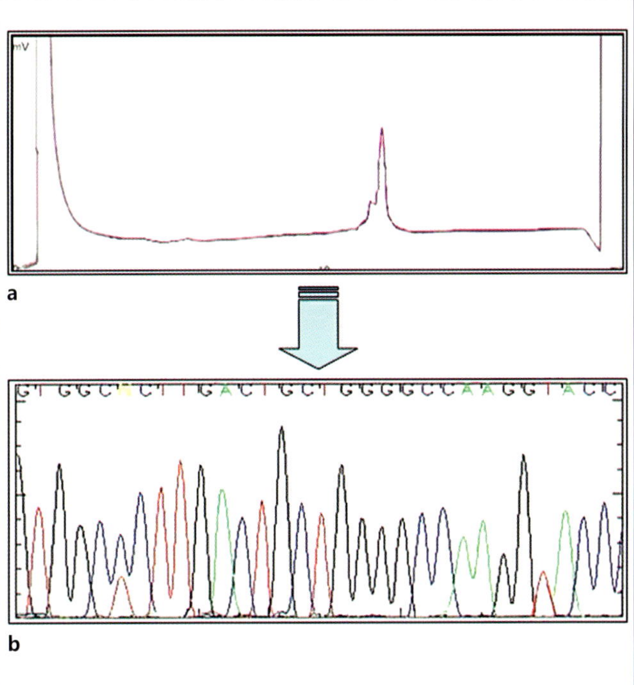

Fig. 17. a Denaturing high-performance liquid chromatography (DHPLC) of the TCRBG amplification products showing single peaks for TCRB (purple) and TCRG (pink), assessing the monoclonality status. **b** Sanger electropherogram of the TCRG amplification product from the same case showing 1 type of sequence corresponding to the Open Reading Frame VG8/JG1 rearrangement, as indicated by Blast analysis in the IMGT® databases.

counterparts. Aberrant phenotypes are also less frequent in T-cell than in B-cell NHL. Therefore, phenotypical tools to assess T-cell clonality are less effective than the B-cell counterparts. As a consequence, T-cell NHL are generally considered when dealing with atypical lymphoid cells that do not express any B cell markers. Mature T cells (CD3+, CD5+, CD10–) generally co-express CD2, CD7 and CD4, or CD8, which are mutually exclusive. Clonal T cells may show a lack of 1 of these antigens; the lack of multiple T cell-associated antigens identifies a null phenotype [20, 41]. Aberrant T-cell phenotypes are not straightforwardly indicative of NHL and need to be assessed in their specific context. For instance, CD10 and CD4/CD8 co-expression may be observed in non-neoplastic T cells at different maturation stages, and the CD4/CD8 ratio is also extremely variable [41]. The CD4+/CD8+ and CD4–/CD8– phenotypes are not specific of a PTCL, as they are also observed in thymus and thymoma lymphoid cells [41]. CD4+CD8+ T cells have also been described in nodular lymphocyte-predominant Hodgkin lymphoma (NLPHL) [48, 49]. Finally, CD4+/CD8+ T cells may be observed in the progressive transformation of germinal centres (PTGC), suggesting a possible relationship between NLPHL and PTGC [49, 50].

FISH/CISH
Clonality can be determined by FISH or CISH (chromogenic in situ hybridization), identifying different and specific chromosomal abnormalities, such as the t(14,18)(q32;q21) translocation in FL or the t(11; 14)(q13;q32) translocation

in MCL, or any breakage involving the IGH locus [37, 38]. Nonetheless, chromosomal abnormalities are usually investigated when a specific NHL type is highly suspected or has already been diagnosed. Moreover, a small number of translocations is shared by different entities; hence, specific chromosomal abnormalities are not routinely employed to determine NHL clonality (Fig. 15).

Immunoglobulin/T-Cell Receptor
Immunoglobulin/T-cell receptor (IG/TCR) PCR assessment is the main procedure and the gold standard for determining NHL clonality since the corresponding neoplastic cells have IG or TCR genes clonally rearranged. This feature has led to the development of different molecular tests to investigate the rearrangement status of these genes, using different primers and gene targets. EuroClonality/ BIOMED-2 have tested and validated primers and PCR systems for IG/TCR clonality testing, and have issued guidelines to interpreting and reporting the results [51]. EuroClo-

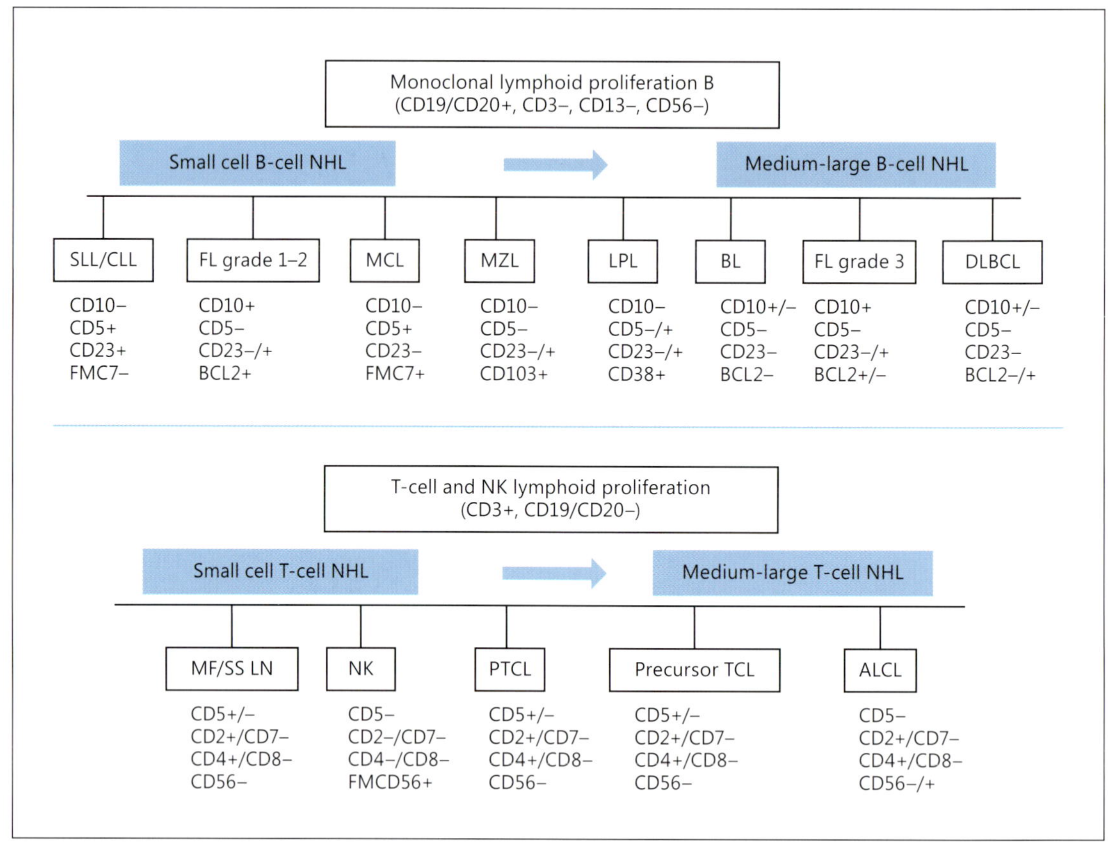

Fig. 18. Basic antibody panel for the diagnosis and classification of B-cell and T-cell NHL.

nality/BIOMED-2 has also validated and standardized PCR for fresh, cryopreserved or formalin-fixed paraffin-embedded tissues or cells [52]. Therefore, IG/TCR PCR clonality can be determined on genetic material obtained from different samples, including FNC (Fig. 16, 17) [53–60].

NHL Differential Diagnosis and Classification

The diagnostic criteria for small cell NHL are different from those for medium and large cell NHL. The differential diagnosis of small B-cell NHL mainly includes benign reactive hyperplasia (BRH), NLPHL, and lymphocyte-rich HL. BRH FNC features are variable. In some cases smears are polymorphous, showing small lymphocytes, follicular centre cells at different stages of maturation, reticular cells, and macrophages with tingible bodies. In specific clinical contexts and with definite ultrasound features (small size, hilum preserved, and oval shape), the FNC diagnosis of BRH is al-

most straightforward. When FNC shows a relatively monomorphous pattern, where small lymphocytes exceed the other components and the heterogeneity of the cellular pattern is lost, the differential diagnosis with small B-cell NHL is almost constantly indicated and mainly depends on clonality assessment by FC, FISH or PCR. The differential diagnosis of small B-cell NHL may also include NLPHL and lymphocyte-rich HL. In these entities, FC shows reactive T cells and polyclonal B cells, but misses the few diagnostic cells that get broken or undetectable among reactive polyclonal cells. Therefore, when these entities are suspected, diagnostic cells may be detected only by ICC, on cell block or de-stained smears, using the usual HL panel (CD30, CD15, CD20, PAX5). As for medium to large NHL, the differential diagnosis is usually indicated with other malignancies with evident nuclear atypia, such as ALCL and lymphocytic depletion HL. This differentiation is extremely difficult on LN-FNC with or without FC, and a definitive diagnosis generally depends on ICC evaluations and a subsequent histological examination. The classification of small B-cell NHL may be attempted by combining cytological features with FC profiles (Fig. 18) [12–15, 17–24, 32, 35, 42, 43, 47, 61, 62]. On the basis of the CD5/CD10 expression, NHL cells can be divided into 4 groups: CD10+/CD5–; CD10-/CD5+; CD10–/CD5–, and CD10+/CD5+ [41, 51]. Each group includes 1 or more histotypes, which may be differentiated through the evaluation of other markers. The CD10+/CD5– group comprises FL, BL, BL-like, and some DLBCL. In this group, the classification may be attempted by combining FC data and cytological features. In fact, FL grade I–II is generally composed of small- to medium-sized monomorphous cells with little atypia, while BL, BL-like, and DLBCL are composed of medium and large cells, respectively, with nuclear atypia and polymorphism, an immature chromatin pattern, and a high mitotic index. The additional evaluation of Ki67 and bcl-2 may be useful in the differential diagnosis of FL (bcl2+, Ki67–/+) and BL (bcl2–, K67++) by ICC. Moreover, FISH can detect the corresponding specific translocations. The second group (CD10–/CD5+) includes SLL/CLL and MCL, which may be cytologically similar. The differential diagnosis may depend on the CD23 and FMC7 expression. CD23 is generally positive in SLL/CLL and negative in MCL, while FMC7 is negative in SLL/CLL and variably expressed in MCL. As for the cytological features, SLL/CLL generally shows small, monomorphous cells with coarse chromatin clumps, while MCL cells are larger, with more dispersed chromatin, nuclear membrane abnormalities, and an occasional moulding arrangement. Additional diagnostic data for MCL are cyclin D1 positivity by ICC and the t(11;14) translocation detected by FISH. The third and fourth groups, CD10–/CD5– and the unusual CD10+/CD5+ phenotype, include small-cell and medium- to large-cell subtypes. MZL is the typical CD10–/CD5– NHL that may be considered by just ruling out other small B-cell NHL. Additional markers for MZL are CD103 and T-Bet that can be tested on cell block. The CD5–, CD10–, CD23– phenotype is also observed in 60–80% of LpcL. In these cases, the expression of

additional markers (CD11c and CD25) and the plasmacytic differentiation may be helpful. Despite these typical phenotypes, a number of cases may show aberrant antigen expressions that significantly hamper the FNC classification. For instance, the reported CD10+/CD5+ phenotype may occur in different NHL subtypes, like DLBCL, FL, and BL, in addition to MCL and SLL/CLL, [32, 41, 45, 62]. CD5 and CD23, which are generally co-expressed in SLL/CLL, may also be mutually exclusive, while CD23 and CD10 may also be expressed in MCL; as well as FL may be CD10– and rarely CD5+. With reference to medium to large NHL, the main diagnostic problem is the identification of DLBCL. DLBCL diagnosis may be helped by the use of some antibodies, such as CD10, MUM1, BCL6, FOXP1, GCET1, and LMO2, which are useful for subtyping DLBCL in the GCB type and non-GCB type [30–32]. In fact, DLBCL may hardly be distinguished from other NHL included in the large cells group, such as FL grade 3, BL, and BL-like and precursor B-cell NHL. FL grade 3 with a nodular growth pattern may be distinguished from the diffuse growth pattern of DLBCL on histological sections, but the same distinction is not possible on FNC. In these cases, when a CD10+ B-cell population is identified by FC, the evaluation of the t(14;18)(q32;q21) translocation by FISH may be useful in establishing the diagnosis of FL, although this translocation may also occur in about 20% of DLBCL [33]. BL also shows a CD10+ FC pattern, but its cytological features are generally different from DLBCL. Moreover, BL FC is CD20/CD19/CD10+ and Bcl2–, MUM1–, and TdT– at ICC. DLBCL-FC may be ineffective or even occur within normal ranges, representing the reactive component only [62]. In fact, very large, atypical, and fragile DLBCL cells may appear outside the usual "lymphoid gate" on FC scattergrams, or may be destroyed or get stuck to the circuits of the cytometer, leading to non-diagnostic FC in DLBCL. Additionally, DLBCL may lack a detectable surface light chain, hampering the confirmation of clonality. Therefore, when DLBCL is suspected by ROSE, ICC in addition to FC may be necessary [63, 64].

References

1 Swerdlow SH, Campo E, Harris NL, Jaffe ES, Pileri SA, Stein H, Thiele J: WHO Classification of Tumours of Haematopoietic and Lymphoid Tissues, ed 4. Lyon, IARC Press, 2017.

2 Crespo M, Bosch F, Villamor N, Bellosillo B, Colomer D, Rozman M, Marcé S, López-Guillermo A, Campo E, Montserrat E: ZAP-70 expression as a surrogate for immunoglobulin-variable-region mutations in chronic lymphocytic leukemia. N Engl J Med 2003;348:1764–1765.

3 Rassenti LZ, Huynh L, Toy TL, Chen L, Keating MJ, Gribben JG, Neuberg DS, Flinn IW, Rai KR, Byrd JC, Kay NE, Greaves A, Weiss A, Kipps TJ: ZAP-70 compared with immunoglobulin heavy-chain gene mutation status as a predictor of disease progression in chronic lymphocytic leukemia. N Engl J Med 2004;351:893–901.

4 Orchard JA, Ibbotson RE, Davis Z, Wiestner A, Rosenwald A, Thomas PW, Hamblin TJ, Staudt LM, Oscier DG: ZAP-70 expression and prognosis in chronic lymphocytic leukaemia. Lancet 2004; 363:105–111.

5 Dürig J, Naschar M, Schmücker U, Renzing-Köhler K, Hölter T, Hüttmann A, Dührsen U: CD38 expression is an important prognostic marker in chronic lymphocytic leukaemia. Leukemia 2002;16:30–35.

6 Del Poeta G, Maurillo L, Venditti A, Buccisano F, Epiceno AM, Capelli G, Tamburini A, Suppo G, Battaglia A, Del Principe MI, Del Moro B, Masi M, Amadori S: Clinical significance of CD38 expression in chronic lymphocytic leukemia. Blood 2001;98:2633–2639.

7 Hamblin TJ, Orchard JA, Ibbotson RE, Davis Z, Thomas PW, Stevenson FK, Oscier DG: CD38 expression and immunoglobulin variable region mutations are independent prognostic variables in chronic lymphocytic leukemia, but CD38 expression may vary during the course of the disease. Blood 2002;99:1023–1029.

8 Ibrahim S, Keating M, Do KA, O'Brien S, Huh YO, Jilani I, Lerner S, Kantarjian HM, Albitar M: CD38 expression as an important prognostic factor in B-cell chronic lymphocytic leukemia. Blood 2001; 98:181–186.

9 Shin HJ, Caraway NP, Katz RL: Cytomorphologic spectrum of small lymphocytic lymphoma in patients with an accelerated clinical course. Cancer 2003;99:293–300.

10 Caraway NP, Wojcik EM, Saboorian HM, Katz RL: Concomitant lymphoma and metastatic carcinoma in a lymph node: diagnosis by fine-needle aspiration biopsy in two cases. Diagn Cytopathol 1997;17:287–291.

11 Zhang YH, Liu J, Dawlett M, Guo M, Sun X, Gong Y: The role of SOX11 immunostaining in confirming the diagnosis of mantle cell lymphoma on fine-needle aspiration samples. Cancer Cytopathol 2014;122:892–897.

12 Dunphy CH, Ramos R: Combining fine-needle aspiration and flow cytometric immunophenotyping in evaluation of nodal and extranodal sites for possible lymphoma: a retrospective review. Diagn Cytopathol 1997;16:200–206.

13 Young NA, Al-Saleem TI, Ehya H, Smith MR: Utilization of fine-needle aspiration cytology and flow cytometry in the diagnosis and sub-classification of primary and recurrent lymphoma. Cancer 1998;84:252–261.

14 Jeffers MD, Milton J, Herriot R, McKean M: Fine needle aspiration cytology in the investigation of non-Hodgkin's lymphoma. J Clin Pathol 1998;51: 189–196.

15 Meda BA, Buss DH, Woodruff RD, et al: Diagnosis and sub-classification of primary and recurrent lymphoma: the usefulness and limitations of combined fine-needle aspiration cytomorphology and flow cytometry. Am J Clin Pathol 2000;113:688–699.

16 Liu K, Stern RC, Rogers RT, Dodd LG, Mann KP: Diagnosis of hematopoietic processes by fine-needle aspiration in conjunction with flow cytometry: a review of 127 cases. Diagn Cytopathol 2001;24: 1–10.

17 Mourad WA, Tulbah A, Shoukri M, Al Dayel F, Akhtar M, Ali MA, Hainau B, Martin J: Primary diagnosis and REAL/WHO classification of non-Hodgkin's lymphoma by fine-needle aspiration: cytomorphologic and immunophenotypic approach. Diagn Cytopathol 2003;28:191–195.

18 Zeppa P, Marino G, Troncone G, Fulciniti F, De Renzo A, Picardi M, Benincasa G, Rotoli B, Vetrani A, Palombini L: Fine-needle cytology and flow cytometry immunophenotyping and subclassification of non-Hodgkin lymphoma: a critical review of 307 cases with technical suggestions. Cancer Cytopathol 2004;102:55–65.

19 Bangerter M, Brudler O, Heinrich B, Griesshammuer M: Fine needle aspiration cytology and flow cytometry in the diagnosis and subclassification of non-Hodgkin's lymphoma based on the World Health Organization classification. Acta Cytol 2007;51:390–398.

20 Barrena S, Almeida J, Del Carmen García-Macias M, López A, Rasillo A, Sayagués JM, Rivas RA, Gutiérrez ML, Ciudad J, Flores T, Balanzategui A, Caballero MD, Orfao A: Flow cytometry immunophenotyping of fine-needle aspiration specimens: utility in the diagnosis and classification of non-Hodgkin lymphomas. Histopathology 2011;58: 906–918.

21 Stacchini A, Carucci P, Pacchioni D, Accinelli G, Demurtas A, Aliberti S, Bosco M, Bruno M, Balbo Mussetto A, Rizzetto M, Bussolati G, De Angelis C: Diagnosis of deep-seated lymphomas by endoscopic ultrasound-guided fine needle aspiration combined with flow cytometry. Cytopathology 2012;23:50–56.

22 Dong HY, Harris NL, Preffer FI, Pitman MB: Fine-needle aspiration biopsy in the diagnosis and classification of primary and recurrent lymphoma: a retrospective analysis of the utility of cytomorphology and flow cytometry. Mod Pathol 2001;14: 472–481.

23 Zeppa P, Vigliar E, Cozzolino I, Troncone G, Picardi M, De Renzo A, Grimaldi F, Pane F, Vetrani A, Palombini L: Fine needle aspiration cytology and flow cytometry immunophenotyping of non-Hodgkin lymphoma: can we do better? Cytopathology 2010;21:300–310.

24 Demurtas A, Accinelli G, Pacchioni D, Godio L, Novero D, Bussolati G, Palestro G, Papotti M, Stacchini A: Utility of flow cytometry immunophenotyping in fine-needle aspirate cytologic diagnosis of non-Hodgkin lymphoma: a series of 252 cases and review of the literature. Appl Immunohistochem Mol Morphol 2010;18:311–322.

25 Sun W, Caraway NP, Zhang HZ, Khanna A, Payne LG, Katz RL: Grading follicular lymphoma on fine needle aspiration specimens: comparison with proliferative index by DNA image analysis and Ki-67 labeling index. Acta Cytol 2004;48:119–126.

26 Jiménez-Heffernan JA, González-Peramato P, Perna C, Alvarez-Ferreira J, López-Ferrer P, Viguer JM: Fine-needle aspiration cytology of extranodal natural killer/T-cell lymphoma. Diagn Cytopathol 2002;27:371–374.

27 Loo CK, Quach HT, Gallo J: Diagnosis of natural killer cell lymphoma by cytology and flow cytometric immunophenotyping: a case report. Acta Cytol 2002;46:877–882.

28 Cho EY, Gong G, Khang SK, Kang YK, Huh J: Fine needle aspiration cytology of CD56-positive natural killer/T-cell lymphoma of soft tissue. Cancer 2002;96:344–350.

29 Wu HH, Ren R, Roepke JE: Fine-needle aspiration cytology of blastic natural killer-cell lymphoma (CD4+ CD56+ hematodermic neoplasm). Diagn Cytopathol 2004;30:268–670.

30 Hans CP, Weisenburger DD, Greiner TC, Gascoyne RD, Delabie J, Ott G, Müller-Hermelink HK, Campo E, Braziel RM, Jaffe ES, Pan Z, Farinha P, Smith LM, Falini B, Banham AH, Rosenwald A, Staudt LM, Connors JM, Armitage JO, Chan WC: Confirmation of the molecular classification of diffuse large B-cell lymphoma by immunohistochemistry using a tissue microarray. Blood 2004; 103:275–282.

31 Visco C, Li Y, Xu-Monette ZY, et al: Comprehensive gene expression profiling and immunohistochemical studies support application of immunophenotypic algorithm for molecular subtype classification in diffuse large B-cell lymphoma: a report from the International DLBCL Rituximab-CHOP Consortium Program Study. Leukemia 2012;26:2103–2113.

32 Cozzolino I, Varone V, Picardi M, Baldi C, Memoli D, Ciancia G, Selleri C, De Rosa G, Vetrani A, Zeppa P: CD10, BCL6, and MUM1 expression in diffuse large B-cell lymphoma on FNA samples. Cancer Cytopathol 2016;124:135–143.

33 Aukema SM, Siebert R, Schuuring E, van Imhoff GW, Kluin-Nelemans HC, Boerma EJ, Kluin PM: Double-hit B-cell lymphomas. Blood 2011;117: 2319–2331.

34 Karube K, Aoki R, Nomura Y, Yamamoto K, Shimizu K, Yoshida S, Komatani H, Sugita Y, Ohshima K: Usefulness of flow cytometry for differential diagnosis of precursor and peripheral T-cell and NK-cell lymphomas: analysis of 490 cases. Pathol Int 2008;58:89–97.

35 Dey P: Role of ancillary techniques in diagnosing and subclassifying non-Hodgkin's lymphomas on fine needle aspiration cytology. Cytopathology 2006;17:275–287.

36 Pai RK, Mullins FM, Kim YH, Kong CS: Cytologic evaluation of lymphadenopathy associated with mycosis fungoides and Sezary syndrome: role of immunophenotypic and molecular ancillary studies. Cancer 2008;114:323–332.

37 Monaco SE, Teot LA, Felgar RE, Surti U, Cai G: Fluorescence in situ hybridization studies on direct smears: an approach to enhance the fine-needle aspiration biopsy diagnosis of B cell non-Hodgkin lymphomas. Cancer Cytopathol 2009; 117:338–348.

38 Zeppa P, Sosa Fernandez LV, Cozzolino I, Ronga V, Genesio R, Salatiello M, Picardi M, Malapelle U, Troncone G, Vigliar E: Immunoglobulin heavy-chain fluorescence in situ hybridization-chromogenic in situ hybridization DNA probe split signal in the clonality assessment of lymphoproliferative processes on cytological samples. Cancer Cytopathol 2012;120:390–400.

39 Zeppa P, Cozzolino I, Peluso AL, Troncone G, Lucariello A, Picardi M, Carella C, Pane F, Vetrani A, Palombini L: Cytologic, flow cytometry, and molecular assessment of lymphoid infiltrate in fine-needle cytology samples of Hashimoto thyroiditis. Cancer 2009;117:174–184.

40 Cozzolino I, Nappa S, Picardi M, De Renzo A, Troncone G, Palombini L, Zeppa P: Clonal B-cell population in a reactive lymph node in acquired immunodeficiency syndrome. Diagn Cytopathol 2009;37:910–914.

41 Craig FE, Foon KA: Flow cytometric immunophenotyping for hematologic neoplasms. Blood 2008; 111:3941–3967.

42 Zardawi IM, Jain S, Bennett G: Flow-cytometric algorithm on fine-needle aspirates for the clinical workup of patients with lymphadenopathy. Diagn Cytopathol 1998;19:274–278.

43 Ohmoto A, Maeshima AM, Taniguchi H, Tanioka K, Makita S, Kitahara H, Fukuhara S, Munakata W, Suzuki T, Maruyama D, Kobayashi Y, Tobinai K: Histopathological analysis of B-cell non-Hodgkin lymphomas without light chain restriction by using flow cytometry. Leuk Lymphoma 2015;56: 3301–3305.

44 Nicol TL, Silberman M, Rosenthal DL, Borowitz MJ: The accuracy of combined cytopathologic and flow cytometric analysis of fine-needle aspirates of lymph nodes. Am J Clin Pathol 2000;114:18–28.

45 Ravoet C, Demartin S, Gerard R, Dehon M, Peny MO, Petit B, Delannoy A, Husson B: Contribution of flow cytometry to the diagnosis of malignant and non malignant conditions in lymph node biopsies. Leuk Lymphoma 2004;45:1587–1593.

46 Liu J, Song B, Fan T, Huang C, Xie C, Li J, Zhong W, Li S, Yu J: Pathological and clinical characteristics of 1,248 non-Hodgkin's lymphomas from a regional cancer hospital in Shandong, China. Asian Pac J Cancer Prev 2011;12:3055–3061.

47 Laane E, Tani E, Björklund E, Elmberger G, Everaus H, Skoog L, Porwit-MacDonald A: Flow cytometric immunophenotyping including Bcl-2 detection on fine needle aspirates in the diagnosis of reactive lymphadenopathy and non-Hodgkin's lymphoma. Cytometry B Clin Cytom 2005;64: 34–42.

48 Rahemtullah A, Reichard KK, Preffer FI, Harris NL, Hasserjian RP: A double-positive CD4+CD8+ T-cell population is commonly found in nodular lymphocyte predominant Hodgkin lymphoma. Am J Clin Pathol 2006;126:805–814.

49 Rahemtullah A, Harris NL, Dorn ME, Preffer FI, Hasserjian RP: Beyond the lymphocyte predominant cell: CD4+CD8+ T-cells in nodular lymphocyte predominant Hodgkin lymphoma. Leuk Lymphoma 2008;49:1870–1878.

50 David JA, Huang JZ: Diagnostic utility of flow cytometry analysis of reactive T cells in nodular lymphocyte-predominant Hodgkin lymphoma. Am J Clin Pathol 2016;145:107–115.

51 Langerak AW, Groenen PJTA, Bruggemann M, et al: EuroClonality/BIOMED-2 guidelines for interpretation and reporting of Ig/TCR clonality testing in suspected lymphoproliferations. Leukemia 2012;26:2159–2172.

52 Berget E, Helgeland L, Molven A, Vintermyr OK: Detection of clonality in follicular lymphoma using formalin-fixed, paraffin-embedded tissue samples and BIOMED-2 immunoglobulin primers. J Clin Pathol 2011;64:37–41.

53 Roepman P, Boots CM, Scheidel KC, Sprong T, de Bruin P, de Weerdt O, Groenen PJ, Kummer JA: Molecular clonality assessment shows high performance to predict malignant B-cell non-Hodgkin's lymphoma using cytological smears. J Clin Pathol 2016;69:1109–1115.

54 Brozic A, Pohar Marinsek Z, Novakovic S, Klobves Prevodnik V: Inconclusive flow cytometric surface light chain results; can cytoplasmic light chains, Bcl-2 expression and PCR clonality analysis improve accuracy of cytological diagnoses in B-cell lymphomas? Diagn Pathol 2015;10:191.

55 Cozzolino I, Vigliar E, Todaro P, Peluso AL, Picardi M, Sosa Fernandez LV, Mignogna MD, Tuccari G, Selleri C, Zeppa P: Fine needle aspiration cytology of lymphoproliferative lesions of the oral cavity. Cytopathology 2014;25:241–249.

56 Vigliar E, Cozzolino I, Picardi M, Peluso AL, Fernandez LV, Vetrani A, Botti G, Pane F, Selleri C, Zeppa P: Lymph node fine needle cytology in the staging and follow-up of cutaneous lymphomas. BMC Cancer 2014;14:8.

57 Maroto A, Martinez M, Martinez MA, de Agustin P, Rodriguez-Peralto JL: Comparative analysis of immunoglobulin polymerase chain reaction and flow cytometry in fine needle aspiration biopsy differential diagnosis of non-Hodgkin B-cell lymphoid malignancies. Diagn Cytopathol 2009;37: 647–653.

58 Barroca H: Fine needle biopsy and genetics, two allied weapons in the diagnosis, prognosis, and target therapeutics of solid pediatric tumors. Diagn Cytopathol 2008;36:678–684.

59 Mayall F, Johnson S: Immunoflow cytometry compared with PCR for the identification of clonality in FNAs of T-cell-rich B-cell lymphomas. Cytopathology 2007;18:117–119.

60 Galindo LM, Garcia FU, Hanau CA, Lessin SR, Jhala N, Bigler RD, Vonderheid EC: Fine-needle aspiration biopsy in the evaluation of lymphadenopathy associated with cutaneous T-cell lymphoma (mycosis fungoides/Sézary syndrome). Am J Clin Pathol 2000;113:865–871.

61 Swart GJ, Wright C, Brundyn K, Mansvelt E, du Plessis M, ten Oever D, Jacobs P: Fine needle aspiration biopsy and flow cytometry in the diagnosis of lymphoma. Transfus Apher Sci 2007;37:71–79.

62 Kalina T, Flores-Montero J, van der Velden VH, Martin-Ayuso M, Böttcher S, Ritgen M, Almeida J, Lhermitte L, Asnafi V, Mendonça A, de Tute R, Cullen M, Sedek L, Vidriales MB, Pérez JJ, te Marvelde JG, Mejstrikova E, Hrusak O, Szczepański T, van Dongen JJ, Orfao A; EuroFlow Consortium (EU-FP6, LSHB-CT-2006-018708): EuroFlow standardization of flow cytometer instrument settings and immunophenotyping protocols. Leukemia 2012;26:1986–2010.

63 Cozzolino I, Rocco M, Villani G, Picardi M: Lymph node fine-needle cytology of non-Hodgkin lymphoma: diagnosis and classification by flow cytometry. Acta Cytol 2016;60:302–314.

64 Bertram HC, Check IJ, Milano MA: Immunophenotyping large B-cell lymphomas: flow cytometric pitfalls and pathologic correlation. Am J Clin Pathol 2001;116:191–203.

Zeppa P, Cozzolino I: Lymph Node FNC. Cytopathology of Lymph Nodes and Extranodal Lymphoproliferative Processes.
Monogr Clin Cytol. Basel, Karger, 2018, vol 23, pp 52–59 (DOI: 10.1159/000478881)

Hodgkin Lymphoma

Hodgkin lymphoma (HL) is a very particular tumour for different reasons: it has a variable geographic, racial, and social epidemiology; it is related to Epstein Barr virus (EBV) infection, but the virus is rarely detectable in tumour cells; its multifactorial pathogenesis overlaps with other inflammatory and neoplastic processes, and it has different pathological features, resulting in different subtypes that may overlap with some NHLs. It has a good prognosis in most cases, but patients may develop reactive lymph node enlargements (LNe) over time, as well as relapses or secondary/iatrogenic neoplasms [1]. Despite these heterogeneities, HL has maintained its name, unicity, and classification over the years. HL-specific aspects affect corresponding fine-needle cytology (FNC) features and this should be kept in mind when dealing with HL. Clinical signs, if present, are nocturnal sweating, itch, fever, weakness, cough, or mediastinal syndrome, when mediastinum is involved. Regarding HL staging, the Cotswolds modification of the Ann Arbor Staging System [2] has maintained the 4 original clinical pathological stages. These are: stage I, single LN group; stage II, multiple LN groups on the same side of the diaphragm; stage III, multiple LN groups on both sides of the diaphragm, and stage IV, multiple extranodal sites or LNs and extranodal disease. The A or B designation is then assigned according to the absence or presence of symptoms (weight loss, fever, drenching night sweats). Moreover, stage X (bulky tumours larger than 10 cm) and stage E (extranodal extension or a single, isolated site of extranodal disease) have been added [2]. HL usually arises in 1 or more adjacent LNs, with cervical LNs being the most frequently involved, followed by supraclavicular and axillary LNs; primary inguinal LNs are involved in roughly 15% of cases [3]. The mediastinum is mainly involved in the case of nodular sclerosis and the spleen in mixed cellularity subtypes [3]. According to the WHO [1], HL is classified as nodular lymphocyte-predominant HL (5%) and classical HL (95%), with lymphocyte-rich (3–5%), nodular sclerosis (60–70%), mixed cellularity (20–25%), and lymphocyte-depleted (5%) HL subtypes. The incidence of the different subtypes is related to staging and prognosis, while treatment mainly depends on staging and clinical features. HL prognosis is favourable in more than 80% of cases [1, 3]. The LN architecture is subverted and characterized by a variable number of scattered large mononucleated cells: Hodgkin cells (HC), lobulated mononucleated cells, "popcorn cells" (lymphocyt-

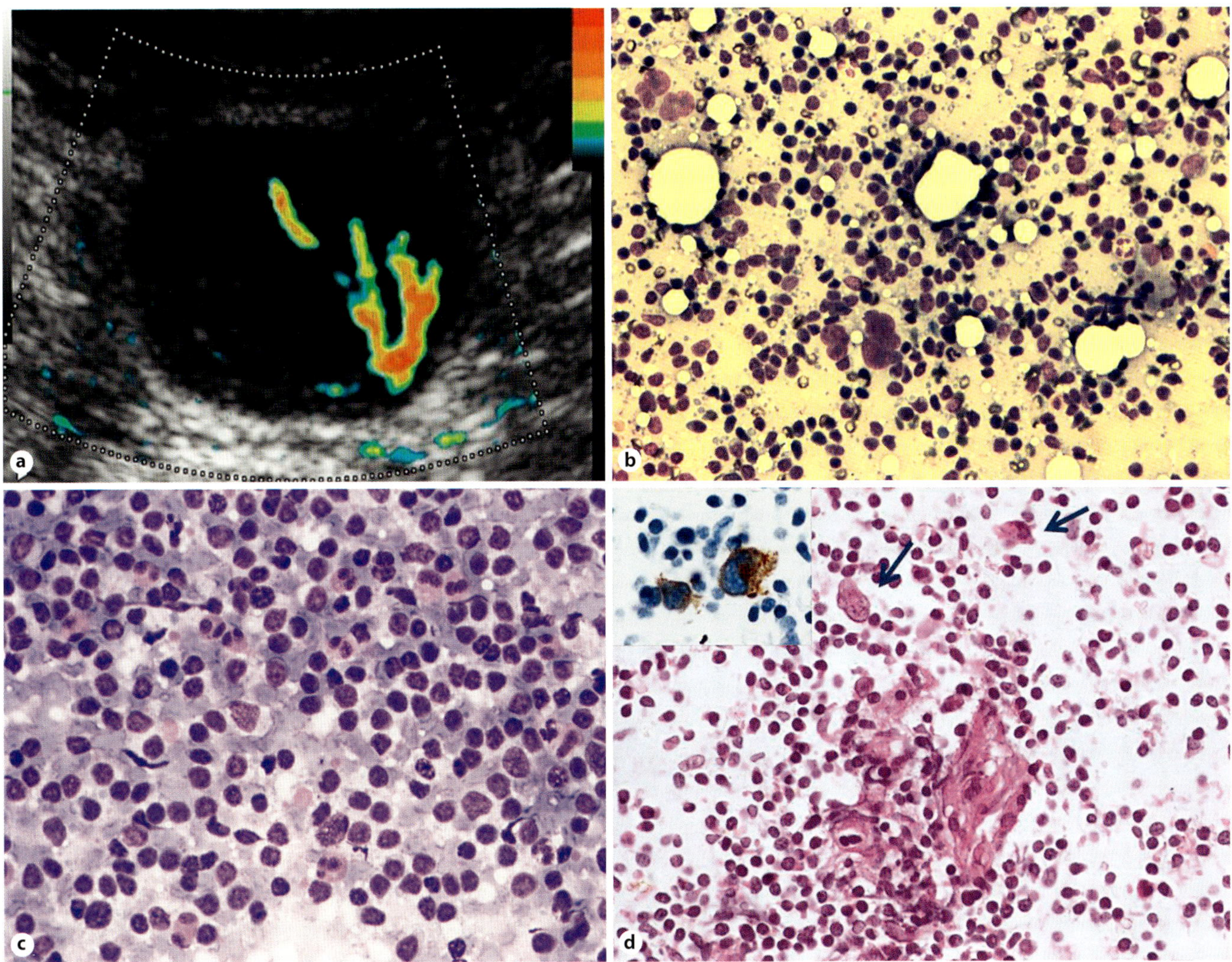

Fig. 1. a Ultrasound imaging of a lymph node with Hodgkin lymphoma: the node is round and hypoechoic, with an abnormal vascular pattern at Power Doppler. **b** FNC showing a polymorphous pattern and RSCs. **c** Numerous eosinophils in the background. **d** Fibrosis in the cell block with diagnostic cells (arrows). **Inset** CD30+ cells.

ic and histiocytic), and multinucleated Reed-Sternberg cells (RSC) [1, 3]. The background is composed of a heterogeneous mixture of fibrous hyaline, birefringent stroma, often with a "woven basket" appearance, lymphocytes, epithelioid cells, neutrophils, and eosinophils (Fig. 1). Affected LNs are generally hard at physical examination, with an irregular shape and surface. At US, LNs are roundish, subverted, and hypoechoic; partial involvement and abnormal vascular patterns may occur (Fig. 1) [4]. FNC cell harvesting may be scanty due to the amount of fibrosis in the LN; therefore, FNC by syringe aspiration would be advisable when dealing with HL. Haemorrhagic, necrotic, or suppurative material

may also occur [5–10]. Rapid on-site evaluation (ROSE) generally shows a variable, polymorphous, or lymphoid background, whereas the purpose of ROSE, and of the final diagnosis, is the search for and the identification of diagnostic cells (Fig. 1). These latter are usually scanty and not always easily detectable; therefore, a careful search for rare and partially hidden diagnostic cells is often required and their cytological variability should also be taken into account. ROSE may suggest the repetition of FNC in cases lacking diagnostic cells, also on a different LN if possible, and obtained material should be used to prepare alcohol-fixed smears or cell blocks.

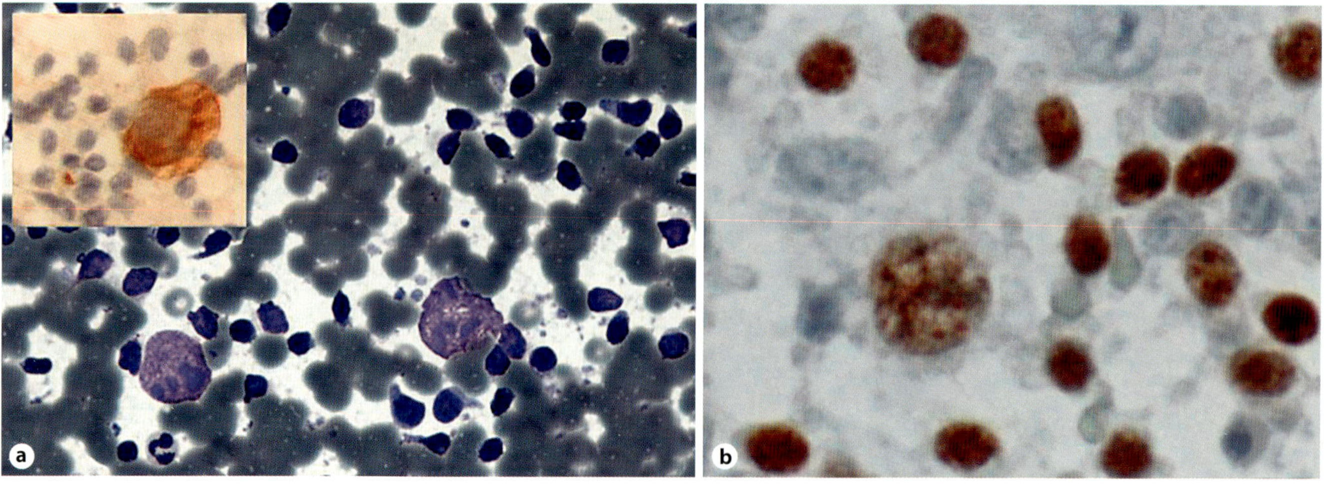

Fig. 2. a Lymphocytic and histiocytic variant of Hodgkin lymphoma. The nuclei are roundish, folded, or multilobulated, the chromatin is vesicular, the nucleoli are usually multiple and smaller than those seen in classical Hodgkin and Reed-Sternberg cells. Lymphocytic and histiocytic cells are CD20+ (**inset**), CD15–, CD30–. **b** PAX5+ in one diagnostic cell and mature B-lymphocytes in the background.

Hodgkin Lymphoma Background

HL FNC smears are generally scantily cellular, but may also show the same cellularity of reactive or NHL LNs. The background is composed of a reactive infiltrate that may vary according to the histological subtype. Fibrosis is the main cause of hypocellular smears; it is generally absent, but small groups or isolated fibroblasts with plump nuclei and elongated cytoplasm may be observed on the smears (Fig. 1). Fibrosis is also responsible for cell distortion and fragility, resulting in lymphoid tangles and crushed nuclei. Eosinophils are frequently but not constantly present in the background; their presence should focus the search for diagnostic cells, but numerous eosinophils may also occur in LNs in the absence of HL, such as in the case of drug-induced or dermatopathic lymphadenopathies, Kimura disease, angiolymphoid hyperplasia with eosinophilia, filaria, or malignancies like eosinophilic myeloid or angioimmunoblastic T-cell NHL [1, 3]. Histiocytes frequently occur in HL smears, both isolated or organized in granuloma. Sometimes the granulomatous pattern largely exceeds the lymphoid component and, together with the paucity of diagnostic cells, may cause FNC false negatives. Conversely, isolated, bi- or multinucleated histiocytes may mimic HCs or RSCs [5–10]. Attention should be paid to the different nuclear and nucleolar features for the differential diagnosis, but definitive differentiation and assessment mainly depend on the phenotype of diagnostic cells by immunocyto-

chemistry (ICC). The background is quite variable; it may be scanty and polymorphous or hypercellular and mainly composed of small lymphocytes. This latter background generally corresponds to the lymphocyte-rich HL subtype or the nodular lymphocyte-predominant variant. These lymphocytes are small, polyclonal, mainly T cells that may hide or hamper the identification of diagnostic cells. The FNC diagnosis of HL is very difficult in cases of the nodular lymphocyte-predominant variant, in which diagnostic cells are large atypical B cells with a scanty or absent cytoplasm (Fig. 2). These cells are CD20+ and CD30–; therefore, ICC may be ineffective for their detection and identification. FC, which is not suitable in the diagnosis of HL, should suggest this possibility when an unsuspected LN-FNC polyclonal, CD2+/CD3+/CD7+, CD4+, CD8+ T-cell population is detected. CD4+/CD8+ has occasionally been observed in HL FC assessment, mainly in nodular lymphocyte predominant HL [11] and considered a possible indirect sign of HL [12], whereas it seems to be the expression of early stages of maturation of the T lineage and has been observed in the progressive transformation of germinal centres and T-cell NHL [10]. A haemorrhagic background may occur as a consequence of an abnormal vascular pattern or a prolonged and energetic aspirations; blood may spoil cytological details and hamper the ICC. Blood presence in the smears may be minimized by a short aspiration and a proper haematological smearing [see Chapter 2, this vol., pp. 14–18]. A suppurative and necrotic background may also

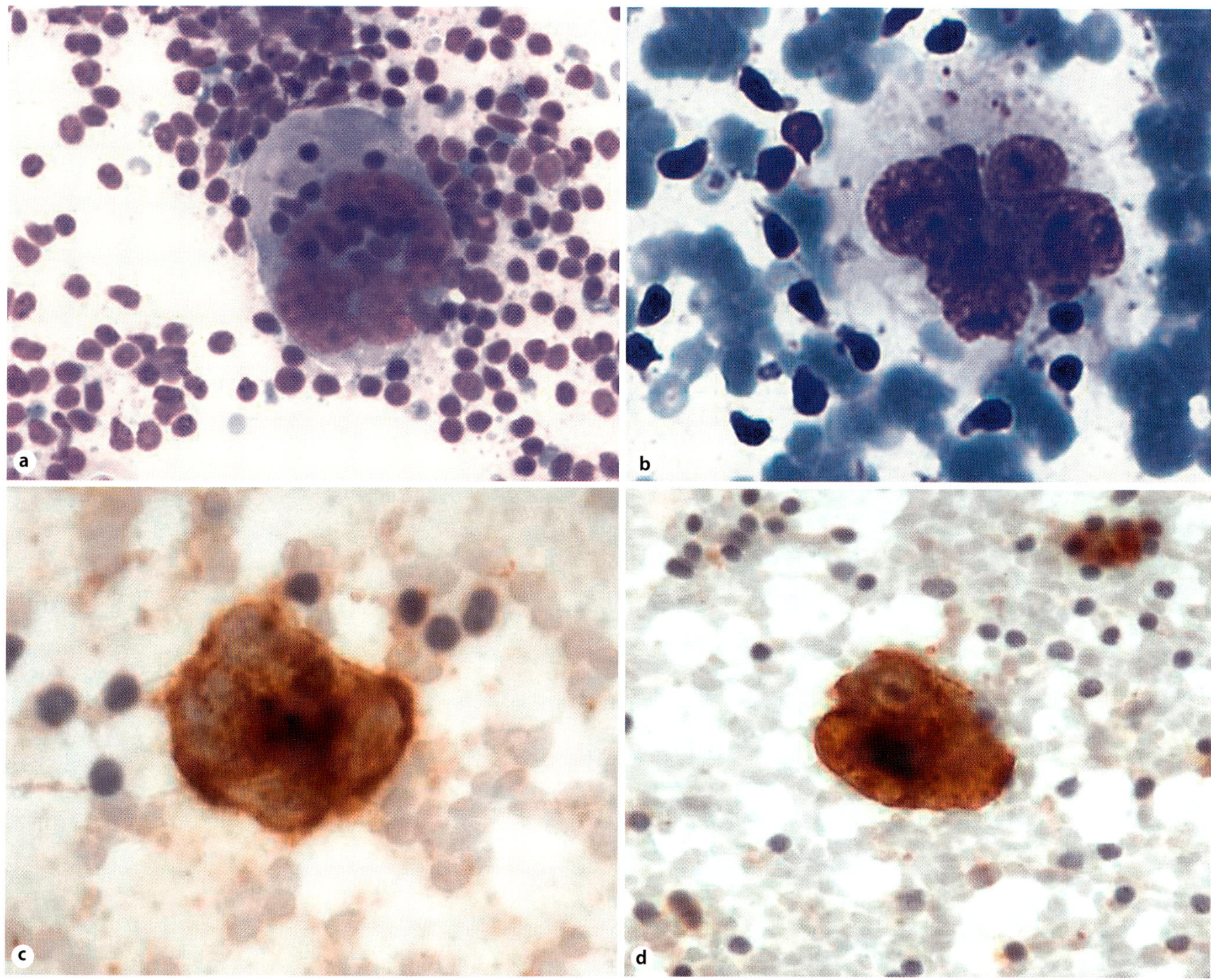

Fig. 3. a, b Classical multinucleated RSCs with lobulated nuclei, clumped chromatin, and large nucleoli. **c, d** CD15+ and CD30+ RS cells on additional smears.

occur, hindering the identification of HCs and RSCs. This evidence has been reported as a possible cause of diagnostic mistakes [13–15].

Hodgkin Lymphoma Diagnostic Cells

Typical RSCs are large with abundant, slightly basophilic cytoplasm and 2 or more nuclear lobes or nuclei. RSCs generally have at least 2 large nucleoli, typically described as resembling owl eyes, which are bluish or reddish in colour, according to the different stains (Fig. 3). Anaplastic, polyp-oid, "mummified" and other variants may also occur (Fig. 4) [5–10, 16, 17]. Mirror cells generally appear as 2 identical, close but separate, round-oval nuclei with similar large nucleoli (Fig. 5); the cytoplasm of mirror cells is often absent. HCs are large atypical mononuclear cells with macronucleoli (Fig. 6). "Lacunar" cells are typical of the histological sections of the nodular sclerosis variant; they are formalin fixation artefacts, and are not observed on smears. The nodular lymphocytic predominant variants show a lymphoid background, and a variable number of large neoplastic mononucleated cells, known as lymphocytic and/or histiocytic RSC variants. These cells show folded or lobulated nuclei.

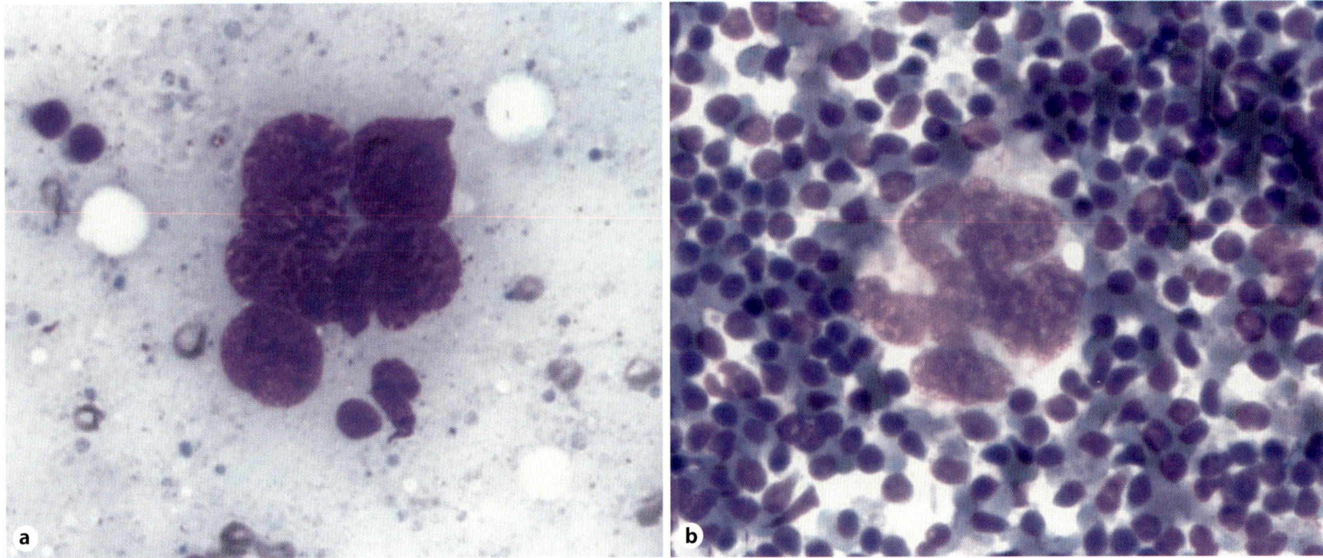

Fig. 4. a Abnormal presentation of RS cells with a condensed cytoplasm and dark nuclei with an abnormal chromatin pattern. **b** Polyploid multinucleated RS cells in a lymphoid background.

The chromatin is mostly vesicular, and nucleoli are usually multiple and smaller than those seen in classical RSCs (Fig. 2). Regarding the number of diagnostic cells, they may be rare or extremely numerous, as in the case of the HL "syncytial" variant [18].

Ancillary Techniques

Provided that the FNC diagnosis of HL mainly depends on the identification of diagnostic cells and their differentiation from HC-like or Reed-Sternberg-like cells, ancillary techniques aim for the identification of their specific phenotypes. RSCs and HCs are defective, clonal B cells that have partially lost the B-cell phenotype; these cells escape apoptosis and develop mechanisms to facilitate survival and activation. HCs and RSCs express specific surface and nuclear antigens, such as CD15, CD30, and PAX5 [5–10]. Conversely, HC-like and RSC-like cells in some NHL express, in variable percentages, CD20, Bcl6, Oct-2, BOB.1, MUM1, and other antigens [1, 3]. The main limitation of ancillary techniques on HL-LN FNC is the frequently scanty number of diagnostic cells and the heterogeneity of the LN cell population. Diagnostic cells are not sufficient to represent a reliable gate on FC; moreover, such cells are fragile and get broken or stick to the FC circuits, and therefore the same FC is not suitable on HL FNC. HC and RSC identification mainly depends on ICC; for this purpose, a reliable support is provided by additional destained Papanicolaou smears or cell blocks in which the presence of diagnostic cells has been previously verified. CD30 is helpful to differentiate diagnostic cells from follicular centre cells and immunoblasts. CD15 is less sensitive but specific enough and benefits from the presence of granulocytes as positive internal controls. PAX5, which is a B-cell lineage-specific activator protein, generally produces less intense, nuclear signals, but the nuclear staining is enhanced by the negativity of T lymphocytes in the background and may identify HCs and RSCs that have lost their cytoplasm. The other mentioned markers are generally used in large panels for complex histological differential diagnoses that require tissue samples and are beyond the tasks of FNC.

Differential Diagnosis and FNC Report

An FNC diagnosis is generally straightforward in the typical HL presentation, while the differential diagnosis has to be performed with other benign and malignant entities that show variable amounts of HC-like and RSC-like cells. The latter may be observed in EBV reactive lymphadenitis, Castleman disease, and other reactive LNs [19, 20] and malignant entities, such as ALCL (anaplastic large cell lymphoma; ALK +/–; Fig. 7), some polymorphous DLBCLs (diffuse large B-cell lymphomas), mediastinal-type DLBCL, T-rich B-cell NHLs, and even nasopharyngeal carcinoma [5–10, 21–23]. An FNC differential diagnosis of HL with all these reactive and malignant entities depends on the microscopic identification of diagnostic cells and their ICC confirmation. HL without further subclassification should be diagnosed and reported only when these criteria are fulfilled. In case of the above-reported malignant entities that may simulate HL, the diagnosis of malignancy may be provided on the basis of the sole cytological features, but the identification of the specific entities and the differential diagnosis may be extremely difficult or almost impossible on FNC samples. In these cases, a timely excision for a histological differential diagnosis is advisable.

LN-FNC Sensitivity and Specificity in HL Diagnosis

It is commonly believed that an FNC diagnosis of HL is easier and less controversial than the diagnosis of NHL but, looking at the reported sensitivity and specificity values, this seems not to be the case [16]. The reason for the low diagnostic sensitivity of FNC mainly lies in the possible lack of identification of diagnostic cells [24]. This possibility is very high in cases of nodular lymphocyte-predominant HL [25]. Atypical sites of onset such as salivary glands, thyroid, or even bone may also hamper the FNC sensitivity [26–30]. The low diagnostic specificity is due to the misdiagnosis of RS-like cells that may be observed in different neoplastic and non-neoplastic processes, as previously discussed. Other reasons are the possible association of HL with other pathological entities [31–33] and the morphological and biological overlaps existing between HL and ALCL [21], some T-cell NHLs, and the T-cell-rich B-cell NHL [5–10, 23], as demonstrated by immunophenotyping and molecular procedures [1, 3]. Finally, the identification of specific HL subtypes is almost impossible on FNC samples [5–10]; therefore, despite its limited clinical value, the HL subclassification is a histological task. The usage and value of an LN-FNC diagnosis of HL depend on the protocols of the different institutions and the clinical context in which the FNC diagnosis is made. When HL is primary diagnosed by FNC, a histological assessment is usually required for confirmation and subtyping. Histological confirmation is also required in negative FNC cases when HL is suspected. In HL follow-up, the FNC diagnosis of HL relapse may be ac-

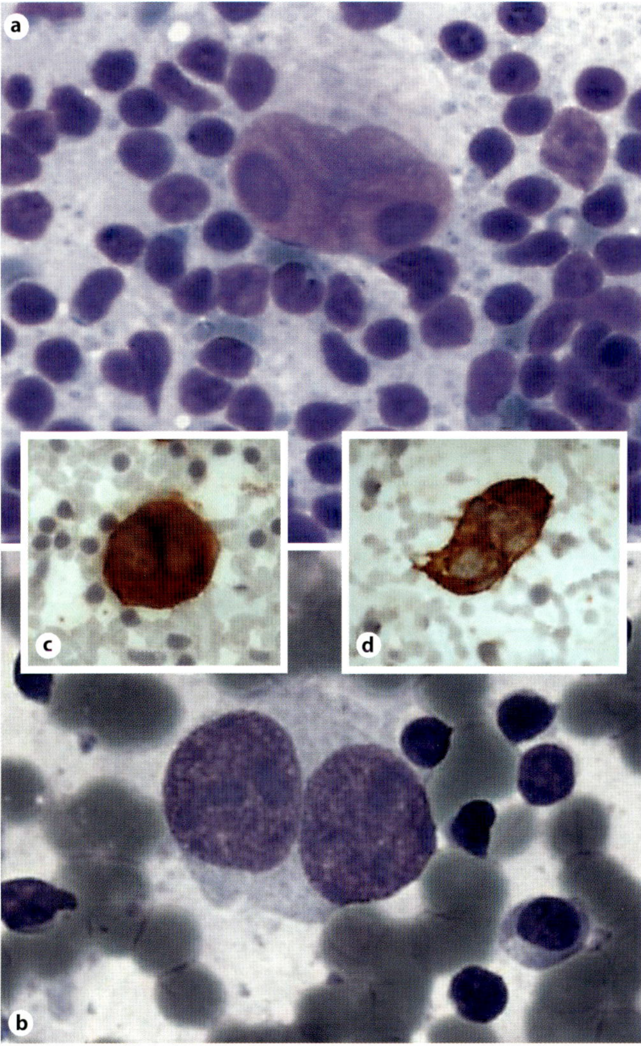

Fig. 5. Reed-Stenberg cells: "mirror" variants with extremely large nucleoli (**a**, **b**); CD30+ and CD15+ on additional smears (**c**, **d**).

cepted by clinicians, but the histological evaluation is required when clinical data diverge or when FNC does not provide an explanation for an LNe. Finally, in the case of secondary neoplasms or other possible pathological processes unrelated to HL [34], further diagnostic procedures should be performed according to the specific clinical contexts.

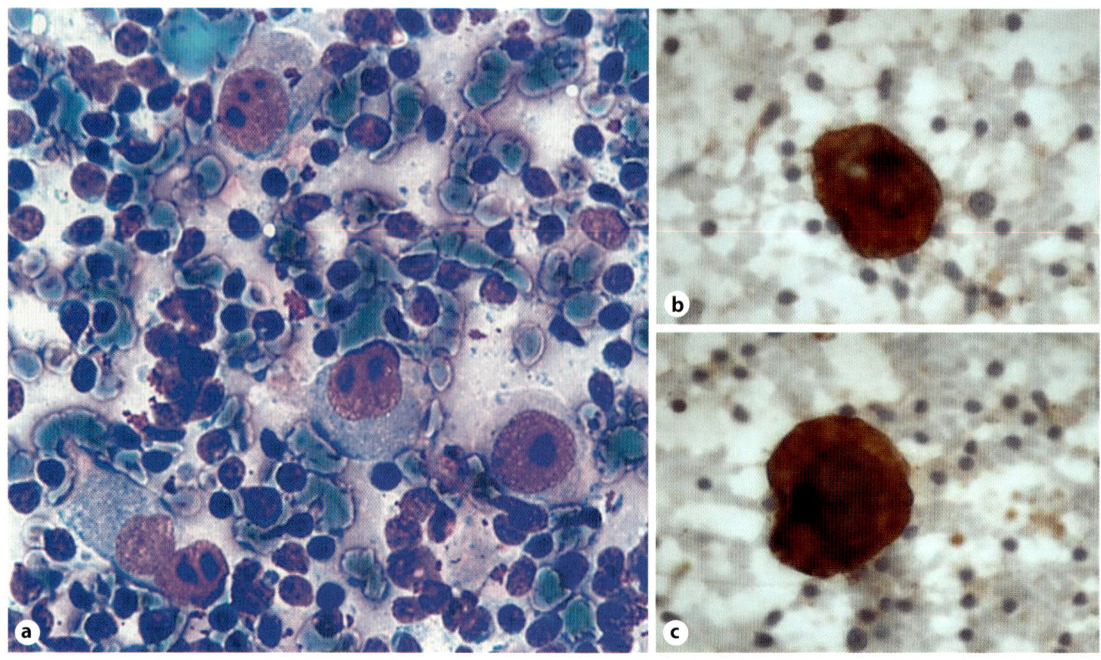

Fig. 6. a Mononucleated HCs with irregular chromatin and large, basophilic nucleoli. **b**, **c** CD15+ and CD30+ on additional smears.

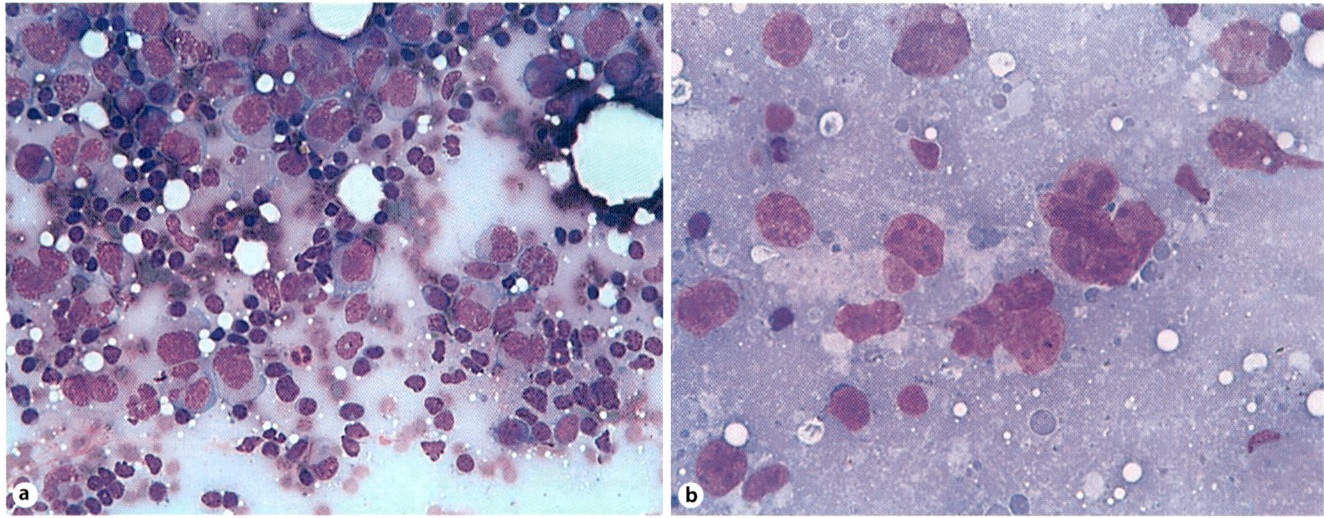

Fig. 7. a HL simulating a large cell or anaplastic lymphoma. **b** Anaplastic lymphoma simulating a HL. A differential diagnosis may be impossible on FNC samples.

References

1 Swerdlow SH, Campo E, Harris NL, Jaffe ES, Pileri SA, Stein H, Thiele J: WHO Classification of Tumours of Haematopoietic and Lymphoid Tissues, ed 4. Lyon, IARC Press, 2017.
2 Lister TA, Crowther D, Sutcliffe SB, Glatstein E, Canellos GP, Young RC, Rosenberg SA, Coltman CA, Tubiana M: Report of a committee convened to discuss the evaluation and staging of patients with Hodgkin's disease: Cotswolds meeting. J Clin Oncol 1989;7:1630–1636.
3 Hodgson DC, Gosporadowicz MK: Clinical evaluation and staging of Hodgkin lymphoma; in Hoppe RT, et al (eds): Hodgkin Lymphoma. Philadelphia, Lippincott, Williams & Wilkins, 2007.
4 Nakase K, Yamamoto K, Hiasa A, Tawara I, Yamaguchi M, Shiku H: Contrast-enhanced ultrasound examination of lymph nodes in different types of lymphoma. Cancer Detect Prev 2006;30: 188–191.
5 Zhang JR, Raza AS, Greaves TS, Cobb CJ: Fine-needle aspiration diagnosis of Hodgkin lymphoma using current WHO classification – re-evaluation of cases from 1999–2004 with new proposals. Diagn Cytopathol 2006;34:397–402.
6 Moreland WS, Geisinger KR: Utility and outcomes of fine-needle aspiration biopsy in Hodgkin's disease. Diagn Cytopathol 2002;26:278–282.
7 Skoog L, Tani E: Lymph nodes; in Gray W, Kocjan G (eds): Diagnostic Cytopathology, ed 3. London, Churchill Livingstone, 2010, pp 409–443.
8 Sheaff MT, Singh N: Lymph nodes; in: Cytopathology. Berlin, Springer, 2012, pp 179–184.
9 Caraway NP, Katz RL: Lymph nodes; in Koss LG, Melamed MR (eds): Koss' Diagnostic Cytology and Its Histopathologic Bases. Philadelphia, Lippincott, Williams & Wilkins, 2006, pp 1186–1228.
10 Wieczorek TJ, Wakely PE: Lymph nodes; in Cibas ES, Ducatman BS (eds): Cytology: Diagnostic Principles and Clinical Correlates, ed 4. Amsterdam, Elsevier, 2014.
11 Rahemtullah A, Harris NL, Dorn ME, Preffer FI, Hasserjian RP: Beyond the lymphocyte predominant cell: CD4+CD8+ T-cells in nodular lymphocyte predominant Hodgkin lymphoma. Leuk Lymphoma 2008;49:1870–1878.
12 Beaty MW, Geisinger KR: Hodgkin lymphoma: flow me? Cytojournal 2005;8;2:13.
13 Tani E, Ersöz C, Svedmyr E, Skoog L: Fine-needle aspiration cytology and immunocytochemistry of Hodgkin's disease, suppurative type. Diagn Cytopathol 1998;18:437–440.
14 Fulciniti F, Zeppa P, Vetrani A, Troncone G, Palombini L: Hodgkin's disease mimicking suppurative lymphadenitis: a possible pitfall in fine-needle aspiration biopsy cytology. Diagn Cytopathol 1989;5:282–285.
15 Florentine BD, Cohen AN: Nodular sclerosing classical Hodgkin lymphoma masquerading as acute suppurative-necrotizing lymphadenitis. Diagn Cytopathol 2014;42:238–241.
16 Das DK, Francis IM, Sharma PN, Sathar SA, John B, George SS, Mallik MK, Sheikh ZA, Haji BE, Pathan SK, Madda JP, Mirza K, Ahmed MS, Junaid TA: Hodgkin's lymphoma: diagnostic difficulties in fine-needle aspiration cytology. Diagn Cytopathol 2009;37:564–573.
17 Srikant N, Yinti SR, Baliga M, Kini H: A rare spindle-cell variant of non-Hodgkin's lymphoma of the mandible. J Oral Maxillofac Pathol 2016;20: 129–132.
18 Park IS, Kim L, Han JY, Kim JM, Chu YC, Choi SJ: Syncytial variant of nodular sclerosis Hodgkin's lymphoma assessed by fine needle aspiration cytology. Cytopathology 2008;19:394–397.
19 Iacobuzio-Donahue CA, Clark DP, Ali SZ: Reed-Sternberg-like cells in lymph node aspirates in the absence of Hodgkin's disease: pathologic significance and differential diagnosis. Diagn Cytopathol 2002;27:335–339.
20 Naik LP, Fernandes G, Mahapatra L: Cytology of Castleman disease hyaline-vascular type: a close differential diagnosis with Hodgkin's lymphoma. Acta Cytol 2010;54(5 suppl):1093–1094.
21 Rosario-Quiñones F, Strauchen JA, Salem F: Anaplastic large cell lymphoma masquerading as classical Hodgkin lymphoma on fine needle aspiration: a potential diagnostic pitfall. Diagn Cytopathol 2015;43:916–919.
22 Lynnhtun K, Varikatt W, Pathmanathan N: B cell lymphoma, unclassifiable, with features intermediate between diffuse large B cell lymphoma and classical Hodgkin lymphoma: diagnosis by fine-needle aspiration cytology. Diagn Cytopathol 2014;42:690–693.
23 Mathur S, Verm K: Peripheral T-cell lymphoma not otherwise specified vs. Hodgkin's lymphoma on fine needle aspiration cytology. Acta Cytol 2005;49:373–377.
24 Chhieng DC, Cangiarella JF, Symmans WF, Cohen JM: Fine-needle aspiration cytology of Hodgkin disease: a study of 89 cases with emphasis on false-negative cases. Cancer 2001;93:52–59.
25 Subhawong AP, Ali SZ, Tatsas AD: Nodular lymphocyte-predominant Hodgkin lymphoma: cytopathologic correlates on fine-needle aspiration. Cancer Cytopathol 2012;120:254–260.
26 Dey B, Goyal V, Bharti JN, Mahajan N, Jain S: A rare cytological diagnosis of primary non-Hodgkin lymphoma of the parotid gland. J Cytol 2016; 33:108–110.
27 Furukawa BS, Bernstein M, Siddiqi N, Pastis NJ: Diagnosing Hodgkin lymphoma from an endobronchial ultrasound core needle biopsy. J Bronchol Interv Pulmonol 2016;23:336–339.
28 Oriot P, Malvaux P, Waignein F, Delcourt A, Doyen C, Rousseau E, Baudry G, Dechambre S: Nodular sclerosing Hodgkin mimicking Riedel's invasivefibrousthyroiditis. Ann Endocrinol (Paris) 2012;73:492–496.
29 Szczepanek-Parulska E, Szkudlarek M, Majewski P, Breborowicz J, Ruchala M: Thyroid nodule as a first manifestation of Hodgkin lymphoma – report of two cases and literature review. Diagn Pathol 2013;8:116.
30 Madan M, Arora R, Singh J: Solitary skeletal lesion as the primary manifestation of Hodgkin's lymphoma: a case report. Acta Cytol 2010; 54(5 Suppl):1035–1038.
31 Das DK, Sheikh ZA, Alansary TA, Amir T, Al-Rabiy FN, Junaid TA: A case of Langerhans' cell histiocytosis associated with Hodgkin's lymphoma: fine-needle aspiration cytologic and histopathological features. Diagn Cytopathol 2016;44: 128–132.
32 Nga ME, Amanuel B: Fine needle aspiration diagnosis of Hodgkin transformation of small lymphocytic lymphoma/chronic lymphocytic leukaemia: a case report. Cytopathology 2013;24: 335–337.
33 Reading FC, Schlette EJ, Stewart JM, Keating MJ, Katz RL, Caraway NP: Fine-needle aspiration biopsy findings in patients with small lymphocytic lymphoma transformed to Hodgkin lymphoma. Am J Clin Pathol 2007;128:571–578.
34 Zeppa P, Picardi M, Cozzolino I, Troncone G, Lucariello A, De Renzo A, Pane F, Rotoli B, Vetrani A, Palombini L: Fine-needle aspiration cytology in the follow-up of Hodgkin lymphoma. Diagn Cytopathol 2008;36:467–472.

Zeppa P, Cozzolino I: Lymph Node FNC. Cytopathology of Lymph Nodes and Extranodal Lymphoproliferative Processes.
Monogr Clin Cytol. Basel, Karger, 2018, vol 23, pp 60–76 (DOI: 10.1159/000478882)

Paediatric Lymphadenopathies

Lymphadenopathies frequently occur in children. Roughly half of children in good health have palpable lymph nodes (LNs), and relevant LN enlargements (LNe) may occur after mild infections and even without a relevant clinical background [1–6]. Reactive LNe account for approximately 75% of paediatric and 25% of adult lymphadenopathies; therefore, the clinical relevance of LNe in children is different compared to adults [3]. Nonetheless, the persistence of LNe in children may worry parents and paediatricians; therefore, enlarged LN are often removed and, in most cases, histology reveals reactive unspecific processes. As in the case of adults, fine-needle cytology (FNC) can diagnose most paediatric lymphadenopathies, provided that the cytopathologists are informed of the clinical data, perform the FNC and rapid on-site evaluation (ROSE) personally, and are aware of the specificities of paediatric pathology.

Clinical Data

LNs larger than 2 cm in children are considered abnormal. Acute lymphadenopathies are generally caused by known or unknown bacterial or viral processes, and should shrink in less than 2 weeks. Subacute or chronic LNe lasting longer than this are most likely caused by chronic infections or malignant processes. Clinical information is mandatory for an accurate LN-FNC, including the pain or tenderness of LNe, fever, malaise, sore throat, upper respiratory tract infections, toothache, ear pain, insect bites or exposure to ani-

mals, exposure to mycobacteria and other infectious agents, vaccinations (smallpox, MMR, diphtheritis, poliomyelitis, typhoid fever) or drug consumption (phenytoin, pyrimethamine, phenylbutazone, isoniazide). All these factors, including storage diseases, may be associated with single or multiple, mild or relevant LNe. The evaluation of the LNe drained area is also important because LNe may be caused by specific pathological processes of corresponding areas, like conjunctivitis or dermatitis [1–6].

Laboratory Evaluation

Neutrophilic leucocytosis is generally associated with bacterial infections and lymphocytic leucocytosis with Epstein-Barr virus (EBV) and other viral infections. Lymphocytic leucocytosis with blasts is indicative of leukaemia; leucopenia, low levels of haemoglobin and platelets may be indicative of neoplastic bone marrow involvement. Lymphopenia with T cell impairment may occur in HIV infections, congenital immunodeficiency disorders, or post-transplantation immunodeficiency. The erythrocyte sedimentation and C-reactive protein levels are evaluated as inflammation and infection indicators, and may help in assessing the patient's response to treatment. High serum levels of lactate dehydrogenase and uric acid are expressions of rapid cell turnover, and are often associated with malignancy. Specific serological data are required in cases of EBV, HIV, cytomegalovirus (CMV), and parvovirus infections. PCR or purified protein

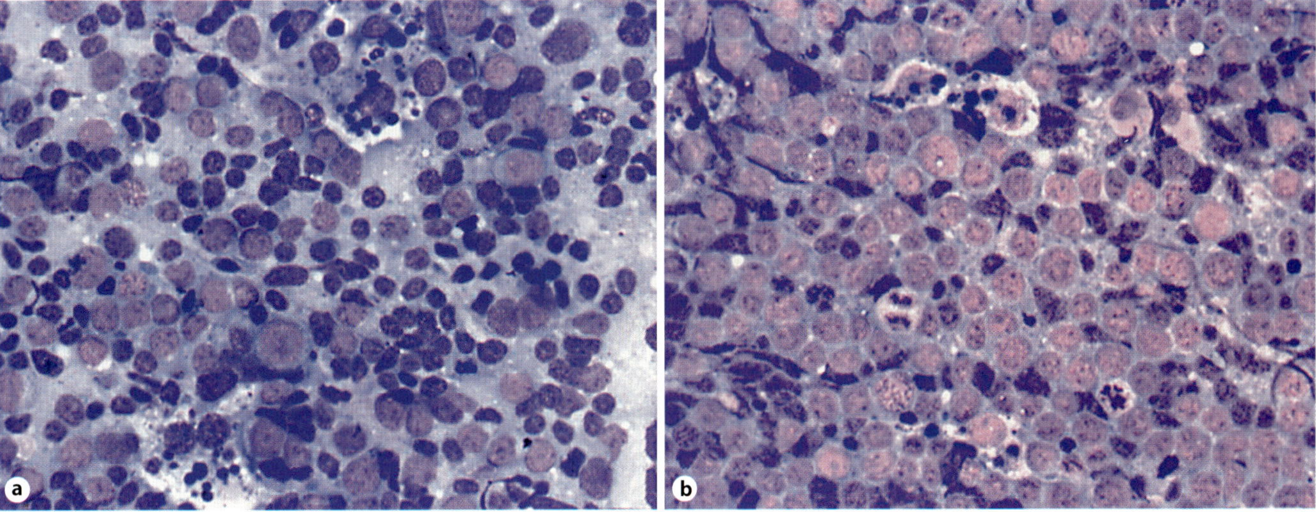

Fig. 1. a Florid reactive hyperplasia showing numerous centrofollicular cells, small lymphocytes, and occasional macrophages. **b** Lymphoblastic lymphoma with monomorphous lymphoblasts and scattered macrophages. Note the numerous mitoses.

Virus-associated LNe generally resolve spontaneously, while bacterial LNe may require specific treatment. Corresponding FNC features are generally unspecific; nonetheless, FNC may be characterized by prevalent cytological patterns, like unspecific reactive hyperplasia with or without a prevalence of follicular cells, granulomatous pattern, histiocytic pattern (with or without haemophagocytosis), follicular pattern with increased plasma cells, or eosinophils and necrotic pattern. These patterns may be indicative of a group of entities or specific entities, if matched with clinical data [9].

Unspecific Reactive Hyperplasia

Unspecific reactive hyperplasia is the most frequent FNC pattern observed in LNe. Reactive LNe rarely exceed 3 cm and the LN structure on US is generally maintained (oval shape, hilum and medulla preserved, cortex expanded, and normal vascularization). FNC shows small lymphocytes, follicular centre cells, plasma cells, and immunoblasts; capillary structures intermingled with lymphoid cells may also be observed. A variable number of macrophages with cytoplasmic tingible bodies are generally present. When follicular cells or immunoblasts are prevalent, the differential diagnosis with lymphoblastic lymphoma (LBL; Burkitt or non-Burkitt) and paediatric, rare, low-grade non-Hodg-

kin lymphoma (NHL; follicular lymphoma [FL], marginal zone lymphoma [MZL], mantle cell lymphoma) may be indicated (Fig. 1). In these cases, flow cytometry (FC) and immunocytochemistry (ICC) assessment show a balanced light chain, a number of CD10+ cells (<50%) [10, 11], and a reasonable mitotic index by Ki67 when compared with LBL. In some cases, groups of lymphocytes, histiocytes, and reticular cells are evident and may be confused with granuloma. Nonetheless, these lymph-histiocytic groups have faint, ill-defined cytoplasm and ovoid eccentric nuclei, while true granulomatous epithelioid cells show elongated curved or bent nuclei and dense and better-defined cytoplasm (Fig. 2).

Drug-Induced Lymphadenopathy

LNe may occur as a hypersensitive reaction to vaccines and drugs, and FNC may show an unspecific reactive hyperplastic pattern, as previously described [see Chapter 3, this vol., pp. 19–33]. In some cases, Reed-Sternberg-like cells and more than occasional eosinophils may occur, suggesting a differential diagnosis with HL. However, these cells should be CD15–, CD30– at ICC on additional slides or cell blocks (Fig. 3).

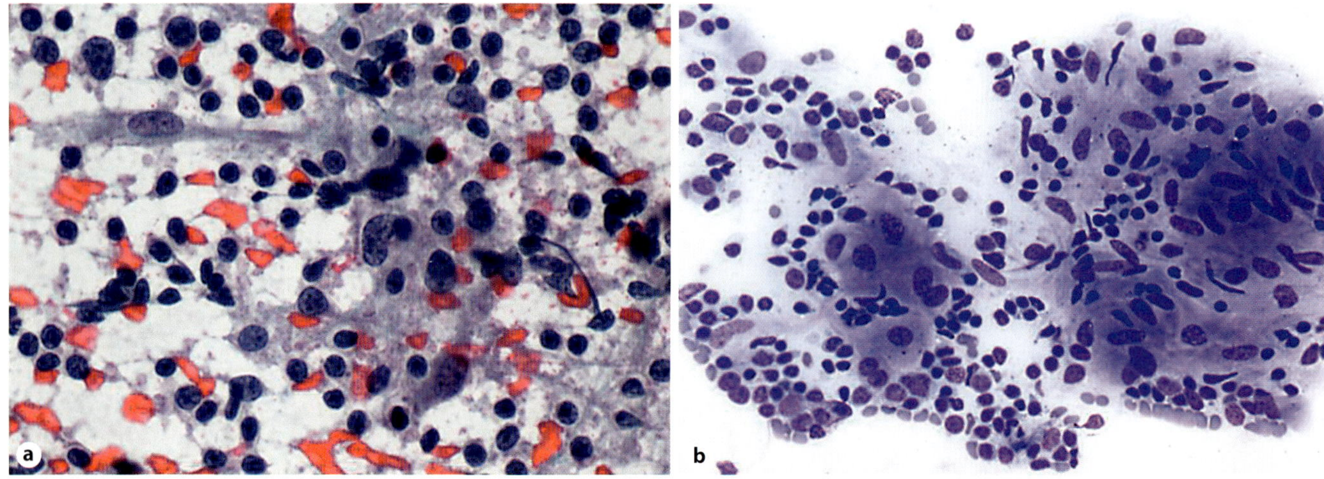

Fig. 2. a Lymphohistiocytic group showing faint, ill-defined cytoplasm and ovoid eccentric nuclei, intermingled with lymphocytes. **b** Epithelioid cells in granulomatous arrangement showing elongated curved or bent nuclei and dense and better-defined cytoplasm.

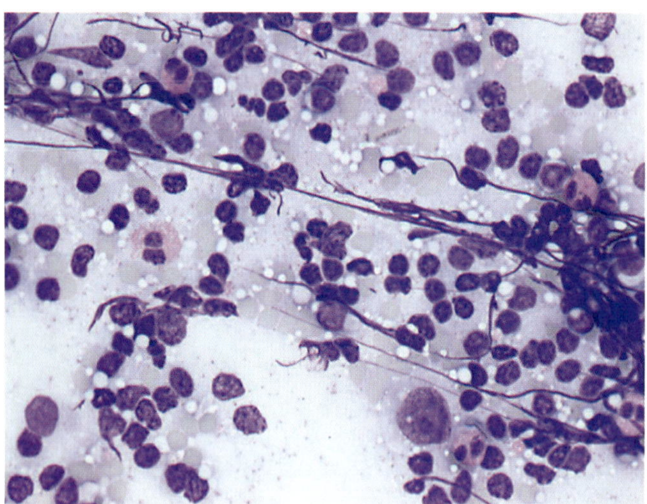

Fig. 3. Reactive LNe caused by a hypersensitive reaction to vaccine. FNC shows lymphocytes, nuclear crushes, eosinophils, and a Hodgkin-like cell that indicated a differential diagnosis with HL. These cells were CD15 and CD30 negatives on ICC.

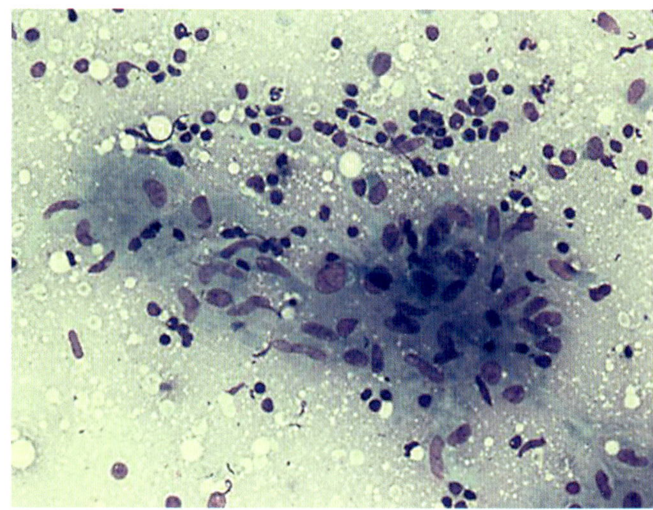

Fig. 4. A granulomatous structure of epithelioid cells with wide, ill-defined cytoplasm and ovaloid or elongated bent nuclei.

Tuberculosis and Sarcoidosis

Granulomatous processes, and tuberculosis (TB) in particular, may cause significant LNe. Cervical LNs are mainly involved, and submandibular stations are often involved in atypical TB. Fistulae and sinus tract formation may occur, showing typical modifications of the skin. US may show round, hypoechoic LNs with no visible hilum, blurred margins, and perinodal oedema; abnormal vascularization, necrosis and calcifications may also exist. FNC is characterized by a granulomatous pattern (with or without necrosis; Fig. 4), as previously described [see Chapter 3, this vol., pp. 19–33]. Asteroid bodies (star shaped) and Schaumann bodies (cytoplasm spherule of calcium or iron) have been tradi-

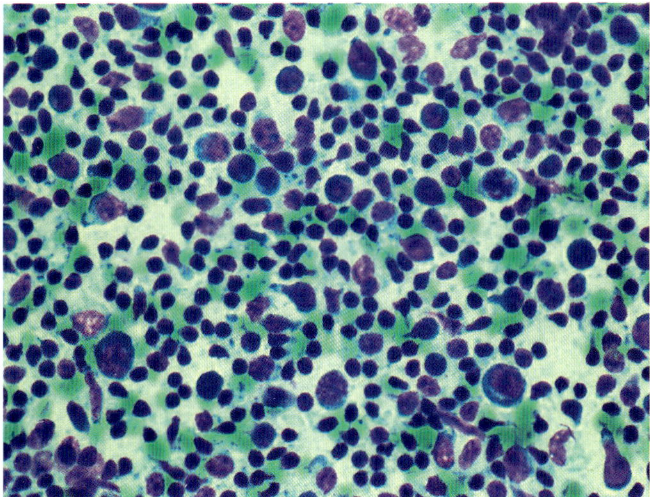

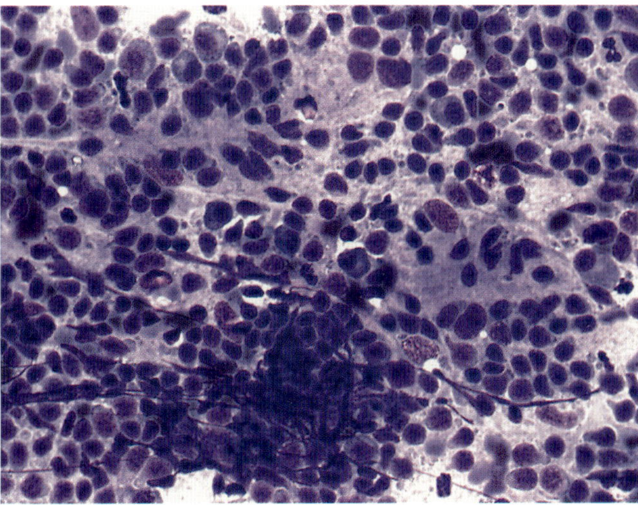

Fig. 5. Cytological features of LN reactive hyperplasia with small lymphocytes and numerous immunoblasts; mitoses are present. A serological test was consistent with mononucleosis.

Fig. 6. LNe from lupus erythematosus showing lymphocytes, numerous plasma cells, and karyorrhectic nuclear debris in the absence of epithelioid cells and neutrophils.

tionally reported in sarcoidosis and occasionally seen on FNC, but they are rare, inconstant, and unspecific. The FNC granulomatous pattern may be predominant, and particular attention should be paid to the infiltrate in the background because HL and high-grade NHL may occur with predominant granulomatous reactions that may blur or even hide the basic lymphomatous process [12–14]. The TB diagnosis has to be confirmed by a skin test or by specific chest X-ray features. TB bacilli may be detected by FNC (Ziehl-Nielsen stain on smears or PCR) [see Chapter 3, this vol., pp. 19–33].

Infectious Mononucleosis

Mononucleosis is caused by EBV infection; patients may experience fever, malaise, sore throat, and LNe. Children younger than 4 years may be asymptomatic, while older children and adolescents may show generalized LNe and hepatosplenomegaly. Some patients may show exudative tonsillitis and palatal petechiae that may blur the clinical presentation. At US, LNe may also show irregular margins, a hypoechoic centre, and absence of hilum. Cytological features are similar to those of the unspecific reactive hyperplasia, but a worrying number of immunoblasts and mitoses may be present (Fig. 5). Ancillary techniques may be needed to assess the polyclonality of the process [15]. The definitive diagnosis of mononucleosis requires serological assessment.

Cat-Scratch Disease

This infection is caused by the inoculation of *Bartonella henselae* through epidermal wounds or cat scratch. The event and the related skin lesion may have been forgotten by the time of the LNe, which generally occurs 1 week or 2 months later. LNe usually occur in the axillary or epitrochlear area, followed by the cervical location. General symptoms such as fever, malaise, and anorexia may be associated. FNC shows a granulomatous process in a necrotic background [16, 17]. The infection may be confirmed by serology and generally heals spontaneously within a few months [for cytological features, see Chapter 3, this vol., pp. 19–33].

Autoimmune Diseases

Autoimmune diseases and autoimmune lymphoproliferative syndrome (ALPS) may show generalized, sometimes unexplained LNe. These latter may herald autoimmune diseases that are frequently accompanied by fever, arthritis, malaise, pruritus, and urticarial rash. LN-FNC of autoimmune diseases generally reveals an unspecific reactive hyperplasia pattern. Some specific features like plasma cells with an eosinophilic cytoplasm, individual cell necrosis, macrophages, karyorrhectic nuclear debris in the absence of

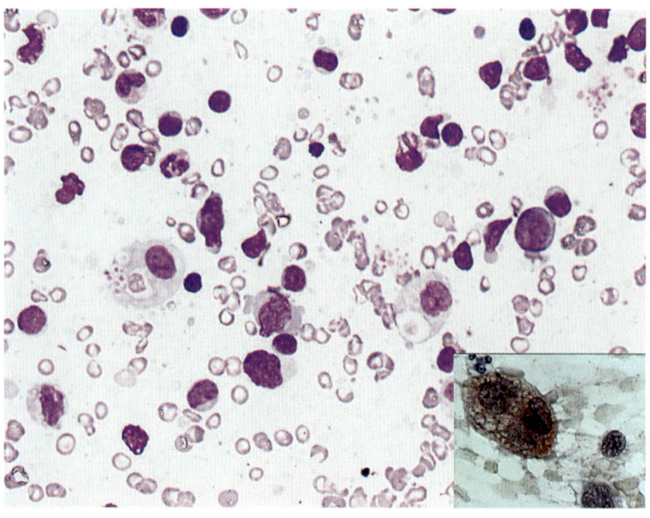

Fig. 7. Haemophagocytosis in LNe; histocytes engulfed with erythrocytes and lymphocytes in the background. **Inset** CD68 ICC positivity.

epithelioid cells, and neutrophils may be consistent with the clinical diagnosis of lupus erythematosus (Fig. 6).

ALPS is a genetic disorder of lymphocyte apoptosis (Fas/CD95), resulting in chronic LNe, splenomegaly, multilineage cytopenia, and an increased risk of NHL. Cytological features are reactive hyperplasia with or without histiocytosis [18]. ALPS is characterized by thymic, immature circulating double-negative T cells (CD3+, CD4–, CD8–) and this feature may be detected by LN-FNC/FC [18].

Haemophagocytic Lymphohistiocytosis

Haemophagocytic lymphohistiocytosis (HLH) is a potentially fatal inflammatory disease, usually occurring in children younger than 4 years. HLH may be associated with the genetic mutation of perforin, munc13-4 disease, or EBV, CMV, or HIV infections [19]. HLH clinically appears with generalized LNe, fever, irritability, maculopapular or petechial rash, hepatosplenomegaly, respiratory distress, and aseptic meningitis. The serology of corresponding patients shows hypertriglyceridemia, hyperferritinaemia, cytopenia, low natural killer cell activity and high soluble CD25 antibody levels. Haemophagocytosis is observed in bone marrow or LNe. A few reports have described FNC features [16, 20, 21] showing histiocytes engulfed with erythrocytes and lymphocytes with evidence of emperipolesis. Histiocytes are usually CD68+, S100+, and CD1a– (Fig. 7).

Kikuchi-Fujimoto disease

Kikuchi-Fujimoto disease (KFD) patients generally complain of fever and localized cervical LNe. Other signs include cutaneous rash, weight loss, night sweats, nausea, and diarrhea. Despite the worrying systemic signs, KFD usually regresses spontaneously. LNe are firm, smooth, tender, and mobile; leucopenia and a high ESR may occur. FNC features include a necrotizing background with nuclear debris, without granulocytes or suppurative features. Macrophages with crescent-shaped nuclei and plasmacytoid dendritic cells have been described (Fig. 8) [16].

Rosai-Dorfman Disease

Rosai-Dorfman disease (RDD) is a massive, cervical, often bilateral LNe of unknown origin. It is caused by an extreme expansion of the medulla with cortical compression or atrophy. Involved LNs generally appear soft and mobile and very large in size. Despite its worrying clinical and US presentation (involved LN are hypoechoic and round, with no hilum and abnormal vascularization), the disease is self-limiting. FNC is characterized by histiocytes engulfed with lymphocytes and erythrocytes by emperipolesis in a lymphoplasmacytic background. Histiocytes are usually CD68+, S100+, and CD1a–. Detailed features and corresponding references have been reported [see Chapter 3, this vol., pp. 19–33].

Langerhans Cell Histiocytosis

Langerhans cell histiocytosis (LCH) includes a group of histiocytic disorders with different clinical presentations and outcomes, caused by a clonal proliferation of Langerhans cells [22]. LCH may arise in the bone, skin, lung, pituitary gland, and LNs. On the basis of the involved organs, LCH may be monosystemic monostotic (involving only 1 bone), polyostotic (involving more than 1 bone), and multisystemic (involving bones and extraosseous sites). Corresponding clinical entities include eosinophilic granuloma, Hand-Schüller-Christian disease, and Letterer-Siwe disease, with different behaviours and prognoses. Despite their clinical differences, all the entities share the same pathological and FNC features characterized by the typical Langerhans cells in a polymorphous inflammatory background, with an eosinophilic predominance. Diagnostic cells show oval and convoluted nuclei with grooves (Fig. 9) and Birbeck granules on electron microscopy. Langerhans cells are CD1a+, CD68+, langerin+, fascin+, and generally S100– (Fig. 9). These features are detectable on FNC of the bones and LNs [23–25] with high diagnostic sensitivity. Differential diagnoses include all the entities caused by the proliferation of histiocytes, such as histiocytoses or RDD, and eosinophilic-rich entities like KFD, HL, and peripheral T-cell lymphoma [23–25].

Hodgkin Lymphoma

HL generally affects adolescents more than children. EBV is involved in a definite percentage of HL, as proven by epidemiological and serum data. In situ hybridization studies have detected EBV genomes in Reed-Sternberg cells. HL develops as an abnormal immunological reaction to "crippled" B cells that escape apoptosis, namely Hodgkin cells and Reed-Sternberg cells in all their variants. As in adults, HL is classified in nodular sclerosis that accounts for 70% of paediatric cases, mixed cellularity, which generally occurs in children younger than 10 years, and lymphocyte predominance, occurring also in younger children [26, 27]. HL FNC features and material management have been previously described [see Chapter 5, this vol., pp. 52–59].

Non-Hodgkin Lymphoma

The single entities of paediatric NHL are the same as in adults, but differ in their incidence rate, the higher occurrence of low-grade NHL types in adults, and the general better prognosis in children [28, 29]. Paediatric NHLs are classified as B-cell NHL represented by Burkitt lymphoma (BL), diffuse large B-cell lymphoma (DLBCL), primary mediastinal, lymphoblastic B-cell NHL (PMLBCL), paediatric FL (PFL), paediatric nodal MZL (PNMZL), grey zone lymphoma intermediate between BL and DLBCL or intermediate between DLBCL and HL, LBL, anaplastic large cell lymphoma (ALCL; ALK+ or ALK–), post-transplant lymphoproliferative diseases (PTLD), and T-cell NHL.

Burkitt Lymphoma

BL accounts for 40% of paediatric NHL. Patients are predominantly male (male:female ratio = 4:1), with a median age of about 9 years. Frequent localizations are abdominal

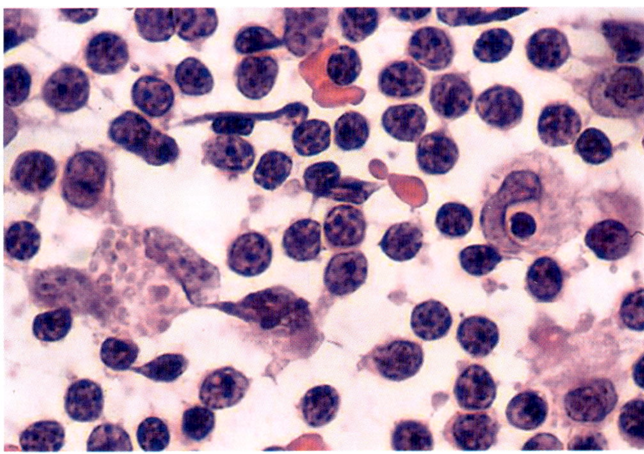

Fig. 8. LNe characterized by macrophages with crescent-shaped nuclei; these cells are typically observed in Kikuchi-Fujimoto disease. Image courtesy of Guido Pettinato, University of Naples Federico II.

and cervical LNs and tonsils. A relevant number of cases are diagnosed in an advanced stage, with bone marrow or central nervous system (CNS) involvement. BL is characterized by the t(8;14)(q24;q32) IGH/MYC, and as a result, MYC is activated by the immunoglobulin gene enhancer. The activation of MYC leads to cell cycle progression, the promotion of cell proliferation, loss of differentiation, genomic instability and alterations of endogenous apoptotic programs. FNC shows medium-sized cells with round nuclei and coarse chromatin and scanty blue cytoplasm. Macrophages with tingible bodies are usually intermingled with the neoplastic population producing the "starry sky pattern" (Fig. 10a) [30–35]. The t(8; 14)(q24;q32) IGH/MYC is detectable by FISH on smears or cell block (Fig. 10b). Material management, and ancillary techniques have been previously described [see Chapters 2, 4, this vol., pp. 14–18, 34–51].

Diffuse Large B-Cell Lymphoma

DLBCL accounts for 20% of all paediatric NHLs. Unlike BL, the median age of DLBCL is higher (11–12 years) and the sex ratio is roughly 2:1 (male:female) [28, 29]. Cervical LN are mainly associated with DLBCL, and CNS and/or bone marrow involvement rarely occurs. Gene expression profiling studies have demonstrated at least 2 different molecular patterns of DLBCL: the activated B-cell-like and the germinal-centre B-cell-like (GCB) subgroups. Each of these subgroups has specific immunophenotypic profiles and GCB is

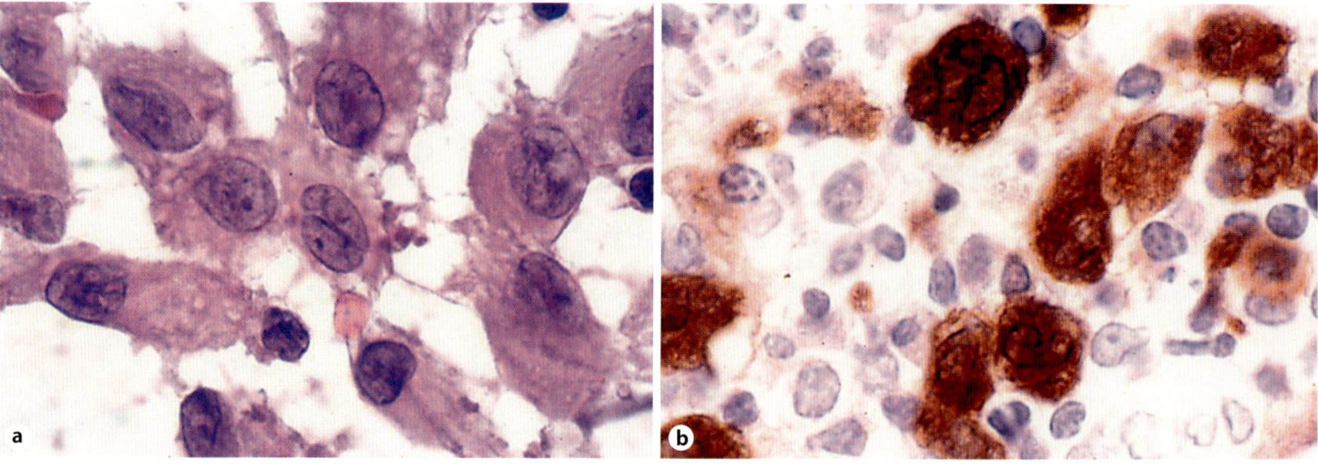

Fig. 9. LN involvement by Langerhans cell histiocytosis. Langerhans cells with oval and convoluted, grooved nuclei (**a**), CD1a+ in a cervical LN of a 9-year-old boy (**b**).

associated with a more favourable outcome in adults [see Chapter 4, this vol., pp. 34–51]. About 75% of paediatric DLBCL are phenotypically GCB type, which might explain their overall better prognosis when compared to adult DLBCL. FNC features, material management, and ancillary techniques have been previously described [see Chapters 2, 4, this vol., pp. 14–18, 34–51].

Primary Mediastinal Lymphoblastic B-Cell Lymphoma

PMLBCL is a rare subtype affecting mainly young adults, predominantly women (female:male ratio = 2:1). PMLBCL clinically shows a large, fast-growing mediastinal mass that infiltrates the chest wall, pleura, lungs, and pericardium, causing pleural and/or pericardial effusion. PMLBCL are rarely found outside the mediastinum; therefore, cytopathologists may deal with PMLBCL mainly on pleural effusions or on transthoracic, CT-guided FNC [36, 37]. Cells are generally medium to large in size, with a fragile cytoplasm. Nuclei are polymorphous with scattered chromatin and evident nucleoli (Fig. 11) [36, 37]. Pleomorphic, binucleated, and multinucleated Reed-Sternberg-like cells, and multilobulated cells like those in DLBCL, may occur. The presence of collagen bands that are thinner than the broad birefringent bands of HL nodular sclerosis are a typical feature of PMLBCL. Fibrosis is not detectable on smears, but hampers FNC and contributes to cell fragility. PMLBCL are positive for pan-B cell antigens (CD19, CD20, CD22); CD15 and CD30 are generally negative, whereas its molecular signature resembles classical HL [36].

Paediatric Follicular Lymphoma

PFL is extremely rare and appears localized in the tonsilla or as cervical LNe. Unlike adult FL, PFL is generally diagnosed at early clinical stages, has a good response to therapy and a better survival than in adults [38–40]. PFL generally lacks *BCL2* abnormalities and has a low proliferative rate; light chain restriction has been reported [38]. No extensive FNC descriptions are currently available.

Paediatric Nodal Marginal Zone Lymphoma

In the WHO classification [22], PNMZL is described as a separate variant of nodal marginal zone lymphoma (NMZL). PNMZL is associated with HIV infections and autoimmune diseases. It has a male predominance and an indolent behaviour. Cervical LNs are the most frequently involved; salivary glands and the orbit are reported as extranodal sites [40]. Histologically, PNMZL shows the disruption of follicles resembling the progressive transformation of follicular centres. At the early stage, PNMZL has no splenic involvement, and has a better prognosis when compared to adult NMZL. No FNC reports are currently available.

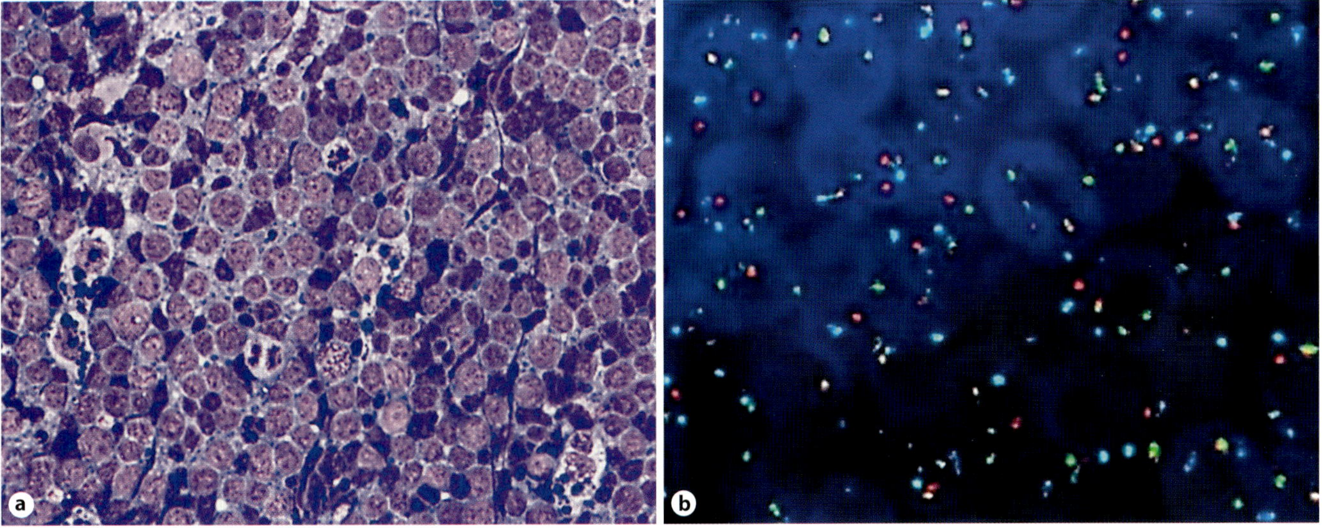

Fig. 10. LN Burkitt lymphoma. **a** A monomorphous of undifferentiated medium-sized cells with numerous mitoses and macrophages scattered in the background. **b** FISH using an IGH-MYC cep8 probe shows MYC in green, IGH in orange, and numerous fusion signals in yellow.

Lymphoblastic Lymphoma

LBL is an aggressive NHL that arises from immature precursor T or B cells. It is the second most common subtype of paediatric NHL [22]. LBL mainly occurs in young adults and adolescents (median age 20 years) with a slight male predominance (male:female ratio = 2:1). LBL arises from T-cell precursors in 85–90% of cases and from immature B cells in the remaining cases [22]. Most LBL show translocations involving the alpha and delta T-cell receptor loci at band 14q11.2, the beta locus at band 7q35, and the gamma locus at band 7p14-15. These translocations cause the juxtaposition of the T-cell receptor promoter and specific enhancers with different transcription factors (HOX11/TLX1, TAL1/SCL, TAL2, *LYL1*), which lead to their high levels of expression in thymic T-cell precursors. LBL is aggressive and has a rapid progression, being diagnosed at stage IV in most of the cases, with bone marrow, spleen, and CNS involvement. In addition to LNe, LBL patients show mediastinal masses in up to 75% of cases. The mediastinal mass is the predominant finding in young adults because of the thymic origin of most LBLs, and it is uncommon in B-cell LBL. Symptoms include fever, night sweats, weight loss and asthenia, anemia and thrombocytopenia, which may cause bleeding and bruising. LBL is closely related to acute lymphoblastic leukaemia (ALL) because peripheral blood involvement is also common, but this event in LBL should be distinguished from ALL. Peripheral LN involvement is present in up to 80% of patients. FNC and pleural effusions show dispersed lymphoblasts, with a high nuclear/cytoplasmic ratio and a scanty basophilic cytoplasm. Nuclei show irregularities in the shape as notches and indentations. The chromatin is condensed or dispersed, depending on the size of the blasts; nucleoli are inconspicuous and mitoses are present [41, 42]. The LBL phenotype: CD3+, TdT+, CD10+, may be assessed by FC or ICC on cell blocks. CD10+ in LBL is not surprising because CD10 is expressed in a subset of immature thymic lymphocytes [41]. Differential diagnosis should consider ALL, BL, HL, germ cell tumours, and thymoma. In the latter, only the demonstration of an epithelial component by ICC may distinguish 2 overlapping phenotypes.

Anaplastic Large Cell Lymphoma

ALCL accounts for approximately 10% of childhood NHL. ALCL are CD30+ and around 90% of cases carry the *ALK* gene chromosomal rearrangement. Similarly to other NHLs, paediatric ALCL prognosis is better than in adults where, more frequently, there is no ALK mutation. Clinically, ALCL may show LNe or extranodal involvement (skin, bone, pleura, gastrointestinal tract, and muscle) and systemic symptoms (such as fever, weight loss, etc.) that may hamper and delay the diagnosis. CNS and bone mar-

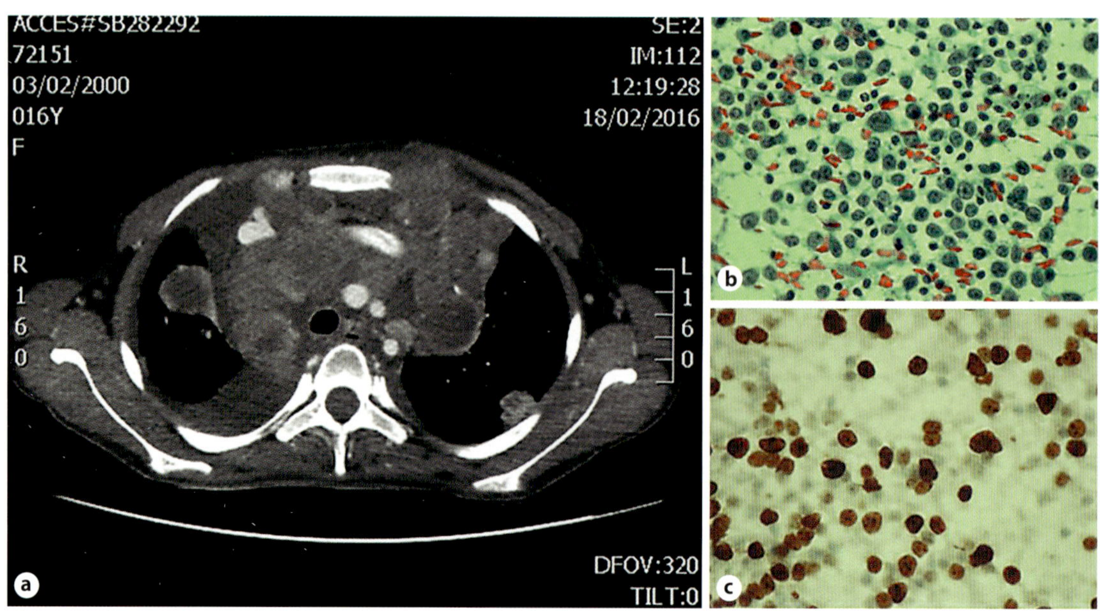

Fig. 11. a Primary mediastinal, lymphoblastic, B-cell lymphoma with diffuse mediastinal involvement. **b** The smear shows undifferentiated medium-sized cells in a haemorrhagic background; FC demonstrated a B-cell phenotype. **c** Ki67 positivity in almost all the cells.

Table 3. Paediatric small round-cell tumours (LCA–) phenotype

	CD56	CD99	MYOD1/ myogenin	CKAE1 AE3	NB84	WT1
Neuroblastoma	+	–/+	–	–	+	–/+
ES/PNET	–	+	–	–/+	+	–
Wilms tumour	+	–	–	–	–	+
RMS	–	–	+	–	–	+(c)
DSRC	+	+/–	–	+/–	–	+(n)

ES/PNET, Ewing sarcoma/primitive neuroectodermal tumours; RMS, rhabdomyosarcoma; DSRC, desmoplastic small round cell tumours.

row involvement is uncommon. FNC show large, pleomorphic, atypical cells with large nuclei and a vacuolated cytoplasm (Fig. 12). Atypical cells are positive for LCA, CD30, CD3, EMA, and ALK (Fig. 12), and negative for CD15 and CD56 (Fig. 10). Molecular analysis of TCRβ and TCRγ genes demonstrated clonal TCR gene rearrangement. A complex karyotype with multiple numerical and structural changes was found on conventional cytogenetics [33, 43–48].

Post-Transplant Lymphoproliferative Diseases

PTLD are a heterogeneous group of self-limiting or aggressive lymphoid processes that represent the complications of solid organ and haematopoietic stem cell transplantation arising in up to 20% of transplant recipients. Infection or reactivation of EBV, in combination with chronic immunosuppression, are the main predisposing factors; in situ hybridization for EBV is positive in up to 70% of cases [49]. The most frequent PTLD subtypes are the self-limiting early lesions: plasmacytic hyperplasia and infectious mononucleosis-like PTLD, the polymorphic PTLD and the monomorphic PTLD mainly represented by post-transplant DLBCL, post-transplant BL (Fig. 13), and post-transplant plasmablastic lymphoma. Despite the similarities with the corresponding non-post-transplantation entities, the reduction or interruption of immunosuppressive therapies determines a reduction or remission of PTLD in many cases. This result is determined by restoring the patient's natural immunity and related repression of proliferating EBV-infected cells [for more details of FNC on PTLD, see Chapter 7, this vol., pp. 77–80].

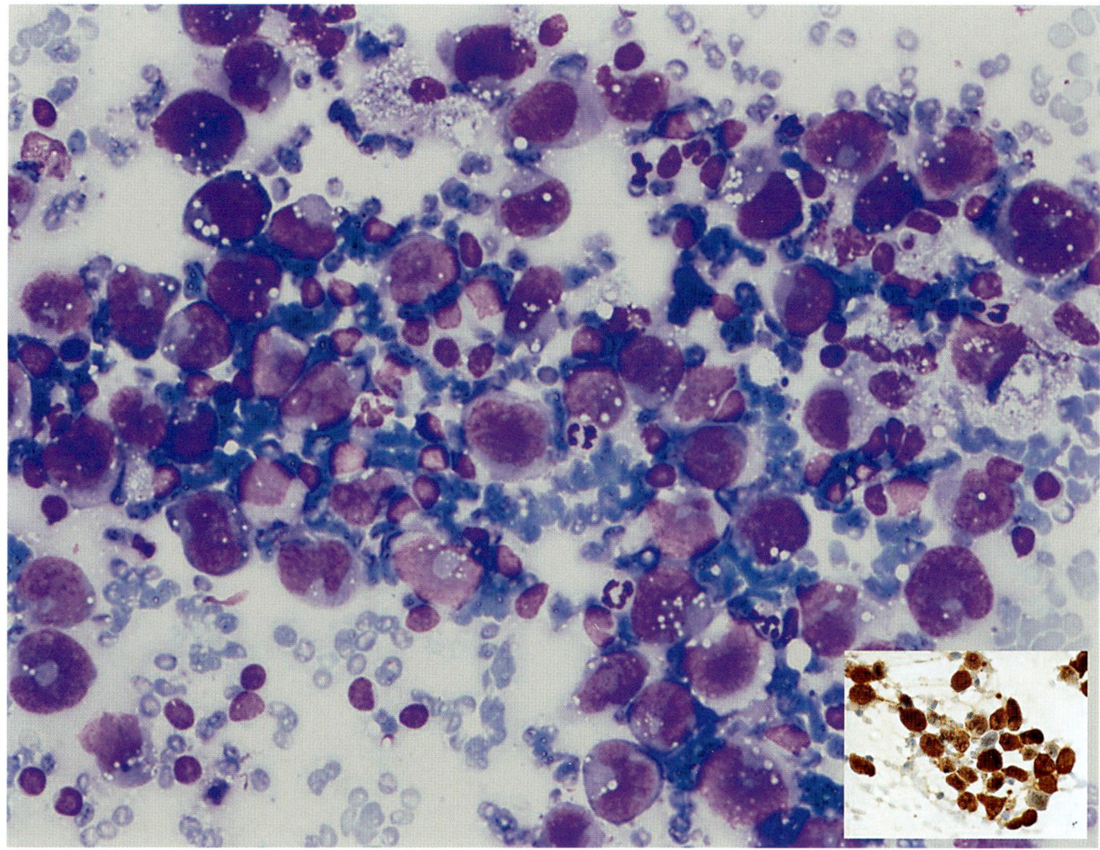

Fig. 12. Anaplastic large cell lymphoma FNC showing large, pleomorphic, atypical cells with irregular nuclei and vacuolated cytoplasm. Note the numerous horseshoe-shaped nuclei. **Inset** Diffuse ALK ICC positivity.

Peripheral T-Cell Lymphoma

Peripheral T-cell lymphoma (PTCL) is rare in paediatric patients (1% of paediatric NHL with the exclusion of cutaneous PTCL). It includes T-cell post-transplant, hepatosplenic T-cell, and not otherwise specified PTCL. Morphological and molecular features of paediatric PTCL differ from adult PTCL, as well as the response to therapy and prognosis [50].

LN Metastatic Paediatric Small Round-Cell Tumours

Paediatric small round-cell tumours (PSRCT) include neuroblastoma, rhabdomyosarcoma (RMS), and Ewing sarcoma/primitive neuroectodermal tumours (ES/PNET) other than NHL. Other malignancies may be considered in the differential diagnosis, such as small-cell osteogenic sarcoma, synovial sarcoma, undifferentiated (anaplastic) hepatoblastoma, granulocytic sarcoma, blastemal-type Wilms tumour, and desmoplastic, small, round-cell tumour of the peritoneum. PSRCT are generally soft-tissue or organ-specific tumours; nonetheless, they may metastasize to LNs or may occur in the head and neck region, simulating LNs [51–56]. It is difficult for cytopathologists to obtain enough experience on this type of neoplasia because of their rarity and because only a few institutions perform FNC in paediatric tumours [51–56]. PSRCT are morphologically similar and many of them do not express specific antigens that might be assessed with ICC, or the same antigens may get lost in poorly differentiated tumours. In addition, cross-reactivity exists among some PSRCT antigens (Table 3). ROSE is a fundamental step in PSRCT FNC; it should prompt the need for additional material to be used with ancillary techniques. FNC of PSRCT, although challenging to perform, can be useful for a primary diagnostic orientation and to document recurrent and/or metastatic diseases.

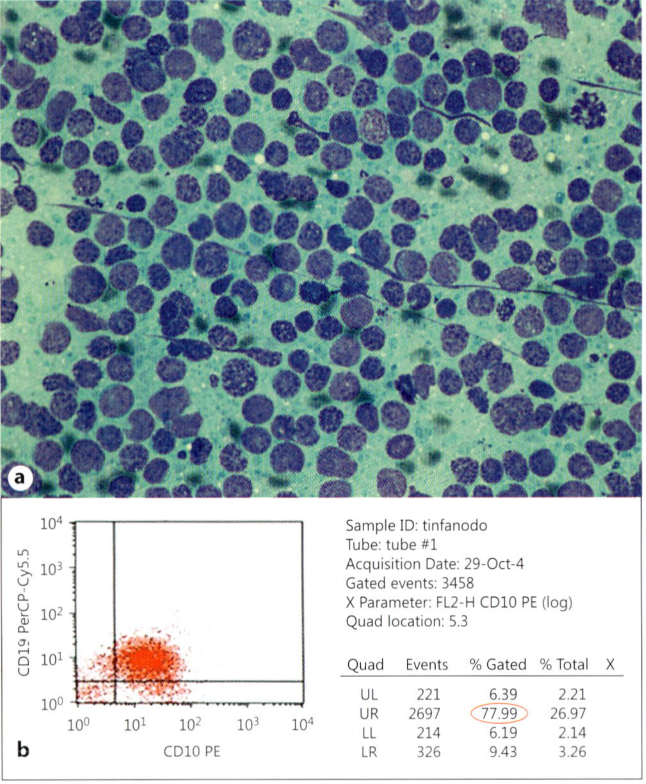

Fig. 13. Burkitt-like post-transplant lymphoproliferative diseases. **a** Undifferentiated medium-sized lymphoid cells with immature, granular chromatin without nucleoli. Note the mitoses and nuclear strips expression of fragility. **b** Flow cytometry shows CD10/CD19 co-expression in almost 80% of the cells.

Neuroblastoma

Well-differentiated neuroblastoma FNC shows dissociated small round cells (Fig. 14a). Moderately or well-formed Homer-Wright rosettes with neuropils in their centres, which stain pink or blue-grey with Giemsa stain, may be observed. Pools of neuropils, outside the rosettes, have been described [51–54]. Poorly differentiated neuroblastoma do not contain rosettes or only have rudimentary ones, similar to those observed in ES/PNET or other PSRCTs [51–54]. A poorly differentiated neuroblastoma may be misinterpreted as an ES/PNET, being morphologically similar and sharing immunoreactivity for NB84 and CD99 [53]. Moreover, an undifferentiated neuroblastoma is composed exclusively of dissociated primitive cells and it is morphologically indistinguishable from undifferentiated blastema cells of a nephroblastoma. As for ICC, NB84 is expressed by neuro-

blastoma but it does not react with nephroblastoma (Fig. 14b). CD56 is not useful since it is positive in both neuroblastoma and nephroblastoma, while WT1 is of limited value, being positive in some cases of neuroblastoma but also in 70% of nephroblastomas (Table 3).

Rhabdomyosarcoma

RMS is the most common soft tissue tumour in children. The RMS subtypes are the embryonal (60% of all cases), which has a better prognosis, and the alveolar RMS (30% of all cases) [53]. Anaplastic foci may occur in both subtypes. FNC cytology of embryonal RMS may harvest highly cellular tissue fragments with moderate or abundant stroma, while the number of dissociated cells varies from a few to many [51–56]. Immature small tumour cells with uniform, slightly oval or round nuclei predominate, while mature rhabdomyoblasts with single or multiple nuclei are rare. Smears from alveolar RMS are usually very cellular with predominantly dissociated cells but small groups without stroma may also be observed [51–54]. The number of mature rhabdomyoblasts is variable from a few to many [53]. Several myogenic markers are positive in RMS with different percentages; recent studies showed that MyoD1 and myogenin appear to be highly specific for RMS (Table 3).

Ewing Sarcoma/Primitive Neuroectodermal Tumours

ES/PNET are composed almost entirely of monomorphous small round cells with a high nuclear/cytoplasmic ratio and hyperchromatic nuclei without evident nucleoli (Fig. 15). Homer Wright rosettes may also be observed; neuropils and ganglion cells are not usually present. In a small percentage of cases, ES/PNET are composed of a mixture of round and oval cells, which vary from small to medium in size. In such a setting, smears can be similar to other PSRCTs, especially to poorly differentiated synovial sarcoma, neuroblastoma, alveolar RMS, desmoplastic small round-cell (DSRC) tumour, and NHL. The differential diagnosis between ES/PNET and neuroblastoma is difficult on the basis of FNC alone, although some microscopic differences exist. Clinical features (e.g., age, primary site, metastatic patterns), catecholamine levels, and cytogenetics are required for an accurate diagnosis [53, 54]. CD99 (Fig. 15), which was considered specific for ES/PNET, may be detected also in other PSRCT. An additional difficulty in ES/PNET diagnosis is its

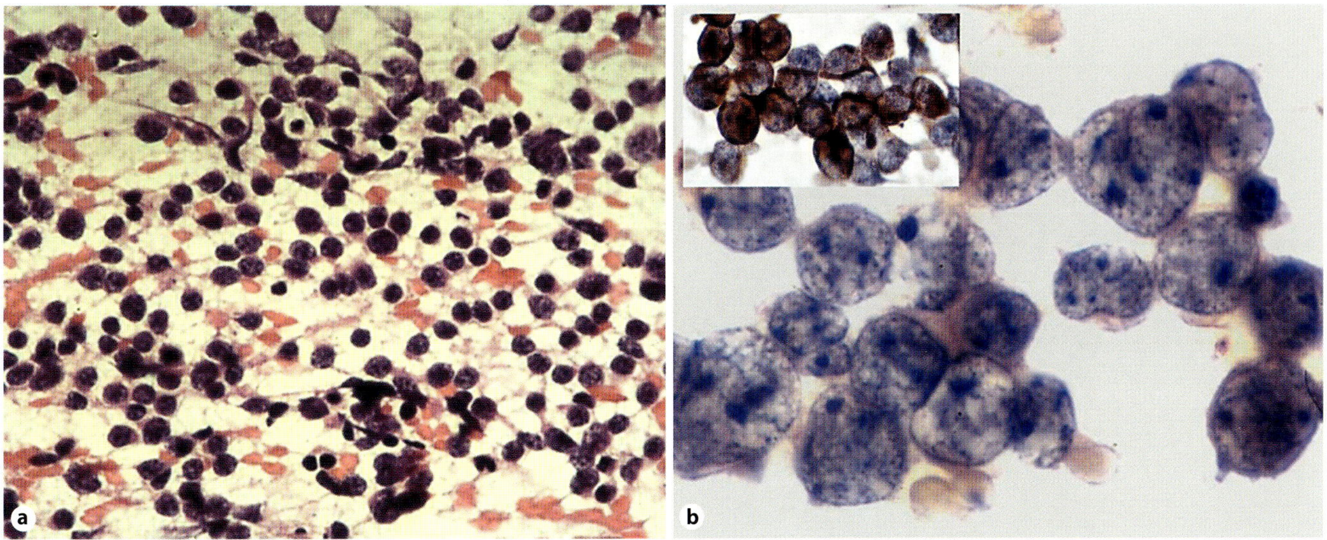

Fig. 14. a LN-FNC of metastatic neuroblastoma almost indistinguishable from other undifferentiated small cell neoplasms showing dispersed undifferentiated cells. **b** Naked nuclei with granular "salt and pepper" chromatin and small nucleoli. **Inset** ICC positivity for NB84. Image courtesy of Guido Pettinato, University of Naples Federico II.

occasional positivity for CK and desmin. CK positivity in ES/PNET increases the diagnostic difficulties when synovial sarcoma and DSRC tumour come into the differential diagnosis. FISH, CISH, and PCR can successfully be performed on FNC in order to demonstrate specific translocations, gene amplifications, and other molecular changes. The most useful translocations in the diagnosis of specific PSRCT are t(11;22)(q24;q12) for ES/PNET (Fig. 15), t(x;18)(p11;q11) for synovial sarcoma, t(11;22)(q13;q12) for DSRC tumour, and t(2;13)(q35;q14) for alveolar RMS.

Serous Effusions

Several malignant neoplasms in children may infiltrate serous cavities and cause effusions [57, 58]. Lymphoma and leukaemia account for more than 50% of paediatric serous effusions [57]. As in adults, serous effusion may be the first presentation of lymphoma or may develop during the course of the disease. Young patients with pleural effusions generally suffer from respiratory distress and require immediate medical treatment, hence a timely cytological diagnosis is crucial. Cytological and immunophenotypical examination of serous effusions by FC or/and ICC may allow a quick diagnosis and classification of NHL. However, cytological diagnosis may be difficult in early stages when effusions may be scanty cellular in the presence of degenerative changes,

and when NHL cells are intermingled with reactive lymphoid and inflammatory cells. The incidence of T- and B-cell NHL in ascites and pleural effusions in children is different. T-NHL are more frequent in pleural effusions, while B-NHL occur more frequently in ascites [59]. Pleural effusions in NHL are frequently caused by lymphatic obstruction, but may also be determined by direct pleural involvement or by a thymic tumour, namely a thymic NHL [60]. Impaired lymphatic drainage seems to be the primary pathogenic mechanism of ascites in B-NHL. ALCL and HL are not uncommon in children, but they are less likely to cause effusions. As for non-lymphomatous neoplasm, neuroblastoma represents the main differential diagnosis to consider in paediatric serous effusions because of the cytological similarities with NHL and because it ranks second to NHL in causing paediatric malignant effusions [61]. Other frequent small round-cell tumours in children, such as Wilms' tumour, gonadal and extragonadal germ cell tumours, bone and soft tissue sarcomas, epithelial neoplasms, and Ewing sarcoma, may also cause the effusions [62].

Cerebrospinal Fluid

Cerebrospinal fluid (CSF) analysis in paediatric patients is generally used to diagnose neurological disorders, including meningitis and brain or spinal cord damage. CSF analysis is

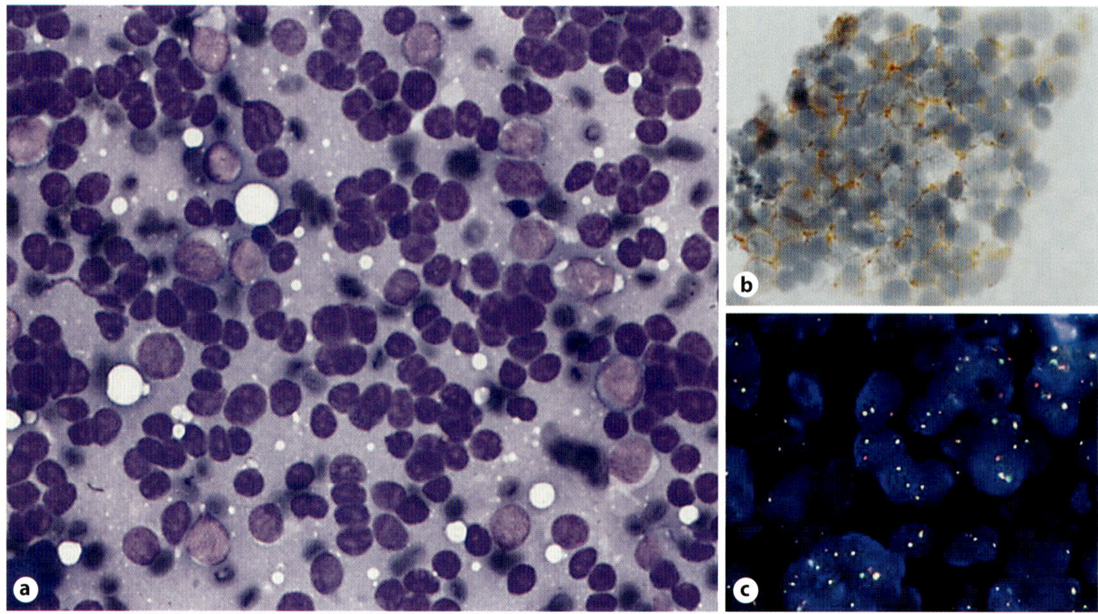

Fig. 15. a Cytological features of LN metastasis from Ewing sarcoma showing small, oval, undifferentiated, mainly dispersed cells. Nuclei had dense coarse chromatin without visible nucleoli. Some cells are larger with a thin cytoplasm. **b** CD99 ICC cytoplasmic positivity on cytospin. **c** FISH using a Dual Color, Break Apart Rearrangement probe for 22q12 showing the green and red probe breaking apart in numerous nuclei confirming the Ewing sarcoma.

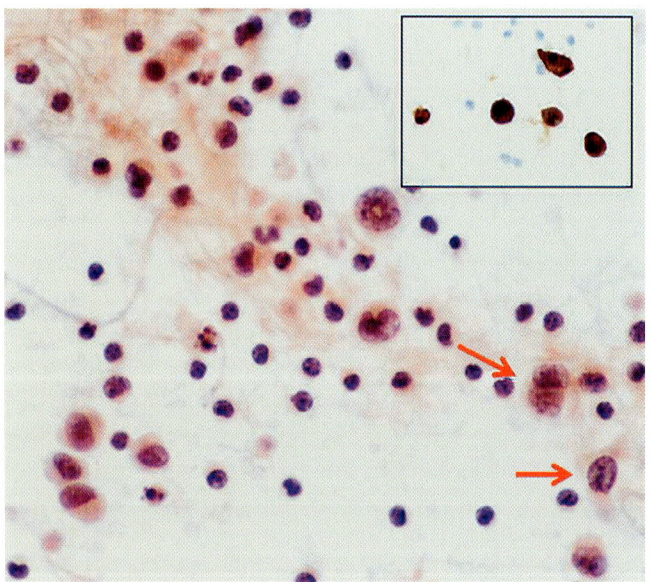

Fig. 16. Leptomeningeal involvement from LCH showing a polymorphous infiltrate with large histiocytic cells with kidney-shaped nuclei and grooves (arrows). **Inset** CD1a ICC positivity.

also performed in cases of leukaemia and NHL, medulloblastoma and other spinal cord tumours. Leukaemia and NHL represent the most frequent paediatric malignancies and both may invade the CNS. Therefore, CSF obtained before prophylactic intrathecal chemotherapy and or for NHL staging is routinely observed. B- and T-cell lymphoblastic NHL, BL, and DLBCL are the most frequent histotypes, whereas other less frequent or rare entities, such as HLH and LCH (Fig. 16), may also occur. The cytological features of these entities have been described [63–65].

References

1 Friedmann AM: Evaluation and management of lymphadenopathy in children. Pediatr Rev 2008; 29:53–60.
2 Herzog LW: Prevalence of lymphadenopathy of the head and neck in infants and children. Clin Pediatr 1983;22:485–487.
3 Monaco SE, Khalbuss WE, Pantanowitz L: Benign non-infectious causes of lymphadenopathy: a review of cytomorphology and differential diagnosis. Diagn Cytopathol 2012;40:925–938.
4 Huyett P, Monaco SE, Choi SS, Simons JP: Utility of fine-needle aspiration biopsy in the evaluation of pediatric head and neck masses. Otolaryngol Head Neck Surg 2016;154:928–935.

5 Soldes OS, Younger JG, Hirschl RB: Predictors of malignancy in childhood peripheral lymphadenopathy. J Pediatr Surg 1999;34:1447–1452.

6 Celenk F, et al: Incidence and predictors of malignancy in children with persistent cervical lymphadenopathy. Int J Pediatr Otorhinolaryngol 2013; 77:2004–2007.

7 Restrepo R, Oneto J, Lopez K, Kukreja K: Head and neck lymph nodes in children: the spectrum from normal to abnormal. Pediatr Radiol 2009;39: 836–846.

8 Ang GA, Gerardo LT: Cervical rib mimicking supraclavicular fossa neoplasia: a case report. Acta Cytol 1994;38:271–274.

9 van de Schoot L, Aronson DC, Behrendt H, Bras J: The role of fine-needle aspiration cytology in children with persistent or suspicious lymphadenopathy. J Pediatr Surg 2001;36:7–11.

10 Zardawi IM, Jain S, Bennett G: Flow-cytometric algorithm on fine-needle aspirates for the clinical workup of patients with lymphadenopathy. Diagn Cytopathol 1998;19:274–278.

11 Cozzolino I, Nappa S, Picardi M, DeRenzo A, Troncone G, Palombini L, Zeppa P: Clonal B-cell population in a reactive lymph node in acquired immunodeficiency syndrome. Diagn Cytopathol 2009;37:910–914.

12 Liu K, Stern RC, Rogers RT, Dodd LG, Mann KP: Diagnosis of hematopoietic processes by fine-needle aspiration in conjunction with flow cytometry: a review of 127 cases. Diagn Cytopathol 2001;24: 1–10.

13 Zardawi IM, Barker BJ, Simons DP: Hodgkin's disease masquerading as granulomatous lymphadenitis on fine needle aspiration cytology. Acta Cytol 2005;49:224–226.

14 Koo V, Lioe TF, Spence RA: Fine needle aspiration cytology (FNAC) in the diagnosis of granulomatous lymphadenitis. Ulster Med J 2006;75:59–64.

15 Silowash R, Pantanowitz L, Craig FE, Simons JP, Monaco SE: Utilization of flow cytometry in pediatric fine-needle aspiration biopsy specimens. Acta Cytol 2016;60:344–353.

16 Monaco SE, Khalbuss WE, Pantanowitz L: Benign non-infectious causes of lymphadenopathy: a review of cytomorphology and differential diagnosis. Diagn Cytopathol 2012;40:925–938.

17 Stastny JF, Wakely PE Jr, Frable WJ: Cytologic features of necrotizing granulomatous inflammation consistent with cat-scratch disease. Diagn Cytopathol 1996;15:108–115.

18 Shah S, Wu E, Rao VK, Tarrant TK: Autoimmune lymphoproliferative syndrome: an update and review of the literature. Curr Allergy Asthma Rep 2014;14:462.

19 Rosado FG, Kim AS: Hemophagocytic lymphohistiocytosis: an update on diagnosis and pathogenesis. Am J Clin Pathol 2013;139:713–727.

20 Rekha TS, Kiran HS, Nandini NM, Murthy S: Cytology of secondary hemophagocytic lymphohistiocytosis masquerading as lymphoma in a non-immunocompromised adult. J Cytol 2014;31: 239–241.

21 Zeppa P, Vetrani A, Ciancia G, Cuccuru A, Palombini L: Hemophagocytic histiocytosis diagnosed by fine needle aspiration cytology of the spleen: a case report. Acta Cytol 2004;48:415–419.

22 Swerdlow SH, Campo E, Harris NL, Jaffe ES, Pileri SA, Stein H, Thiele J: WHO Classification of Tumours of Haematopoietic and Lymphoid Tissues, ed 4. Lyon, IARC Press, 2017.

23 Patne SC, Dwivedi S, Katiyar R, Gupta V, Gupta AK: Langerhans cell histiocytosis diagnosed by FNAC of lymph nodes. J Cancer Res Ther 2015;11: 1028.

24 Handa U, Kundu R, Punia RS, Mohan H: Langerhans cell histiocytosis in children diagnosed by fine-needle aspiration. J Cytol 2015;32:244–247.

25 Fassina A, Olivotto A, Cappellesso R, Vendraminelli R, Fassan M: Fine-needle cytology of cutaneous juvenile xanthogranuloma and langerhans cell histiocytosis. Cancer Cytopathol 2011;119:134–140.

26 Chen Y, Savargaonkar P, Fuchs A, Wasserman P: Role of flow cytometry in the diagnosis of lymphadenopathy in children. Diagn Cytopathol 2002; 26:5–9.

27 Monaco SE, Teot LA: Cytopathology of pediatric malignancies: where are we today with fine-needle aspiration biopsies in pediatriconcology? Cancer Cytopathol 2014;122:322–336.

28 Allen CE, Kelly KM, Bollard CM: Pediatric lymphomas and histiocytic disorders of childhood. Pediatr Clin North Am 2015;62:139–165.

29 Cairo MS, Pinkerton R: Childhood, adolescent and young adult non-Hodgkin lymphoma: state of the science. Br J Haematol 2016;173:507–530.

30 Das DK, Gupta SK, Pathak IC, Sharma SC, Datta BN: Burkitt-type lymphoma: diagnosis by fine needle aspiration cytology. Acta Cytol 1987;31: 1–7.

31 Meda BA, Buss DH, Woodruff RD, Cappellari JO, Rainer RO, Powell BL, Geisinger KR: Diagnosis and subclassification of primary and recurrent lymphoma: the usefulness and limitations of combined fine-needle aspiration cytomorphology and flow cytometry. Am J Clin Pathol 2000;113:688–699.

32 Troxell ML, Bangs CD, Cherry AM, Natkunam Y, Kong CS: Cytologic diagnosis of Burkitt lymphoma. Cancer 2005;105:310–318.

33 Ali AE, Morgen EK, Geddie WR, Boerner SL, Massey C, Bailey DJ, da Cunha Santos G: Classifying B-cell non-Hodgkin lymphoma by using MIB-1 proliferative index in fine-needle aspirates. Cancer Cytopathol 2010;118:166–172.

34 Mann G, Attarbaschi A, Steiner M, Simonitsch I, Strobl H, Urban C, Meister B, Haas O, Dworzak M, Gadner H; Austrian Berlin-Frankfurt-Münster (BFM) Group: Early and reliable diagnosis of non-Hodgkin lymphoma in childhood and adolescence: contribution of cytomorphology and flow cytometric immunophenotyping. Pediatr Hematol Oncol 2006;23:167–176.

35 da Cunha Santos G, Ko HM, Geddie WR, Boerner SL, Lai SW, Have C, Kamel-Reid S, Bailey D: Targeted use of fluorescence in situ hybridization (FISH) in cytospin preparations: results of 298 fine needle aspirates of B-cell non-Hodgkin lymphoma. Cancer Cytopathol 2010;118:250–258.

36 Minard-Colin V, Brugières L, Reiter A, Cairo MS, Gross TG, Woessmann W, Burkhardt B, Sandlund JT, Williams D, Pillon M, Horibe K, Auperin A, Le Deley MC, Zimmerman M, Perkins SL, Raphael M, Lamant L, Klapper W, Mussolin L, Poirel HA, Macintyre E, Damm-Welk C, Rosolen A, Patte C: Non-Hodgkin lymphoma in children and adolescents: progress through effective collaboration, current knowledge, and challenges ahead. J Clin Oncol 2015;33:2963–2974.

37 Wakely PE Jr, Kornstein MJ: Aspiration cytopathology of lymphoblastic lymphoma and leukemia: the MCV experience. Pediatr Pathol Lab Med 1996;16:243–252.

38 Agrawal R, Wang J: Pediatric follicular lymphoma: a rare clinicopathologic entity. Arch Pathol Lab Med 2009;133:142–146.

39 Schmidt J, Gong S, Marafioti T, Mankel B, Gonzalez-Farre B, Balagué O, Mozos A, Cabeçadas J, van der Walt J, Hoehn D, Rosenwald A, Ott G, Dojcinov S, Egan C, Nadeu F, Ramis-Zaldívar JE, Clot G, Bárcena C, Pérez-Alonso V, Endris V, Penzel R, Lome-Maldonado C, Bonzheim I, Fend F, Campo E, Jaffe ES, Salaverria I, Quintanilla-Martinez L: Genome-wide analysis of pediatric-type follicular lymphoma reveals low genetic complexity and recurrent alterations of TNFRSF14 gene. Blood 2016;128:1101–1111.

40 Quintanilla-Martinez L, Sander B, Chan JK, Xerri L, Ott G, Campo E, Swerdlow SH: Indolent lymphomas in the pediatric population: follicular lymphoma, IRF4/MUM1+ lymphoma, nodal marginal zone lymphoma and chronic lymphocytic leukemia. Virchows Arch 2016;468:141–157.

41 Bhaker P, Das A, Rajwanshi A, Gautam U, Trehan A, Bansal D, Varma N, Srinivasan R: Precursor T-lymphoblastic lymphoma: speedy diagnosis in FNA and effusion cytology by morphology, immunochemistry, and flow cytometry. Cancer Cytopathol 2015;123:557–565.

42 Patel RA, Sheehan AM, Finch CJ, Lopez-Terrada D, Hernandez VS, Curry CV: Fine-needle aspiration cytology of T-lymphoblastic lymphoma associated FGFR1 rearrangement myeloproliferative neoplasm. Diagn Cytopathol 2014;42:45–48.

43 Das P, Iyer VK, Mathur SR, Ray R: Anaplastic large cell lymphoma: a critical evaluation of cytomorphological features in seven cases. Cytopathology 2010;21:251–258.

44 Rekhi B, Sridhar E, Viswanathan S, Shet TM, Jambhekar NA: ALK+ anaplastic large cell lymphoma with cohesive, perivascular arrangements on cytology, mimicking a soft tissue sarcoma: a report of 2 cases. Acta Cytol 2010;54:75–78.

45 Muzzafar T, Wei EX, Lin P, Medeiros LJ, Jorgensen JL: Flow cytometric immunophenotyping of anaplastic large cell lymphoma. Arch Pathol Lab Med 2009;133:49–56.

46 Rapkiewicz A, Wen H, Sen F, Das K: Cytomorphologic examination of anaplastic large cell lymphoma by fine-needle aspiration cytology. Cancer 2007;111:499–507.

47 Ng WK, Ip P, Choy C, Collins RJ: Cytologic and immunocytochemical findings of anaplastic large cell lymphoma: analysis of ten fine-needle aspiration specimens over a 9-year period. Cancer 2003; 99:33–43.

48 Bogdanic M, Ostojic Kolonic S, Kaic G, Kardum Paro MM, Lasan Trcic R, Kardum-Kelin I: Fine-needle aspiration cytology yield as a basis for morphological, molecular, and cytogenetic diagnosis in alk-positive anaplastic large cell lymphoma with atypical clinical presentation. Diagn Cytopathol 2017;45:51–54.

49 Nose K, Oki T, Banno E, Sugimoto K, Nishioka T, Ochiai K, Maekura S: The efficacy of EBER in situ hybridization (ISH) stain in PTLD (malignant diffuse large B-cell lymphoma) about 4 years after ABO-incompatible kidney transplantation: a case report. Int J Clin Exp Pathol 2012;5:359–362.

50 Al Mahmoud R, Weitzman S, Schechter T, Ngan B, Abdelhaleem M, Alexander S: Peripheral T-cell lymphoma in children and adolescents: a single-institution experience. J Pediatr Hematol Oncol 2012;34:611–616.

51 Silverman JF, Joshi VV: FNA biopsy of small round cell tumors of childhood: cytomorphologic features and the role of ancillary studies. Diagn Cytopathol 1994;10:245–255.

52 Cole CD, Wu HH: Fine-needle aspiration in pediatric patients 12 years of age and younger: a 20-year retrospective study from a single tertiary medical center. Diagn Cytopathol 2014;42:600–605.

53 Pohar-Marinsek Z: Difficulties in diagnosing small round cell tumours of childhood from fine needle aspiration cytology samples. Cytopathology 2008;19:67–79.

54 Silverman JF, Berns LA, Holbrook CT, Neill JS, Joshi VV: Fine needle aspiration cytology of primitive neuroectodermal tumors: a report of these cases. Acta Cytol 1992;36:541–550.

55 Klijanienko J, Caillaud JM, Orbach D, Brisse H, Lagacé R, Vielh P, Couturier J, Fréneaux P, Theocharis S, Sastre-Garau X: Cyto-histological correlations in primary, recurrent and metastatic rhabdomyosarcoma: the institut Curie's experience. Diagn Cytopathol 2007;35:482–487.

56 Klijanienko J, Couturier J, Bourdeaut F, Fréneaux P, Ballet S, Brisse H, Lagacé R, Delattre O, Pierron G, Vielh P, Sastre-Garau X, Michon J: Fine-needle aspiration as a diagnostic technique in 50 cases of primary Ewing sarcoma/peripheral neuroectodermal tumor. Institut Curie's experience. Diagn Cytopathol 2012;40:19–25.

57 Wong JW, Pitlik D, Abdul Karim FW: Cytology of pleural, peritoneal and pericardial fluids in children: a 40-year summary. Acta Cytol 1997;41:467–473.

58 Hallman JR, Geisinger KR: Cytology of fluids from pleural, peritoneal and pericardial cavities in children: a comprehensive survey. Acta Cytol 1994;38:209–217.

59 Shen H, Tang Y, Xu X, Wang L, Wang Q, Xu W, Song H, Zhao Z, Wang J: Rapid detection of neoplastic cells in serous cavity effusions in children with flow cytometry immunophenotyping. Leuk Lymphoma 2012;53:1509–1514.

60 Das DK: Serous effusions in malignant lymphomas: a review. Diagn Cytopathol 2006;34:335–347.

61 Gupta H, Conrad J, Khoury JD, et al: Significance of pleural effusion in neuroblastoma. Pediatr Blood Cancer 2007;49:906–908.

62 Gautam U, Srinivasan R, Rajwanshi A, et al: Comparative evaluation of flow-cytometric immunophenotyping and immunocytochemistry in the categorization of malignant small round cell tumors in fine-needle aspiration cytologic specimens. Cancer Cytopathol 2008;114:494–503.

63 Damiani D, Suciu V, Andreiuolo F, Calderaro J, Vielh P: Young investigator challenge: cytomorphologic analysis of cerebrospinal fluid in 70 pediatric patients with medulloblastoma and review of the literature focusing on novel diagnostic and prognostic tests. Cancer Cytopathol 2015;123:644–649.

64 Gassas A, Krueger J, Alvi S, Sung L, Hitzler J, Lieberman L: Diagnosis of central nervous system relapse of pediatric acute lymphoblastic leukemia: Impact of routine cytological CSF analysis at the time of intrathecal chemotherapy. Pediatr Blood Cancer 2014;61:2215–2217.

65 Wehle K, Göbel U, Pfitzer P: The cytodiagnosis of meningeal involvement in familial haemophagocytic lymphohistiocytosis. Cytopathology 1995;6:30–38.

Zeppa P, Cozzolino I: Lymph Node FNC. Cytopathology of Lymph Nodes and Extranodal Lymphoproliferative Processes.
Monogr Clin Cytol. Basel, Karger, 2018, vol 23, pp 77–80 (DOI: 10.1159/000478883)

Immunodeficiency-Associated Lymphoproliferative Disorders

Immunodeficiencies may be congenital or acquired. There are over 80 recognized congenital immunodeficiency syndromes that are generally classified by an absent or defective component of the immune system, namely humoral, cellular, or combined immunity, the phagocytic cells, and the complement proteins. Most primary immunodeficiencies are hereditary, autosomal recessive, or X-linked, such as the common variable immunodeficiency (humoral immunodeficiency), the DiGeorge syndrome, the ZAP-70 deficiency, the X-linked lymphoproliferative syndrome (T-cell immunodeficiency), the Ataxia-telangiectasia, the Wiskott-Aldrich syndrome (combined humoral and cellular immunodeficiency), the Chédiak-Higashi syndrome (phagocytic cell defects), and the C1 or C2 deficiencies (complement deficiencies). Acquired immunodeficiencies may be caused by different agents and conditions, such as prolonged serious illness, diabetes, cytotoxic chemotherapy, HIV infection, bone marrow ablation before transplantation, radiation therapy, and malnutrition. Most acquired immunodeficiencies are only of clinical interest and histopathologists or cytopathologists are rarely involved in their diagnosis and clinical management. This is the case when immunodeficiencies cause lymph node enlargements (LNe) and carry a high risk of lymphoproliferative processes or other neoplasms. In this perspective, HIV-related and post-transplant lymphoproliferative diseases (PTLD) are those of main interest to cytopathologists.

HIV-Related Lymphoma

Combined antiretroviral therapies in HIV patients have improved the immune function and reduced the risk of developing AIDS, Kaposi sarcoma and lymphoma. Nonetheless, HIV patients have a higher risk of developing lymphoma compared to the HIV-negative population [1, 2], and lymphomas are still the most common malignancies in HIV patients [3]. Meanwhile, LNe frequently occur in HIV patients, with reactive processes being the most frequent cause. LN-FNC of lymphadenitis and lymphadenopathies was previously described [see Chapter 3, this vol., pp. 19–33]. With reference to lymphomas, approximately 95% of HIV-associated lymphomas are the same non-Hodgkin lymphoma (NHL) and Hodgkin lymphoma (HL) occuring in non-HIV patients whereas with different incidences of the single entities. There is a significantly higher occurrence of primary central nervous system NHL, primary effusion lymphoma, and plasmablastic lymphoma of the oral cavity type in HIV patients. Burkitt lymphoma (BL) and diffuse large B-cell lym-

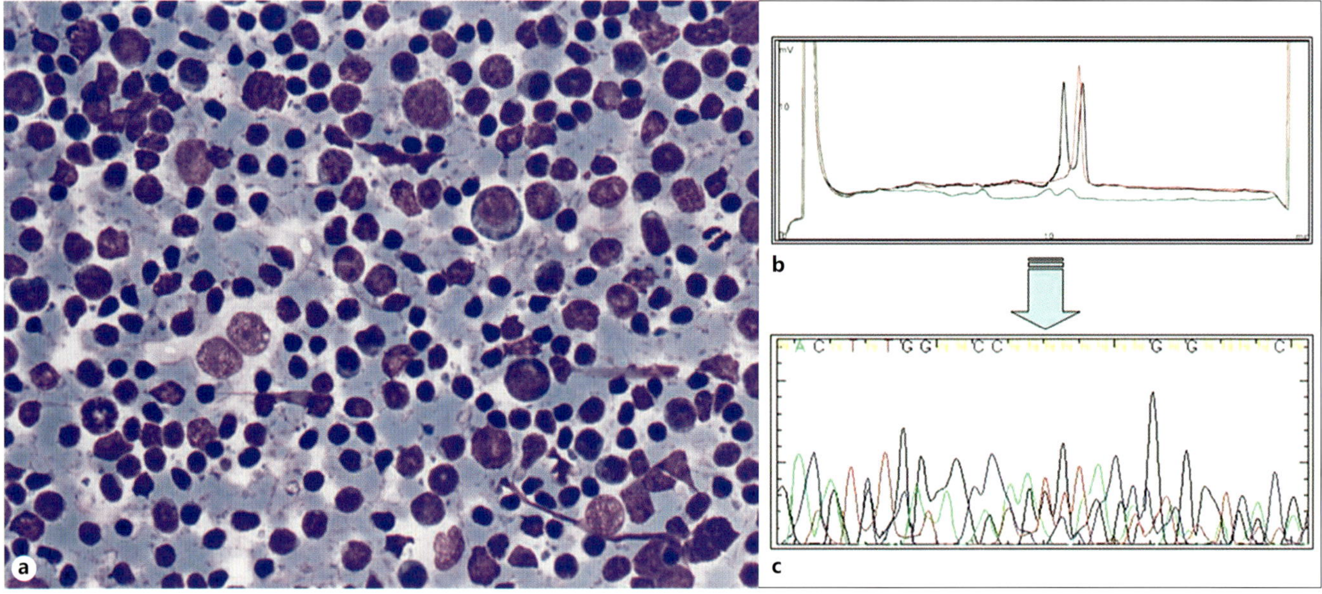

Fig. 1. a LN-FNC of a post-transplant lymphoproliferative disease (PTLD): the smear is polymorphous showing small lymphocytes, plasma cells, centroblasts, and immunoblasts. **b** DHPLC chromatograms of the IGHK amplification products of the case, showing multiple peaks for IGH (green) and not reproducible peaks for IGK (black and red) assessing a psudoclonality status. **c** Sanger electropherogram of the IGK amplification product from the same case showing multiple sequences that did not correspond to any VH-DH-JH rearrangement, as indicated by Blast analysis in the IMGT® databases. Histological control revealed an early lesion "mononucleosis-like" PTLD.

phoma (DLBCL) are the most frequent HIV-related NHL [1, 2]. BL accounts for up to 30–40% of all HIV-associated NHLs, showing the same morphological and cytogenetical features as the non-HIV-related BL [see Chapter 4, this vol., pp. 34–51]. DLBCL frequently has a non-germinal centre B-cell (non-GCB) phenotype (CD10–, BCL6–, MUM1+, CD138+), lacking *BCL6* rearrangement in most cases [4]. Also, HL has a higher incidence when compared to the non-HIV population, with a prevalence of unfavourable subtypes [5].

Post-Transplant Lymphoproliferative Diseases

PTLD are a heterogeneous group of reactive and malignant lymphoproliferative processes that share some common aspects, including emergence in post-transplanted immuno-depressed patients, a strong relationship with Epstein-Barr virus (EBV), and possible regression through the reduction of immunosuppressive therapy [6, 7]. After primary infections, EBV is incorporated and replicates into the host DNA of transformed, circulating B cells and remains in a latent state; its expansion is controlled by EBV-specific cytotoxic T cells. Their inhibition due to anti-EBV T-cell immunity and anti-EBV-specific CD8+ action, as occurs in post-transplant immunosuppression, promotes the proliferation of EBV-infected cells, increases the expression of BCRF1 and BARF1 proteins that help cells to escape the immune control, and enhances LMP1 and LMP2 proteins that promote their growth and escape from apoptosis [1, 2]. Depending on the transplanted organ, the risk of PTLD ranges from 1 to 15% among transplanted patients, with bone marrow and the kidney representing the lowest risk, and the intestine associated with the highest risk of PTLD. Young age, serum negativity for EBV at the time of transplant, and specific therapies are additional risk factors for PTLD [1, 2]. PTLD classification is based on clinical, histologic, cell type, cytogenetic, immunoglobulin gene rearrangement, and virological features. The WHO [2] classifies PTLD in early lesions (plasmacytic hyperplasia and infectious mononucleosis-like PTLD), polymorphic PTLD (DLBCL-like and HL-like), monomorphic PTLD (DLBCL immunoblastic type, plasmacytoma) and PTLD HL. Early lesions are polyclonal and maintain the LN architecture. Polymorphic PTLD may be monoclonal and polyclonal, with loss of the LN architecture in both cases. Monomorphic PTLD are monoclonal with loss of the LN architecture.

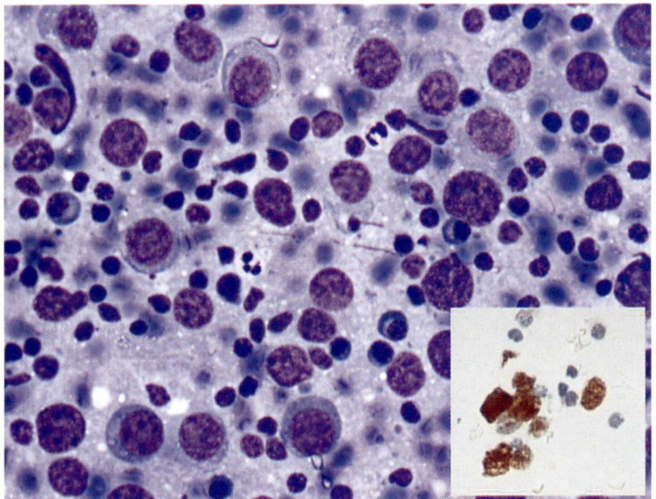

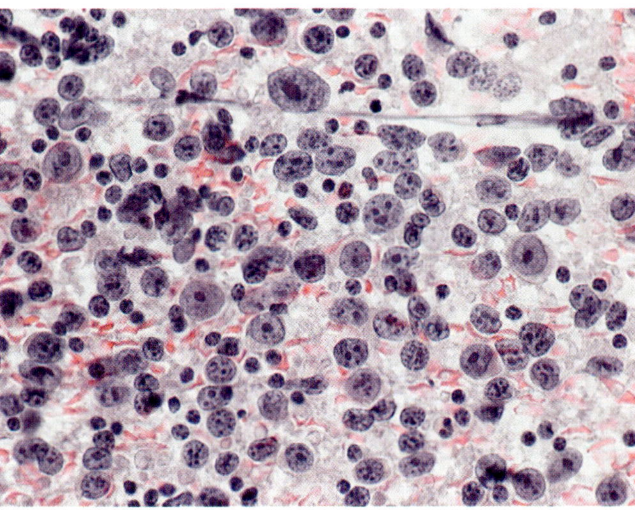

Fig. 2. LN-FNC of a post-transplant lymphoproliferative disease (PTLD) showing small- and medium-sized lymphoid cells, numerous centroblasts, immunoblasts, and plasma cells. **Inset** Nuclear positivity for EBER in situ hybridization. Histological control revealed a polymorphic PTLD.

Fig. 3. LN-FNC of a post-transplant lymphoproliferative disease (PTLD) showing large immunoblasts with dispersed chromatin and 1–2 central, large nucleoli. Small lymphocytes are scattered in the background. The histological control revealed an immunoblastic-type monomorphic PTLD.

Early Lesions

Plasmacytic hyperplasia is characterized by the preservation of the LN structure, with numerous plasma cells and occasional immunoblasts. Mononucleosis-like PTLD also preserves the LN structure with paracortex expansion and numerous immunoblasts and plasma cells. Flow cytometry (FC) shows the proportional B- and T-cell rate and balanced light chain [1, 2, 8]. FNC is polymorphous, showing small lymphocytes, plasma cells, centroblasts, and immunoblasts. The IGHK molecular analisys of PTLD may be pseudoclonal or polyclonal (Fig. 1).

Polymorphic PTLD

DLBCL-like and HL-like PTLD show the effacement of the LN structure with a polymorphous cell population characterized by immunoblasts, plasma cells, and medium-sized lymphoid cells with irregular nuclei. Necrosis may also be present. FNC may show small- and medium-sized lymphoid cells, numerous centroblasts, immunoblasts, and plasma cells (Fig. 2). Light chain restriction and IGH mutation may also be detected. In some cases, Hodgkin-like PTLD, Reed-Sternberg and Hodgkin-like cells (CD30+, CD20+, CD15–) are observed [1, 2, 8].

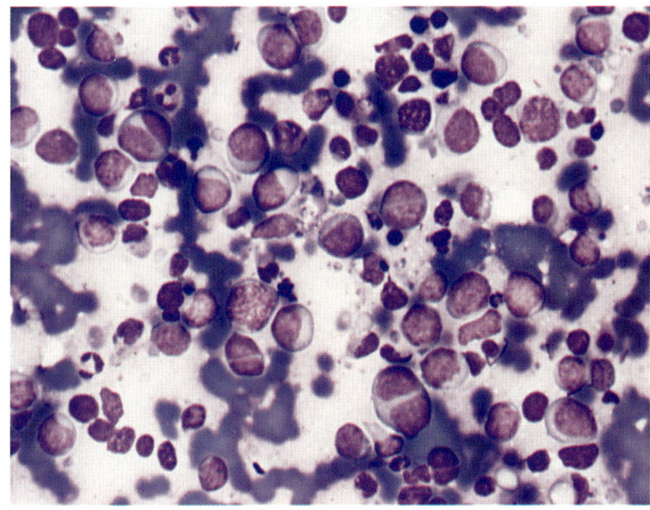

Fig. 4. LN-FNC of a post-transplant lymphoproliferative disease (PTLD) showing medium and large lymphoid cells with evident nuclear irregularities and numerous "polylobulated" nuclei. The histological control revealed a T-cell type monomorphic PTLD.

Monomorphic PTLD

Monomorphic PTLD (DLBCL immunoblastic type, plasmacytoma) show microscopic and genetic features similar to their non-PTLD counterparts [1, 2, 8]. Immunoblastic-type FNC generally reveals numerous large immunoblasts with dispersed chromatin and 1–2 central, large nucleoli. Small lymphocytes are scattered in the background (Fig. 3). T-cell NHL rarely occur [1, 2, 8]; FNC may be similar to non-PTLD counterparts (Fig. 4).

PTLD HL

Microscopic features are similar to HL in non-PTLD patients, whereas most cases are EBV(+) [2].

The diagnosis, classification, and management of all these entities is extremely complex and mainly depends on the histological, phenotypical, and molecular evaluation of LNs, in addition to clinical and serological data. Surgical excision of LNs in immunodepressed patients is generally hampered by the specific clinical context and FNC may be required as a first-line diagnostic procedure. Moreover, cytopathologists may come across PTLD because extranodal PTLD are generally more common than LN PTLD [1, 2]. Only a few studies have dealt with PTLD FNC [9–14] to diagnose reactive processes and/or opportunistic infections, PTLD, non-lymphomatous tumours [15], or clinically unclear nodules or swelling [16]. Therefore, cytopathologists should have a basic knowledge of PTLD as well as of the corresponding cytological features (Fig. 1), and utilize proper ancillary techniques (EBER [EBV-encoded RNA], FC, PCR) to obtain basic information that may be useful in the complex and multidisciplinary PTLD diagnostic process.

References

1 Ioachim HL: Medeiros LJ: Ioachim's Lymph Node Pathology, ed 4. Philidelphia, Lippincott, Williams & Wilkins, 2009.

2 Swerdlow SH, Campo E, Harris NL, Jaffe ES, Pileri SA, Stein H, Thiele J: WHO Classification of Tumours of Haematopoietic and Lymphoid Tissues, ed 4. Lyon, IARC Press, 2017.

3 Grogg KL, Miller RF, Dogan A: HIV infection and lymphoma. J Clin Pathol 2007;60:1365–1372.

4 Morton LM, Kim CJ, Weiss LM, Bhatia K, Cockburn M, Hawes D, Wang SS, Chang C, Altekruse SF, Engels EA, Cozen W: Molecular characteristics of diffuse large B-cell lymphoma in human immunodeficiency virus-infected and -uninfected patients in the pre-highly active antiretroviral therapy and pre-rituximab era. Leuk Lymphoma 2014; 55:551–557.

5 Martis N, Mounier N: Hodgkin lymphoma in patients with HIV infection: a review. Curr Hematol Malig Rep 2012;7:228–234.

6 Raymond E, Tricottet V, Samuel D, Reynès M, Bismuth H, Misset JL: Epstein-Barr virus-related localized hepatic lymphoproliferative disorders after liver transplantation. Cancer 1995;76:1344–1351.

7 Lones MA, Kirov I, Said JW, Shintaku IP, Neudorf S: Post-transplant lymphoproliferative disorder after autologous peripheral stem cell transplantation in a pediatric patient. Bone Marrow Transplant 2000;26:1021–1024.

8 Bezerra AM, Pasqualin DC, Guerra JC, Colombini MP, Velloso ED, Silveira PA, Mangueira CL, Kanayama RH, Nozawa ST, Correia R, Apelle AC, Pereira Wde O, Garcia RG, Bacal NS: Correlation between flow cytometry and histologic findings: ten year experience in the investigation of lymphoproliferative diseases. Einstein (Sao Paulo) 2011;9:151–159.

9 Gattuso P, Castelli MJ, Peng Y, Reddy VB: Posttransplant lymphoproliferative disorders: a fine-needle aspiration biopsy study. Diagn Cytopathol 1997;16:392–395.

10 Hecht JL, Cibas ES, Kutok JL: Fine-needle aspiration cytology of lymphoproliferative disorders in the immunosuppressed patient: the diagnostic utility of in situ hybridization for Epstein-Barr virus. Diagn Cytopathol 2002;26:360–365.

11 Gattuso P, Manosca F: Fine-needle aspiration of posttransplant lymphoproliferative disorders: a review. Diagn Cytopathol 2005;33:273–178.

12 Balachandran I, Walker JW Jr, Broman J: Fine needle aspiration cytology of ALK1(−), CD30+ anaplastic large cell lymphoma post renal transplantation: a case report and literature review. Diagn Cytopathol 2010;38:213–216.

13 Zhao X, Gong Y: Fine needle aspiration diagnosis of an early-onset post-transplant lymphoproliferative disorder. Diagn Cytopathol 2011;39:788–790.

14 Ponder TB, Collins BT, Bee CS, Grosso LE, Dunphy CH: Fine needle aspiration biopsy of a post-transplant lymphoproliferative disorder with pronounced plasmacytic differentiation presenting in the face: a case report. Acta Cytol 2002;46:389–394.

15 Chen X, Lagana SM, Poneros J, Kato T, Remotti F, He H, Kaminsky D, Hamele-Bena D: Cytological diagnosis of angiosarcoma arising in an immunosuppressed patient 6 years after multi-visceral transplantation: a case report and literature review. Diagn Cytopathol 2014;42:884–889.

16 Siddiqui MT, Reddy VB, Castelli MJ, Gattuso P: Role of fine-needle aspiration in clinical management of transplant patients. Diagn Cytopathol 1997;17:429–435.

Zeppa P, Cozzolino I: Lymph Node FNC. Cytopathology of Lymph Nodes and Extranodal Lymphoproliferative Processes.
Monogr Clin Cytol. Basel, Karger, 2018, vol 23, pp 81–92 (DOI: 10.1159/000478884)

Extranodal Lymphoproliferative Processes

The diagnosis of primitive extranodal (EN) non-Hodgkin lymphoma (NHL), as well as their classification and proper treatment, are a common challenge in the routine assessment of lymphoproliferative processes. The term "primitive" is used to distinguish EN-NHL from secondary involvements of EN sites by nodal NHL [1]. EN-NHL may display a variety of morphological features, molecular alterations, and clinical presentations. They can arise in different usual or unusual sites, including the salivary glands (SG) and oral cavity, lung and upper respiratory tract, thyroid, breast, gastrointestinal tract, bone and soft tissues, orbit, and central nervous system [1]. The organ of EN-NHL onset, other than the specific entities, is important for the natural history and prognosis of the disease. EN-NHL is often related to different aetiologies and molecular mechanisms, and may be indolent or aggressive; the corresponding organ of onset shows distinct histopathological features, requires specific staging, follows specific patterns of dissemination and relapse, and requires different treatments [2]. The two most common histotypes are EN marginal zone lymphoma (MZL), also called "mucosa-associated lymphoid tissue" (MALT), and diffuse large B-cell lymphoma (DLBCL) [1]. MALT accounts for 5–8% of all NHL and is characterized by the acquisition of lymphoid tissue in organs that do not contain it physiologically, such as the stomach, conjunctiva, skin, thyroid, and SG [3]. This is often due to autoimmune diseases, in particular Hashimoto's thyroid-

itis and Sjögren's syndrome, or bacterial infections responsible for chronic inflammations, such as *Helicobacter pylori* [1]. Associations between *Borrelia burgdorferi* infections and cutaneous NHL or *Chlamydophila psittaci* infection and ocular adnexal NHL are also known. MALT is usually a self-limiting disease – only in rare cases, and after a long duration, does it disseminate to other distant organs [1]. The median age of MALT onset is the sixth decade; patients have a good performance status and the prognosis is generally favourable, with a 75–80% survival at 10 years. MALT arising in the thyroid or the stomach is associated with a better prognosis than when it affects the SGs or the lungs [3]. The treatment for MALT depends on the organ involved; there are many treatments available, such as local therapy, surgery, radiation therapy, chemotherapy alone or combined with biological or antimicrobial therapies. DLBCL clinically appears as nodules or masses with a short clinical history [2]. Like the MALT counterpart, DLBCL is a mainly localized process, although in some localizations (ocular globe, testis, kidney, and paranasal sinuses), it can disseminate to the brain, hence requiring a timely diagnosis and specific prophylaxis to prevent this complication [4]. EN-NHL requires different diagnostic approaches based on the localization, whereas not all sites can be evaluated by fine-needle cytology (FNC). The SG, thyroid, lung, breast, soft tissues, and orbit are the anatomical sites most frequently investigated by FNC [5].

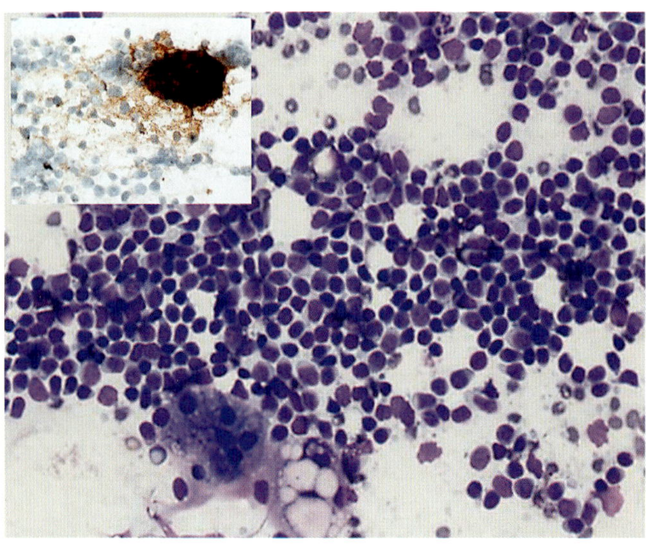

Fig. 1. Myoepithelial sialoadenitis showing monomorphous small lymphocytes with residual acinar cell on the bottom. **Inset** A dense tridimensional group of cytokeratin-positive epithelial-myoepithelial cells are present.

Salivary Gland

SG NHL account for about 3% of all SG tumours [6, 7]. The parotid gland is the most commonly involved one, accounting for about 80% of cases, followed by the submandibular (16%), sublingual (2%), and minor SG (2%) [6]. SG NHL mainly occurs in adults, with a female prevalence [7]. In some cases, it may present with facial paralysis and pain, although it appears most often as a slow growing and painless mass [6]. About 20% of SG NHL patients have a history of Sjögren's syndrome, with benign lymphoepithelial lesion (LEL) or myoepithelial sialoadenitis (MESA) [7]. MESA is considered a precursor of NLH [7] with a risk of developing B-cell NHL 40-fold higher in affected patients. MESA is generally characterized by a lymphoid infiltrate and islands of epithelial-myoepithelial cells [6, 8]. The latter are nests of ductal and occasional acinar cells intermingled with small lymphocytes (Fig. 1). Hyaline material of the basal lamina is often present. In minor SG, the cellular components are similar, although the epithelial-myoepithelial islands may be absent. Over time, the lymphoid infiltrate progressively replaces the acinar tissue, sparing some of the ducts. This results in a complete atrophy of the gland and the formation of organized lymphoid tissue with reactive follicles. Most cases of EN NHL arising in the SG are low-grade NHL (MALT) and DLBCL [8, 9]. For a long time, SG MALT was underdiagnosed compared to DLBCL, which is more easily recognizable by its cytological atypia; however, with the advent of the immunocytochemistry (ICC) and molecular methods, the diagnosis of SG MALT in the context of MESA has increased [8]. FNC of SG MALT is generally performed at the time of full development of the process. Smears show a relatively polymorphous cell population of small lymphocytes, follicular centre cells and histiocytes (Fig. 2). Fibroblasts and endothelial cells may also occur. The small lymphocytes generally have dense, compact chromatin, and nucleoli are absent. Monocytoid features and nuclear membrane irregularities are seldom observed, clear cytoplasm may be observed (Fig. 3), and mitoses are absent. The SG MALT FNC diagnosis mainly depends on the clonality assessment by flow cytometry (FC) or molecular testing, otherwise an FNC diagnosis is almost impossible. SG DLBLC FNC shows cytological features corresponding to the nodal counterpart [see Chapter 5, this vol., pp. 52–59] and the application of ancillary techniques leads to similar results. EN DLBCL cytological atypia is generally evident and the diagnosis of malignancy may be straightforward. Conversely, the differential diagnosis with poorly differentiated carcinoma or other malignancies may be difficult and depends on ICC or FC.

Thyroid

Thyroidal lymphoid infiltrate mainly occurs in Hashimoto thyroiditis (HT). Long-standing HT causes shrinking and atrophy of the thyroid with progressive follicle loss. HT generally shows high levels of serum antiperoxidase and anti-thyroglobulin autoantibodies; an increase in serum thyroid-stimulating hormone indicates concomitant hypothyroidism. During its evolution, HT may also lead to diffuse, symmetrical or asymmetrical enlargement of the gland and eventually to the formation of nodules, which may be requested for FNC. Primary thyroidal NHL (PTL) is a possible and rare complication of HT, whereas half of PTLs arise without an HT background [10–12]. MALT and DLBCL are the most frequent subtypes. DLBCL roughly comprises half of all cases and MALT approximately 20% of PTLs [10–12]. Other rare PTL subtypes are follicular lymphoma, small lymphocytic lymphoma/chronic lymphocytic leukaemia (SLL/CLL) and Hodgkin lymphoma (HL) [2, 10–12]. MALT and DLBLC FNC show cytological features corresponding to the LN counterpart [see Chapter 5, this vol., pp. 52–59] and the application of ancillary techniques is also similar.

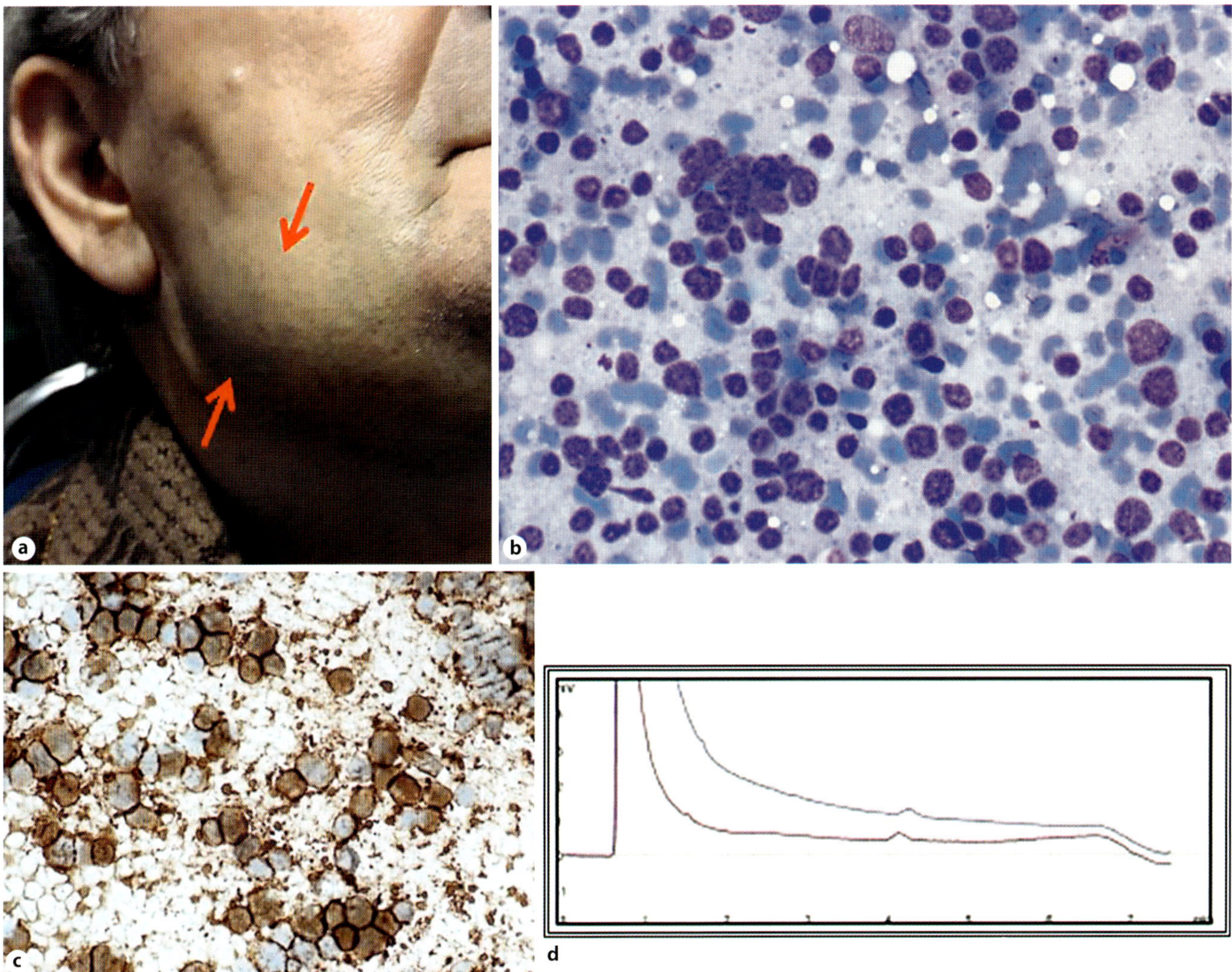

Fig. 2. a SG low-grade NHL (MALT) in an elderly patient showing a slow-growing, soft mass in the right parotid area. **b** FNC showed a relatively polymorphous population of small- and medium-sized CD20-positive lymphocytes (**c**). **d** DHPLC analysis showed IGHK monoclonality.

Differential diagnoses involve florid HT (Fig. 4) and anaplastic thyroid carcinoma, respectively [13–16]. MALT FNC should be suspected when dealing with a long-standing HT that slowly and progressively grows rather than shrinks. FNC of thyroidal MALT generally show a monomorphous population of lymphocytes, whereas more polymorphous presentations may occur (Fig. 5). Hurthle or follicular cells are absent. The FNC diagnosis mainly depends on FC detection of a quantitatively relevant light chain restriction or on molecular testing [13–15]. Thyroidal DLBCL generally has an increasingly worsening clinical presentation and the clinical differential diagnosis with anaplastic thyroid carcinoma is indicated, mainly when dealing with older patients [16]. Thyroidal DLBCL FNC does not show specific cytological features and the diagnosis depends on an ICC or FC assessment of lymphoid differentiation.

Breast

The breast may be involved through primary, EN, lymphoproliferative processes or by secondary localizations of leukaemia or systemic NHL [17–24]. Intramammary LN can also be involved by NHL, but this is a rare event [25, 26].

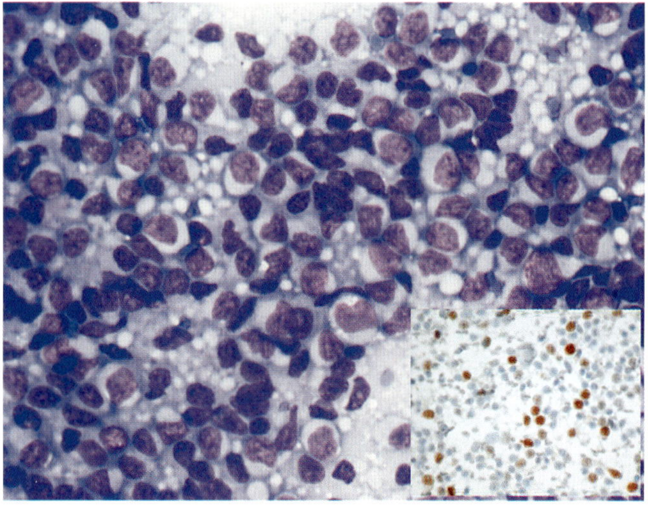

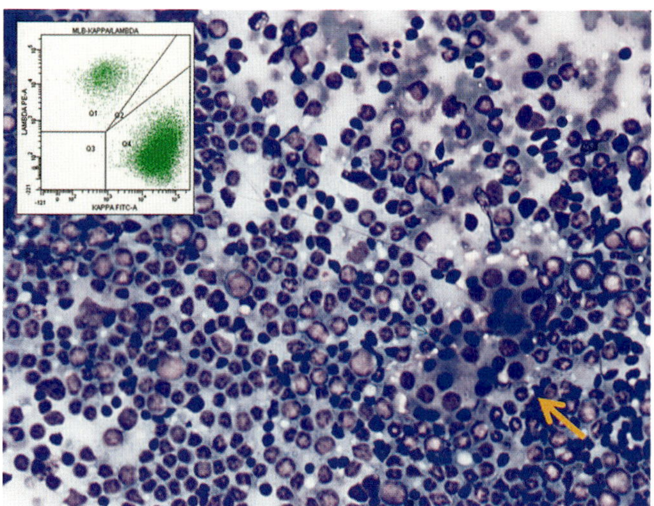

Fig. 3. SG MALT "monocytoid" variant showing medium-sized, monomorphous lymphocytes with irregular monocytoid nuclei and evident, clear cytoplasm. **Inset** Nuclear positivity for T-bet.

Fig. 4. Florid HT showing relatively polymorphous lymphoid cells. Follicular cells and Hurtle cells are variably present (arrow). **Inset** FC balanced light chain.

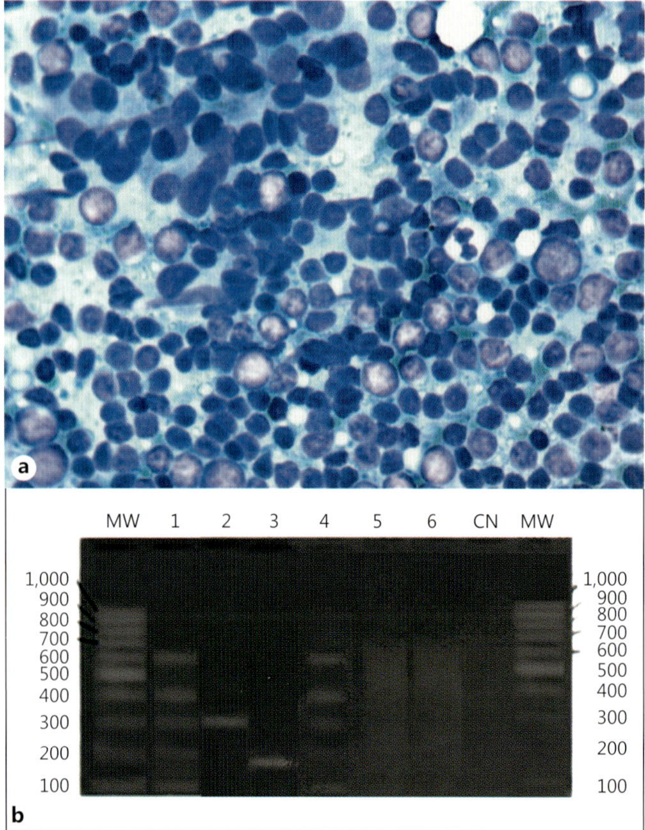

Breast implant-associated anaplastic large-cell lymphoma (BI-ALCL) may rarely arise around breast implants. Non-lymphomatous reactive processes that may occur in the breast are reactive intramammary LN and, more rarely, sclerosing lobulitis [27, 28]. As for NHL, the diagnosis of primary breast lymphoma (PBL) is limited to patients without evidence of other localizations of the disease; these represent 2% of EN NHL and less than 1% of all breast malignancies [17–24]. Conversely, secondary NHL involving the breast (SBL) is more common [17–24]. The clinical presentation and imaging of reactive processes and NHL of the breast are quite variable [29]. Intramammary LN has typical ultrasound features but may be confused with fibroadenoma (Fig. 6) [29]. The rare sclerosing lobulitis typically associated with diabetes mellitus has a variable presentation, with either monolateral or bilateral lumps, with or without an ill-

Fig. 5. a PTL smear showing a polymorphous population of small and large lymphoid cells. Thyroid follicular cells are absent. **b** HD analysis of IGHK multiplex PCR. Lanes 1–3: present case, Gene Control Multiplex PCR (lane 1), IGH monoclonality (lane 2), IGK monoclonality (lane 3). Lanes 4–6: reactive case control: Multiplex PCR (lane 4), IGH polyclonality (lane 5), IGK polyclonality (lane 6). CN lane: negative controls (no DNA in PCR reactions).

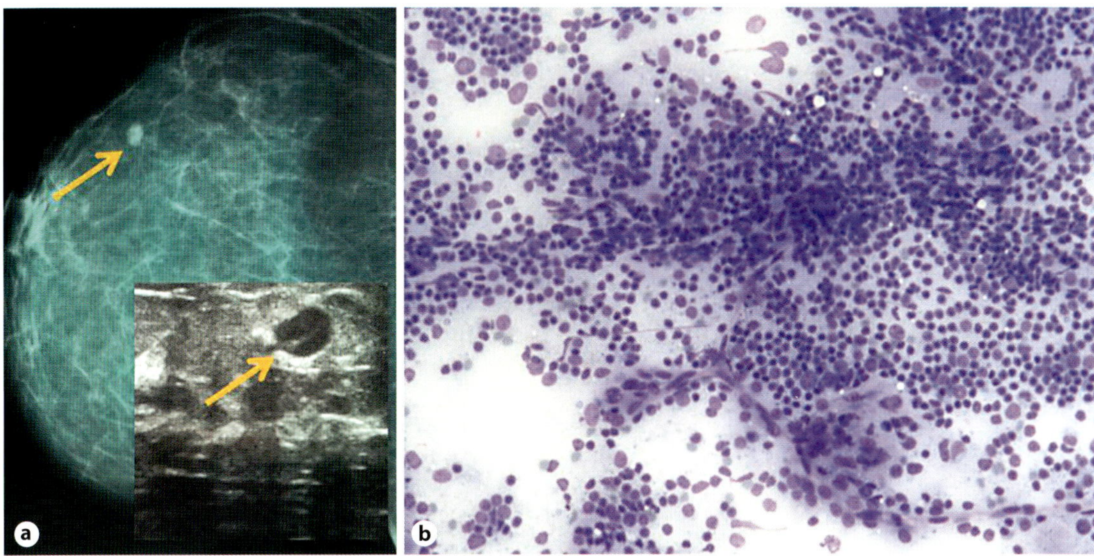

Fig. 6. a Mammographic and ultrasound (**inset**) features of intramammary lymph nodes; in both presentations it may simulate a fibroadenoma, mainly when roundish with an ill-represented hilum (arrow). **b** FNC shows a polymorphous lymphoid population and capillary structures consistent with a reactive hyperplasia.

defined mass. Corresponding smears show relative polymorphous lymphoid cells similar to those observed in intramammary LN with the presence of occasional small groups of benign ductal cells (Fig. 7). Finally, PBL and SBL imaging can be similar to that of breast carcinoma, showing hypoechoic lesions that may also overlap with medullary carcinoma. Moreover, PBL and SBL may show calcifications and/or speculated borders on mammography, which add further diagnostic difficulties [29]. FNC features of the different entities reported above should be evaluated once more in close connection with clinical and imaging data. For instance, the FNC of a clinically and ultrasound suspected fibroadenoma, showing lymphocytes and follicular centre cells, is most likely a reactive intramammary LN. Or a rapid bilateral breast enlargement likely occurs in patients suffering from leukaemia or NHL, mainly myeloid leukaemia and Burkitt NHL, respectively. Cytological features of breast involvement from NHL have been rarely reported and described as similar to the LN counterparts [24]. Attention should be paid to DLBCL, as it may simulate a breast carcinoma at the clinical and mammography evaluation. BI-ALCL rarely occurs in women with breast implants. BI-ALCL may be clinically subtle because it is associated with late seroma that is a benign reactive process in many cases that may occur in BI. BI-ALCL grows by infiltrating the periprosthetic capsule; the cytological and phenotypical fea-

tures are those of T-cell or null, CD30+, AlK-negative ALCL [see Chapter 4, this vol., pp. 34–51]. Cytological identification of diagnostic cells may be challenging because of the peculiar anatomical context and the intermingled inflammatory reactive cells [30–32].

Orbit

Lymphoproliferative lesions are the most common primary orbital tumours in older adults, with a slight female prevalence [2, 33–37]. These lesions represent a spectrum of disorders that include inflammatory pseudotumours, typical and atypical lymphoid hyperplasia, and NHL [2, 33–37]. The latter more frequently arise from the lachrymal glands, with MALT being the most frequent histotype. Corresponding diagnoses depend on a multidisciplinary approach that includes clinical data, imaging and pathology. Orbital lymphoproliferative lesions may be secondary or may arise primarily in the orbit [37]. Possible presentations are palpable masses, proptosis, and mildly restricted ocular motility; pain is an uncommon symptom in orbital NHL, at variance with the pseudotumour, which manifests with acute pain. Most lesions are unilateral (>50% of cases) and are often extraconal. Lacrimal glands are involved by lymphoproliferative processes in nearly 40% of cases [34–37]. At CT or MR imaging, approximately half the lesions are diffuse and ill defined, with the other half appearing as a smooth, circumscribed mass; uniform enhancement at MR is characteristic. An atypical feature of lymphoproliferative processes is their tendency to mould around the globe, the optic nerve, and orbital wall. The NHL shaped around the latter may result

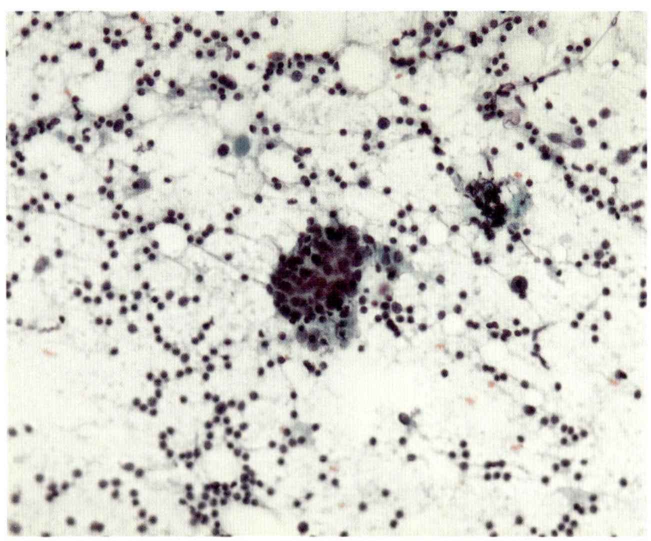

Fig. 7. Sclerosing lobulitis smear showing small lymphocytes and few large follicular cells scattered in a proteinaceous background. Note the group of benign ductal cells in the middle.

in bone remodeling; osseous erosion is quite rare, although it may occasionally occur with DLBCL. FNC may be performed beneath the roof or below the floor of the orbit to reach the lachrymal gland area or the conus, respectively, and all the other localizations according to their anatomical growth with a transconjunctival or transcutaneous approach. The procedure has to be performed by an ophthalmologist (Fig. 8); the role of the cytopathologist should be focused on smearing, ROSE, and material management. FNC of orbital lymphoproliferative lesions shows a variable monomorphism depending on the different corresponding lesions. Pseudotumour FNC may be variably cellular; smears are generally polymorphous showing lymphocytes, plasma cell histiocytes, and fibroblasts (Fig. 8). Eosinophils and vascular fragments may be present [38]. NHL shows the cytological features of the corresponding LN entities. Cytological criteria and ancillary techniques are almost the same as those described for LN, with the significant additional limitation of generally scanty diagnostic material mainly when obtained from posterior lesions.

Lung

Primary pulmonary lymphoma (PPL) refers to the presence of clonal lymphoid proliferations affecting 1 or both lungs and/or bronchi in a patient without evidence of extrapul-

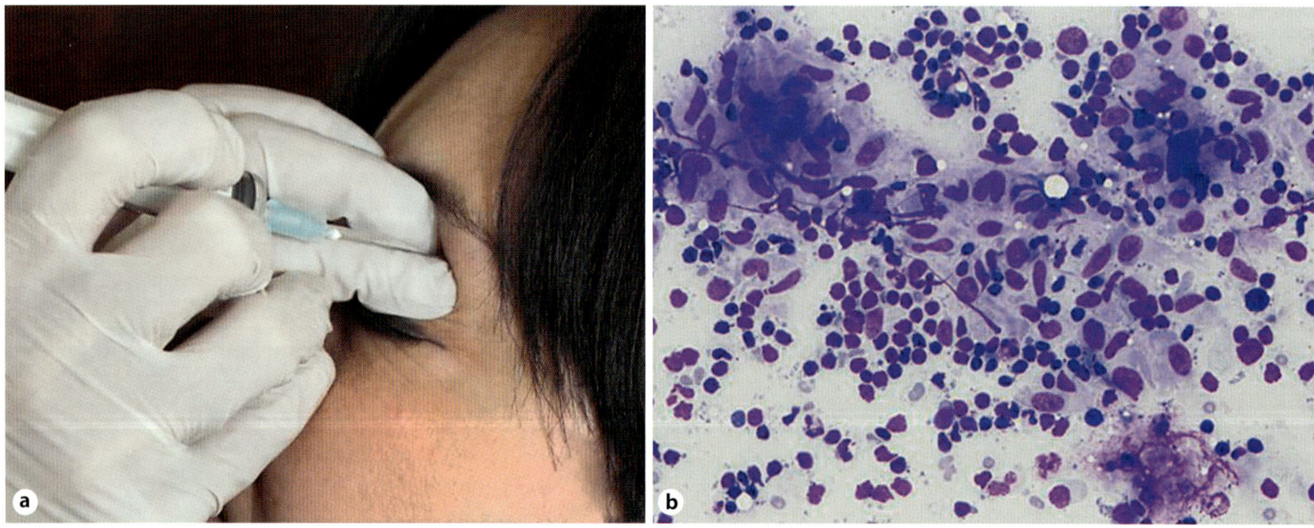

Fig. 8. a Orbital FNC performed beneath the roof or below the floor of the orbit to reach the lachrymal gland area or the conus, respectively. The procedure has to be performed by an ophthalmologist. **b** Cellular inflammatory pseudotumour FNC showing epithelioid cells, fibroblasts, and lymphocytes.

monary NHL at diagnosis or during the subsequent 3 months. PPL are mainly classified into 2 categories: pulmonary marginal lymphoma (PML) and DLBCL (PDLBCL) [1]. PML is the most common primary lung NHL, representing 70–90% of all PPL, whereas it accounts for less than 0.5–1% of all primary lung neoplasms [1]. Because nearly half the patients are asymptomatic and are identified incidentally at imaging, the diagnosis of PML is usually made at a late stage [39, 40]. CT-guided FNC is routinely used to diagnose lung nodules, masses or thickening and PPL may occur [39]. PML FNC has been described as a bland lymphoid proliferation represented by small- to medium-sized lymphocytes with slightly irregular nuclei and dispersed chromatin. Monocytoid cells with pale cytoplasm, plasma cells and a few follicular centres are also present. LEL, previously described in the Salivary Gland section of this chapter, here

are represented by bronchial cells intermingled with lymphocytes, and typical of MZL of other districts, may be scanty or absent in PML. Epithelioid and multinucleated cells in a granulomatous pattern may occur [39]. The FNC diagnosis of PML can be difficult or even impossible because of the similarities with reactive lymphoid hyperplasia and complexity in detecting LEL. Therefore, ROSE and material management for ancillary techniques are essential. In the absence of defined cytological atypia, clonality assessment by FC or PCR is indispensable for malignancy assessment of these lesions. Regarding classification, trisomy of chromosome 3 detectable by FISH (Fig. 9) is an effective procedure on FNC, followed by CD43/CD20 co-expression (Fig. 9). Cytokeratin 7 ICC may be helpful to reveal LEL [39, 41]. PDLBCLs represent a small percentage of PPLs; affected patients complain of respiratory and/or systemic symptoms

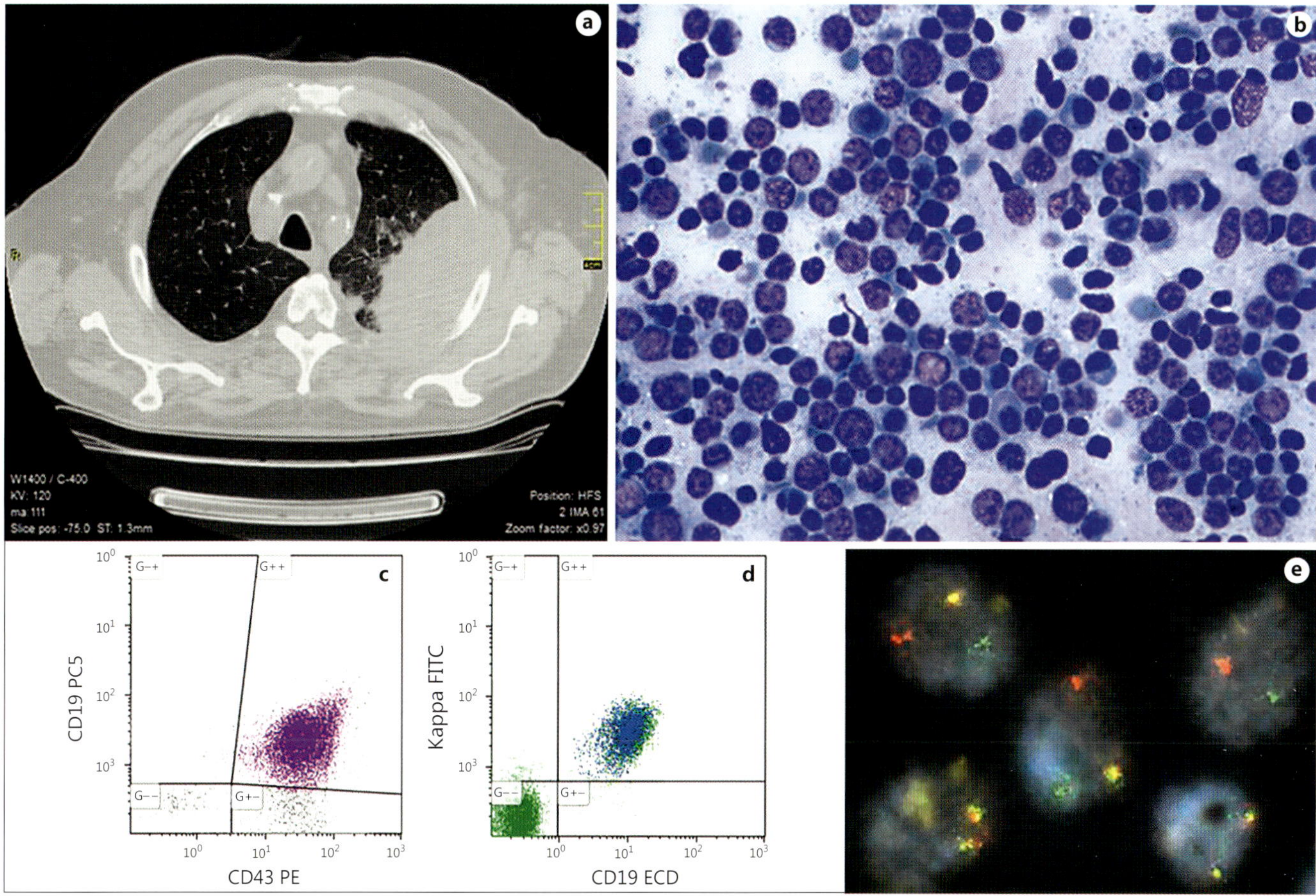

Fig. 9. a CT appearance of a primary lung NHL of the left lobe; the lesion was suspected to be a carcinoma before FNC. **b** ROSE showed a monomorphous population of small- to medium-sized, immature lymphocytes and numerous plasma cells. **c, d** FC histograms showing CD19/CD43 co-expression and kappa light chain restriction. **e** FISH on FNC of another case of lung NHL showing trisomy of chromosome 3 (case and image courtesy of Gilda da Cunha Santos, Toronto, ON, Canada).

[1]. FNC features are similar to those previously described in other locations, and the differential diagnosis is not made with reactive lesions but with lung carcinoma or other malignancies. The diagnosis must be based on ROSE and cell block techniques for an appropriate ICC panel. Other histotypes, such as small lymphocytic pulmonary lymphoma or pulmonary HL, are rare entities; only single cases or small series have been reported in the literature [42, 43].

Effusions and Lymphoproliferative Processes

Pleural, peritoneal and, more rarely, pericardial effusions occur in approximately half of patients with lymphoma. With the exception of the rare primary effusion lymphoma (PEL), they unusually represent the first clinical manifestation of lymphoma [44–46]. The main causes of effusions in lymphoma are infections caused by disease-related or iatrogenic immunodeficiency and serous involvement from NHL or leukaemia. Mediastinal LN enlargements (LNe), increased vascular permeability, and postradiation fibrosis that hamper lymphatic drainage may also cause effusion in lymphoma patients. Other causes are congestive heart failure, kidney or liver deficiencies, and even secondary neoplasms [46]. Pleural effusions represent 80% of serous involvement by NHL, followed by peritoneal (15%) and pericardial (5%), with PEL being extremely rare. In order of incidence, lymphoma-related effusions are NHL, leukaemia, myeloma, very rarely HL, with a high incidence of high-grade and T-cell NHL and a low-incidence of HL when compared to their epidemiologic incidence [46–60]. A cytological diagnosis of lymphoma-related effusions may be difficult because high cellularity and nuclear atypia do not necessarily correlate with serous involvement by NHL; in fact, reactive lymphocytosis in effusions may be highly cellular and may show nuclear atypia. Conversely, NHL-related effusions may be less cellular and with mild or absent cytological atypia. Therefore, effusions with lymphocytosis in NHL patients cannot be diagnosed without ancillary techniques.

Reactive Effusions
Different reactive processes, mainly viral infections, may cause effusions with serosal lymphocytosis. Corresponding cytological samples (cytospin or cell block) generally show a variable number of mesothelial cells, histiocytes, and lymphocytes. Reactive effusions with lymphocytosis may be extremely cellular and warningly monomorphous when com-

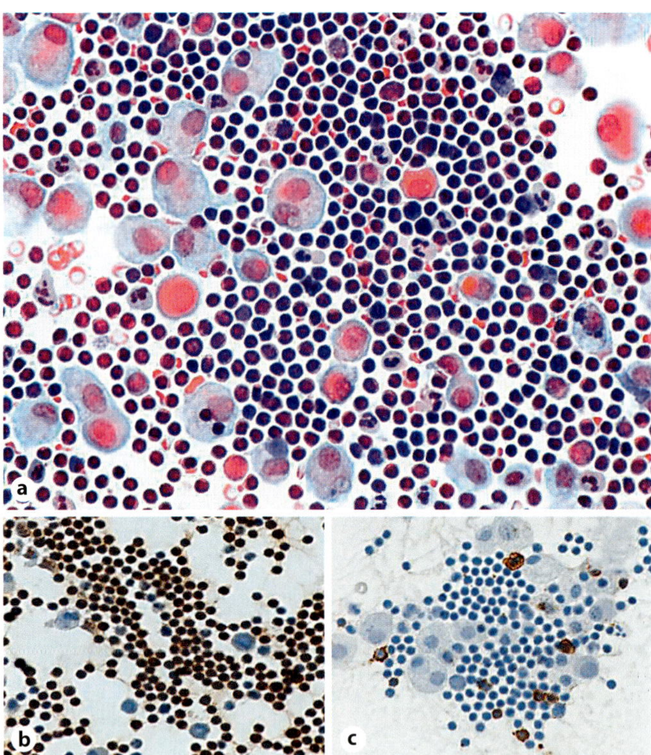

Fig. 10. a Reactive lymphocytosis in an effusion showing small monomorphous lymphocytes and scattered mesothelial cells. **b** CD3-positive T lymphocytes are preponderant with only a few B lymphocytes on cytospins (**c**).

pared to the polymorphism of the reactive LNe counterparts. Reactive lymphocytes are mainly T cells, showing the corresponding phenotype (CD3+, CD4/CD8+, CD5+) by FC or ICC on cell blocks or cytospins (Fig. 10) [46, 61–63].

B-Cell NHL-Related Effusions
SLL/CLL is a frequent cause of effusion, and the cytological features have previously been described [see Chapter 4, this vol., pp. 34–51]. Corresponding cytological samples show a variable number of mesothelial cells intermingled between SLL/CLL cells. The cell phenotype by ICC on cytospins or by FC is CD5+, CD19+, CD23+, CD10–, FMC7–, with light chain restriction. CD19/CD5 co-expression and specific cytological features are the clue to the diagnosis (Fig. 11). Secondary tumour cells (mainly from lung tumour) causing effusions may be hidden by the concomitant SLL/CLL cells [64, 65]. FL, MZL, and mantle cell lymphoma (MCL) may also cause effusions (Fig. 12) [44–47; see Chapter 4, this vol., pp. 36–39]. DLBCL and BL have a high incidence of effu-

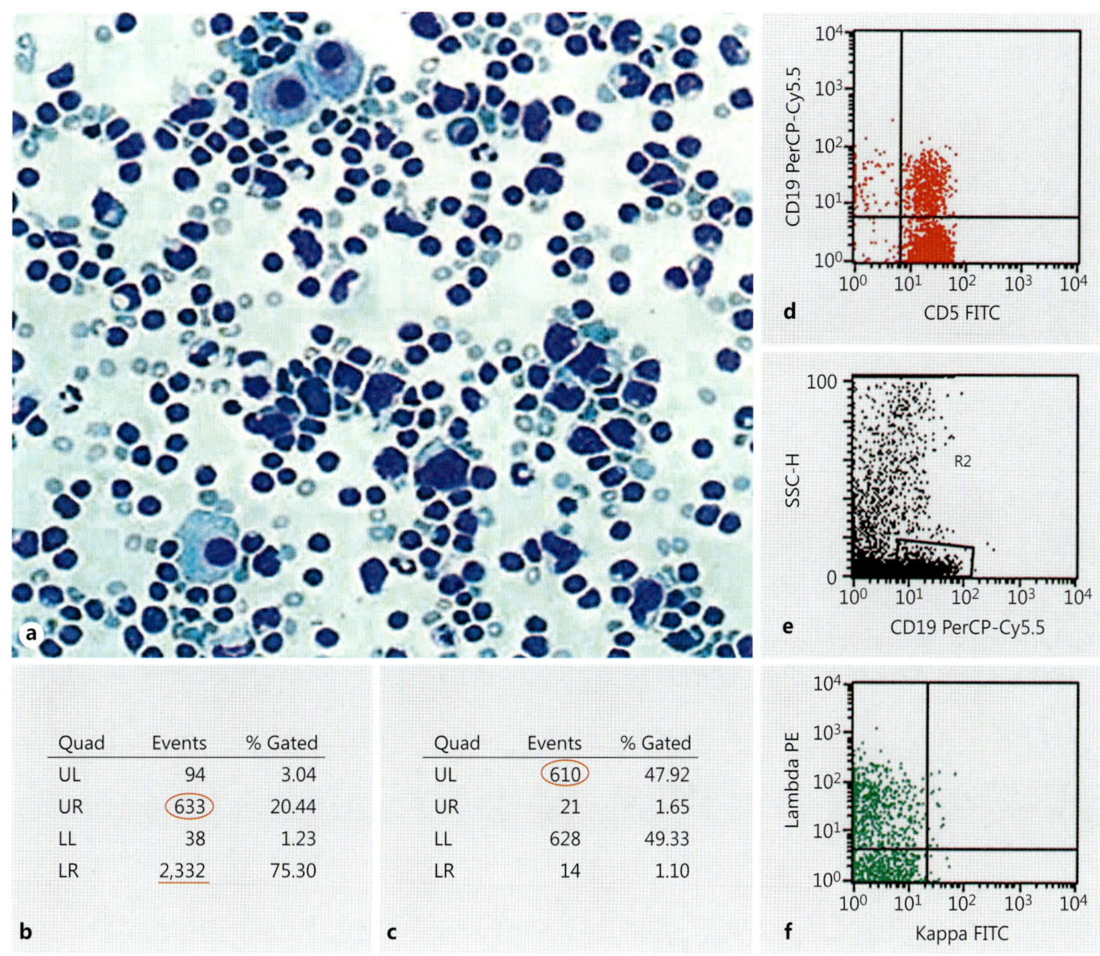

Quad	Events	% Gated
UL	94	3.04
UR	633	20.44
LL	38	1.23
LR	2,332	75.30

b

Quad	Events	% Gated
UL	610	47.92
UR	21	1.65
LL	628	49.33
LR	14	1.10

c

Fig. 11. a Pleural effusion from an SLL/CLL showing small irregular lymphocytes, granulocytes, small mature lymphocytes, and scattered mesothelial cells. The first gating selected 2,332 events, but 633 only showed CD5/CD19 co-expression in upper right (UR) quadrant (**b**) as shown on the histogram (**d**). A second gate (R2) on the CD5/CD19 events (**e**) selected 610 events in upper left (UL) quadrant (**c**) with lambda light chain restriction (**f**).

sion, which may reach 35% in BL [51, 53; see Chapter 4, this vol., pp. 34–51]. Because of their specific cytological features, a cytological diagnosis may not necessarily require ancillary techniques (Fig. 13).

T-Cell NHL-Related Effusions
T-cell NHL determines serous effusions more frequently than B-cell NHL [46]. This high incidence is maintained by precursor T-lymphoblastic lymphoma and leukaemia. Conversely, peripheral T-cell NHL rarely causes effusions [54–56]. Corresponding cytological features and diagnostic criteria have been previously described [see Chapter 4, this vol., pp. 34–51].

Primary Effusion Lymphoma
PEL is an extremely rare NHL, mainly reported in immunodepressed patients, without nodal or EN masses [66]. PEL mainly occurs in AIDS patients and is caused by HHV8 superinfection [67]. It is considered to be of B-cell origin, with unexpressed B-cell and T-cell markers. Activation markers (CD30) and plasma cell differentiation (CD138) may be expressed. Like other high-grade NHL, FC may be ineffective and a cytological diagnosis will rely on microscopic features and leucocyte common antigen positivity on cell block [68].

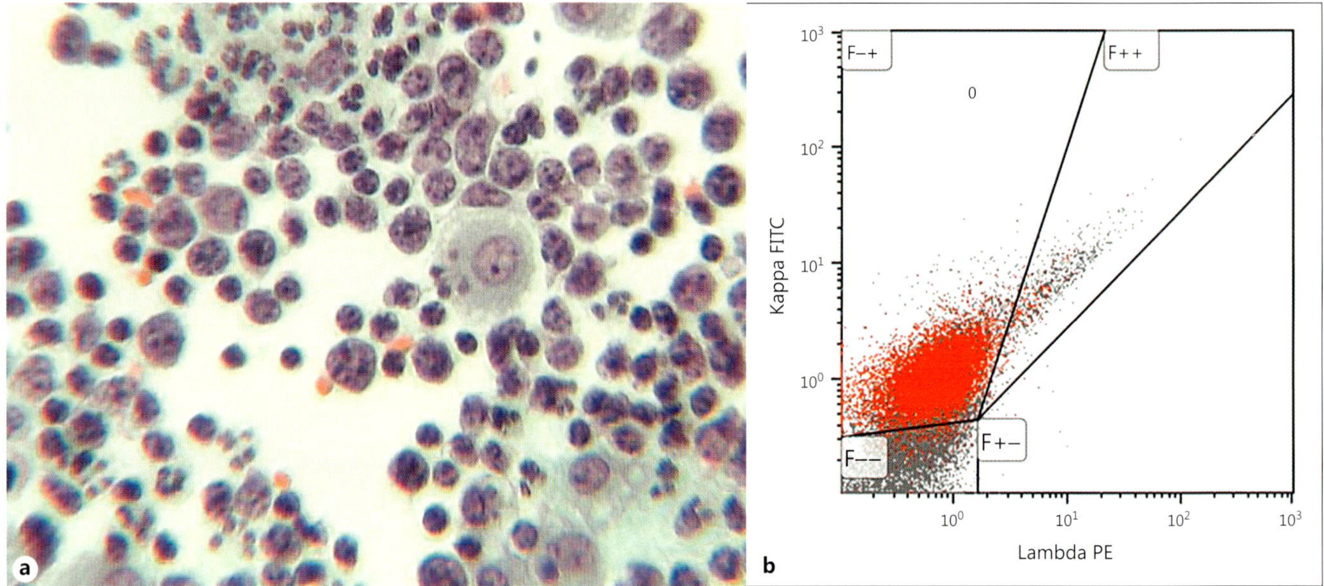

Fig. 12. a Pleural effusion from follicular lymphoma showing medium-sized, irregular lymphocytes with clumped chromatin. A few mesothelial cells and histocytes are scattered. FC showed CD10/CD19 co-expression and kappa light chain restriction (**b**).

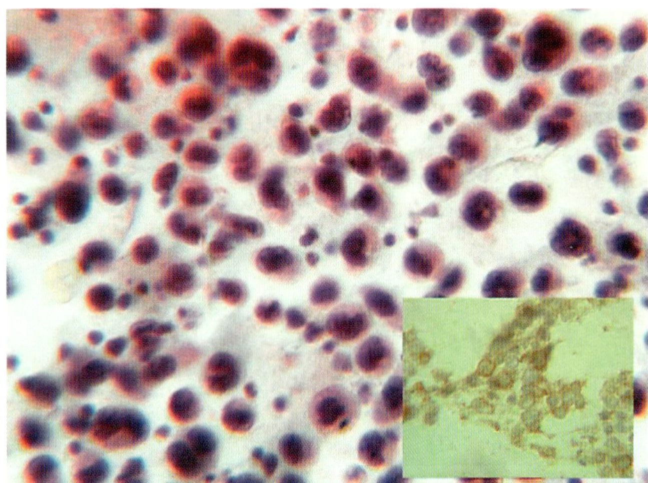

Fig. 13. Pleural involvement from DLBCL. Large isolated scattered cells with highly irregular nuclei. FC was not effective. **Inset** Leucocyte common antigen immunostain positivity on cytospin.

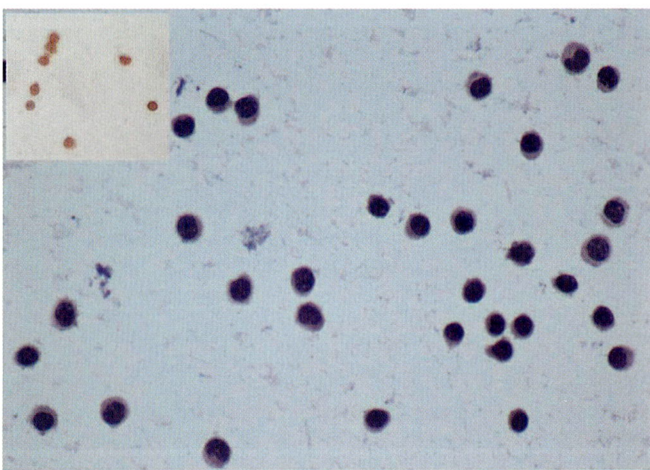

Fig. 14. Monomorphous dispersed population of small lymphocytes with light nuclear irregularities and thin cytoplasmic rhymes. **Inset** CD20 ICC positivity on cytospin.

Cerebrospinal Fluid and Lymphoproliferative Processes

Malignant involvement of the subarachnoid space occurs in 5–8% of patients with malignancies [69] and the cytological evaluation of cerebrospinal fluid (CSF) is an essential step for the diagnosis of leptomeningeal involvement. The most common malignancies that cause leptomeningeal involvement are lung and breast cancer, melanoma, NHL, and leukaemia. Inconclusive diagnoses on CSF are often due to scant cellularity or poor preservation or blood contamination of the sample. Leptomeningeal involvement occurs in 5–10% of patients with NHL, either at presentation, at a later stage of the disease course, or at relapse [69]. Leptomeningeal involvement is more common than parenchymal brain involvement by NHL [70]. The features generally observed are a monomorphous dispersed population of atypical cells larger than normal lymphocytes, irregular nuclear contours, abnormal chromatin, and nucleoli. The differential diagnosis is a reactive lymphocytosis composed of small, mature lymphocytes and larger, activated, so-called atypical lymphocytes. In some cases, a definitive diagnosis is not possible without lymphoid marker evaluation by ICC on cytospins (Fig. 14) or FC [71, 72]. In patients with acute leukaemia, either lymphoid or myeloid, it may be sufficient to identify the presence of blasts in CSF; further phenotypization (lymphoid vs. myeloid) can be performed on peripheral blood and bone marrow. PCR may be useful in selected cases and can be performed on archival and fresh CSF samples [73].

References

1 Swerdlow SH, Campo E, Harris NL, Jaffe ES, Pileri SA, Stein H, Thiele J: WHO Classification of Tumours of Haematopoietic and Lymphoid Tissues, ed 4. Lyon, IARC Press, 2017.

2 Campo E, Chott A, Kinney MC, Leoncini L, Meijer CJ, Papadimitriou CS, Piris MA, Stein H, Swerdlow SH: Update on extranodal lymphomas: conclusions of the workshop held by the EAHP and the SH in Thessaloniki, Greece. Histopathology 2006;48:481–504.

3 Rao DS, Daid JW: Small lymphoid proliferations in extranodal locations. Arch Pathol Lab Med 2007;131:383–396.

4 Vitolo U, Seymour JF, Martelli M, Illerhaus G, Illidge T, Zucca E, Campo E, Ladetto M; ESMO Guidelines Committee: Extranodal diffuse large B-Cell Lymphoma (DLBCL) and primary mediastinal B-cell lymphoma: ESMO Clinical Practice Guidelines for diagnosis, treatment and follow-up. Ann Oncol 2016;27(suppl 5):v91-v102.

5 Cibas ES, Ducatam BS: Cytology: Diagnostic Principles and Clinical Correlates, ed 4. Philadelphia, Elsevier Saunders, 2014.

6 Barnes L, Myers EN, Prokopakis EP: Primary malignant lymphoma of the parotid gland. Arch Otolaryngol Head Neck Surg 1998;124:573–577.

7 Daniels T: Benign lymphoepithelial lesion and Sjogren's syndrome; in Ellis GL, Auclair PL, Gnepp DR (eds): Surgical Pathology of the Salivary Glands. Philadelphia, WB Saunders, 1991, pp 1–83.

8 Hyjek E, Smith WJ, Isaacson PG: Primary B-cell lymphoma of salivary glands and its relationship to myoepithelial sialadenitis. Hum Pathol 1988; 19:766–776.

9 Royer B, Cazals-Hatem D, Sibilia J, et al: Lymphomas in patients with Sjogren's syndrome are marginal zone B-cell neoplasms, arise in diverse extranodal and nodal sites, and are not associated with viruses. Blood 1997;90:766–775.

10 Wang SA, Rahemtullah A, Faquin WC, Roepke J, Harris NL, Hasserjian RP: Hodgkin's lymphoma of the thyroid: a clinicopathologic study of five cases and review of the literature. Mod Pathol 2005;18:1577–1584.

11 Derringer GA, Thompson LD, Frommelt RA, Bijwaard KE, Heffess CS, Abbondanzo SL: Malignant lymphoma of the thyroid gland: a clinicopathologic study of 108 cases. Am J Surg Pathol 2000,24:623–639.

12 Widder S, Pasieka JL: Primary thyroid lymphomas. Curr Treat Options Oncol 2004;5:307–313.

13 Zeppa P, Cozzolino I, Peluso AL, Troncone G, Lucariello A, Picardi M, Carella C, Pane F, Vetrani A, Palombini L: Cytologic, flow cytometry, and molecular assessment of lymphoid infiltrate in fine-needle cytology samples of Hashimoto thyroiditis. Cancer 2009;117:174–184.

14 Caleo A, Vigliar E, Vitale M, Di Crescenzo V, Cinelli M, Carlomagno C, Garzi A, Zeppa P: Cytological diagnosis of thyroid nodules in Hashimoto thyroiditis in elderly patients. BMC Surg 2013; 13(suppl 2):S41.

15 Zeppa P, Vitale M: Fine needle cytology and flow cytometry in Hashimoto thyroiditis and primary thyroid lymphoma. Acta Cytol 2014;58:318.

16 Vigliar E, Caleo A, Vitale M, Di Crescenzo V, Garzi A, Zeppa P: Early cytological diagnosis of extranodal stage I, primary thyroid Non-Hodgkin lymphoma in elderly patients: report of two cases and review of the literature. BMC Surg 2013;13(suppl 2):S49.

17 Provenzano E, Pinder SE: Pre-operative diagnosis of breast cancer in screening: problems and pitfalls. Pathology 2009;41:3–17.

18 Wong WW, Schild SE, Halyard MY, Schomberg PJ: Primary non-Hodgkin lymphoma of the breast: the Mayo Clinic Experience. J Surg Oncol 2002;80:19–26.

19 Baker R, Slayden G, Jennings W: Multifocal primary breast lymphoma. South Med J 2005;98: 1045–1048.

20 Jennings WC, Baker RS, Murray SS, Howard CA, Parker DE, Peabody LF, Vice HM, Sheehan WW, Broughan TA: Primary breast lymphoma: the role of mastectomy and the importance of lymph node status. Ann Surg 2007;245:784–789.

21 Domchek SM, Hecht JL, Fleming MD, Pinkus GS, Canellos GP: Lymphomas of the breast: primary and secondary involvement. Cancer 2002;94:6–13.

22 Duncan VE, Reddy VV, Jhala NC, Chhieng DC, Jhala DN: Non-Hodgkin's lymphoma of the breast: a review of 18 primary and secondary cases. Ann Diagn Pathol 2006;10:144–148.

23 Jeanneret-Sozzi W, Taghian A, Epelbaum R, Poortmans P, Zwahlen D, Amsler B, Villette SP, Krengli M, Raad RA, Ozsahin M, Mirimanoff RO: Primary breast lymphoma: patient profile, outcome and prognostic factors: a multicentre Rare Cancer Network study. BMC Cancer 2008;8:86.

24 Vigliar E, Cozzolino I, Fernandez LV, Di Pietto L, Riccardi A, Picardi M, Pane F, Vetrani A, Troncone G, Zeppa P: Fine-needle cytology and flow cytometry assessment of reactive and lymphoproliferative processes of the breast. Acta Cytol 2012; 56:130–138.

25 Dey P, Al Jassar A, Amir T, Jogai S: Fine needle aspiration cytology of an intramammary reactive lymph node. Acta Cytol 2007;51:119–120.

26 Venizelos ID, Tatsiou ZA, Vakalopoulou S, Mandala E, Garipidou V: Primary non-Hodgkin's lymphoma arising in an intramammary lymph node. Leuk Lymphoma 2005;46:451–455.

27 Lammie GA, Bobrow LG, Staunton MD, Levison DA, Page G, Millis RR: Sclerosing lymphocytic lobulitis of the breast – evidence for an autoimmune pathogenesis. Histopathology 1991;19: 13–20.

28 Tomaszewski JE, Brooks JS, Hicks D, Livolsi VA: Diabetic mastopathy: a distinctive clinicopathologic entity. Hum Pathol 1992;23:780–786.

29 Mason HS, Johari V, March DE, Crisi GM: Primary breast lymphoma: radiologic and pathologic findings. Breast J 2005;11:495–496.

30 Granados R, Lumbreras EM, Delgado M, Aramburu JA, Tardío JC: Cytological diagnosis of bilateral breast implant-associated lymphoma of the ALK-negative anaplastic large-cell type: clinical implications of peri-implant breast seroma cytological reporting. Diagn Cytopathol 2016;44:623–627.

31 Talagas M, Uguen A, Charles-Petillon F, Conan-Charlet V, Marion V, Hu W, Amice J, De Braekeleer M: Breast implant-associated anaplastic large-cell lymphoma can be a diagnostic challenge for pathologists. Acta Cytol 2014;58:103–107.

32 Roden AC, Macon WR, Keeney GL, Myers JL, Feldman AL, Dogan A: Seroma-associated primary anaplastic large-cell lymphoma adjacent to breast implants: an indolent T-cell lymphoproliferative disorder. Mod Pathol 2008;21:455–463.

33 Vega F, Lin P, Medeiros LJ: Extranodal lymphomas of the head and neck. Ann Diagn Pathol 2005; 9:340–350.

34 Woolf DK, Ahmed M, Plowman PN: Primary lymphoma of the ocular adnexa (orbital lymphoma) and primary intraocular lymphoma. Clin Oncol 2012;24:339–344.

35 Watkins LM, Carter KD, Nerad JA: Ocular adnexal lymphoma of the extraocular muscles: case series from the University of Iowa and review of the literature. Ophthal Plast Reconstr Surg 2011;27: 471–476.

36 Nutting CM, Jenkins CD, Norton AJ, Cree I, Rose GE, Plowman PN: Primary orbital lymphoma. Hematol J 2002;3:14–16.

37 Valvassori GE, Sabnis SS, Mafee RF, Brown MS, Putterman A: Imaging of orbital lymphoproliferative disorders. Radiol Clin North Am 1999;37: 135–150.

38 Zeppa P, Tranfa F, Errico ME, Troncone G, Fulciniti F, Vetrani A, Bonavolontà G, Palombini L: Fine needle aspiration (FNA) biopsy of orbital masses: a critical review of 51 cases. Cytopathology 1997;8:366–372.

39 Ko HM, Geddie WR, Boerner SL, Rogalla P, da Cunha Santos G: Cytomorphological and clinicopathological spectrum of pulmonary marginal zone lymphoma: the utility of immunophenotyping, PCR and FISH studies. Cytopathology 2014; 25:250–258.

40 Borie R, Wislez M, Thabut G, et al: Clinical characteristics and prognostic factors of pulmonary MALT lymphoma. Eur Respir J 2009;34:1408–1416.

41 Chhieng DC: Cytology of bronchial associated lymphoid tissue lymphoma. Diagn Cytopathol 2008;36:723–728.

42 Sprague RI, deBlois GG: Small lymphocytic pulmonary lymphoma: diagnosis by transthoracic fine needle aspiration. Chest 1989;96:929–930.

43 Kumar R, Sidhu H, Mistry R, Shet T: Primary pulmonary Hodgkin's lymphoma: a rare pitfall in transthoracic fine needle aspiration cytology. Diagn Cytopathol 2008;36:666–669.

44 Das DK: Serous effusions in malignant lymphomas: a review. Diagn Cytopathol 2006;34:335–347.

45 Gilbert CR, Lee HJ, Skalski JH, Maldonado F, Wahidi M, Choi PJ, Bessich J, Sterman D, Argento AC, Shojaee S, Gorden JA, Wilshire CL, Feller-Kopman D, Ortiz R, Nonyane BA, Yarmus L: The use of indwelling tunneled pleural catheters for recurrent pleural effusions in patients with hematologic malignancies: a multicenter study. Chest 2015;148:752–758.

46 Bode-Lesniewska B: Flow cytometry and effusions in lymphoproliferative processes and other hematologic neoplasias. Acta Cytol 2016;60:354–364.

47 Podder S, Mora M, Patel V, Sivamurthy S: A rare case of bilateral chylothorax: a diagnostic challenge – follicular lymphoma versus primary effusion lymphoma. BMJ Case Rep 2015;2015: bcr2015211935.

48 Yonal I, Ciftcibasi A, Gokturk S, Yenerel M, Akyuz F, Karaca C, Demir K, Besisik F, Kalayoglu Besisik S: Massive ascites as the initial manifestation of Mantle cell lymphoma: a challenge for the gastroenterologist. Case Rep Gastroenterol 2012;6:803–809.

49 Keklik M, Yildirim A, Keklik E, Ertan S, Deniz K, Ozturk F, Ileri I, Cerci I, Camlica D, Cetin M, Eser B: Pericardial, pleural and peritoneal involvement in a patient with primary gastric Mantle cell lymphoma. Scott Med J 2015;60:e21–e24.

50 Meykler S, Baloch ZW, Barroeta JE: A case of marginal zone lymphoma with extensive emperipolesis diagnosed on pleural effusion cytology with immunocytochemistry and flow cytometry. Cytopathology 2016;27:70–72.

51 Chen Y-P, Huang H-Y, Lin K-P, Medeiros LJ, Chen T-Y, Chang K-C: Malignant effusions correlate with poorer prognosis in patients with diffuse large B-cell lymphoma. Am J Clin Pathol 2015; 143:707–715.

52 Haddad MG, Silverman JF, Joshi VV, Geisinger KR: Effusion cytology in Burkitt's lymphoma. Diagn Cytopathol 1995;12:3–7.

53 Bhaker P, Das A, Rajwanshi A, Gautam U, Trehan A, Bansal D, Varma N, Srinivasan R: Precursor T-lymphoblastic lymphoma: speedy diagnosis in FNA and effusion cytology by morphology, immunochemistry, and flow cytometry. Cancer Cytopathol 2015;123:557–565.

54 Ameri M, Parekh T, Qian Y-W, Elghetany MT, Schnadig V, Nawgiri R: A case of peripheral T-cell lymphoma, not otherwise specified in a HCV and HTLV-II-positive patient, diagnosed by abdominal fluid cytology. J Gastrointest Oncol 2016; 7:S96–S99.

55 Kesler M, Paranjape G, Asplund S, McKenna R, Jamal S, Kroft S: Anaplastic large cell lymphoma: a flow cytometric analysis of 29 cases. Am J Clin Pathol 2007;128:314–322.

56 Hunter B, Dhakal S, Voci S, Goldstein NPN, Constine L: Pleural effusions in patients with Hodgkin lymphoma: clinical predictors and associations with outcome. Leuk Lymphoma 2014;55:1822–1826.

57 Keklik M, Sivgin S, Pala C, Eroglu C, Akyol G, Kaynar L, Koker MY, Camlica D, Unal A, Cetin M, Eser B: Flow cytometry method as a diagnostic tool for pleural fluid involvement in a patient with multiple myeloma. Mediterr J Hematol Infect Dis 2012;4:e2012063.

58 Marchesi F, Masi S, Summa V, Gumenyuk S, Merola R, Orlandi G, Cigliana G, Palombi F, Pisani F, Romano A, Spadea A, Papa E, Canfora M, De Bellis C, Conti L, Mengarelli A, Cordone I: Flow cytometry characterization in central nervous system and pleural effusion multiple myeloma infiltration: an Italian national cancer institute experience. Br J Haematol 2016;172:980–982.

59 Wang Z, Xia G, Lan L, Liu F, Wang Y, Liu B, Ding Y, Dai L, Zhang Y: Pleural effusion in multiple myeloma. Intern Med 2016;55:339–345.

60 Faiz SA, Bashoura L, Lei X, Sampat KR, Brown TC, Eapen GA, Morice RC, Ferrajoli A, Jimenez CA: Pleural effusions in patients with acute leukemia and myelodysplastic syndrome. Leuk Lymphoma 2013;54:329–335.

61 Tong LC, Ko HM, Saieg MA, Boerner S, Geddie WR, da Cunha Santos G: Subclassification of lymphoproliferative disorders in serous effusions: a 10-year experience. Cancer Cytopathol 2013;121: 261–270.

62 Yu GH, Vergara N, Moore EM, King RL: Use of flow cytometry in the diagnosis of lymphoproliferative disorders in fluid specimens. Diagn Cytopathol 2014;42:664–670.

63 Iqbal J, Liu T, Mapow B, Swami VK, Hou JS: Importance of flow cytometric analysis of serous effusions in the diagnosis of hematopoietic neoplasms in patients with prior hematopoietic malignancies. Anal Quant Cytol Histol 2010;32:161–165.

64 Sur N, Silverman JF: Synchronous malignancies detected by effusion cytology. Diagn Cytopathol 1998;18:184–187.

65 Vrettos I, Kamposioras K, Peridis S, Aninos D, Kazika S, Spathis A, Karakitsos P, Papadopoulos A: Concurrent pleural infiltration by chronic lymphocytic leukemia and adenocarcinoma of unknown primary site diagnosed by effusion cytology. Diagn Cytopathol 2014;42:151–155.

66 Campo E, Swerdlow S, Harris N, Pileri S, Stein H, Jaffe E: The 2008 WHO classification of lymphoid neoplasms and beyond: evolving concepts and practical applications. Blood 2011;117:5019–5032.

67 Grogg KL, Miller RF, Dogan A: HIV infection and lymphoma. J Clin Pathol 2007;60:1365–1372.

68 Mihaescu A, Gebhard S, Chaubert P, Rochat M-C, Braunschweig R, Bosman F, Delacrétaz F, Benhattar J: Application of molecular genetics to the diagnosis of lymphoid-rich effusions: study of 95 cases with concomitant immunophenotyping. Diagn Cytopathol 2002;27:90–95.

69 Chamberlain MC, Nolan C, Abrey LE: Leukemic and lymphomatous meningitis: incidence, prognosis and treatment. J Neurooncol 2005;75:71–83.

70 Scott BJ, Douglas VC, Tihan T, Rubenstein JL, Josephson SA: A systematic approach to the diagnosis of suspected central nervous system lymphoma. JAMA Neurol 2013;70:311–319.

71 Ahluwalia MS, Wallace PK, Peereboom DM: Flow cytometry as a diagnostic tool in lymphomatous or leukemic meningitis: ready for prime time? Cancer 2012;118:1747–1753.

72 Tani E, Costa I, Svedmyr E, Skoog L: Diagnosis of lymphoma, leukemia, and metastatic tumor involvement of the cerebrospinal fluid by cytology and immunocytochemistry. Diagn Cytopathol 1995;12:14–22.

73 Liu L, Cao F, Wang S, Zhou J, Yang G, Wang C: Detection of malignant B lymphocytes by PCR clonality assay using direct lysis of cerebrospinal fluid and low volume specimens. Int J Lab Hematol 2015;37:165–173.

Zeppa P, Cozzolino I: Lymph Node FNC. Cytopathology of Lymph Nodes and Extranodal Lymphoproliferative Processes.
Monogr Clin Cytol. Basel, Karger, 2018, vol 23, pp 93–101 (DOI: 10.1159/000478885)

Metastases

Biology of Lymph Node Metastasis

Metastases are the most common non-haematopoietic cause of malignant lymph node (LN) enlargement. Metastatic LN (MLN) may occur in patients with a history of cancer or as a primary clinical manifestation of a neoplastic disease, and fine-needle cytology (FNC) plays a different role in the 2 clinical settings. In the case of a known primary tumour, FNC may confirm the diagnosis and contribute to the clinical staging and prognostic evaluations [1–5]. In cases of unknown primary tumour, FNC may identify or suggest the possible origin of the metastasis [6, 7]. Any malignant tumour can metastasize to LNs, but this occurrence varies greatly on the basis of the tumour type and the different clinical contexts [8]. Carcinoma most frequently produces MLNs, followed by melanoma and germ-cell tumours [6, 7]. Sarcoma rarely causes MLN, and central nervous system tumours almost never lead to such an occurrence. Relationships exists between the primary tumour and the MLN in the related anatomical district and the time interval between the primary tumour and MLNs. For instance, papillary thyroid carcinoma (PTC) may produce early anterior cervical MLN, while prostatic carcinoma usually leads to late inguinal-crural MLN. Cytopathologists dealing with LN-FNC should be aware of these aspects and should take into account the clinical history of the patient, including the spe-

cific histotypes in cases of known primary tumours. Nonetheless, in the clinical practice, many exceptions exist to the general rules concerning the site and the timing of MLNs. For instance, the possibility of a second neoplasm was considered exceptional in the past, but nowadays it is not an infrequent occurrence, especially in the elderly or long survival patients from primary-treated tumours. Therefore, cytopathologists dealing with MLN should also be open minded towards any possible occurrence and FNC diagnosis.

LN Topography and Cytological Features

MLN from an unknown primary tumour is an uncommon event. In these cases, the anatomic location of the MLN may contribute to the identification of the primary tumour; for instance, high-cervical (jugular and posterior) LNs may be the site of metastases from carcinoma of the tongue and the floor of the mouth, as well as from nasopharyngeal and tonsillar carcinoma. Anterior mid-cervical MLNs may be caused by PTC. Scalene LNs are usually the sites of metastases from intrathoracic neoplasms (Fig. 1, 2) and, on the left side, from abdominal tumours too (Fig. 3). Most supraclavicular MLNs originate from lung or breast tumours, whereas they may also originate from gastric, pancreatic, and prostatic carcinoma and testis tumours, mainly when locat-

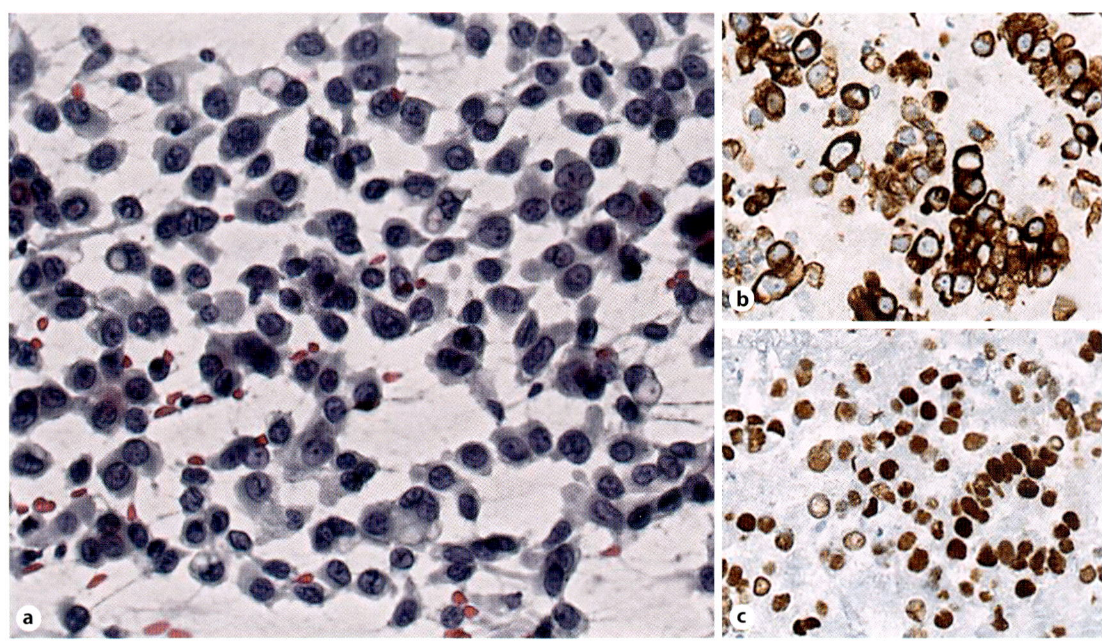

Fig. 1. LN metastasis from adenocarcinoma of the lung. **a** Dispersed medium-sized cells with round-oval nuclei, dispersed chromatin, and small nucleoli. Nuclear grooves, ill-defined cytoplasm, and occasional vacuoles are present. **b** CK7 positivity and TTF1 positivity (**c**) on cell block.

ed on the left side. In adult females, most axillary MLNs are ipsilateral to breast carcinoma or malignant melanoma; lung carcinoma should also be considered when dealing with axillary MLNs. Inguinal LNs often originate from carcinoma of the external genitalia, melanoma of the extremities, and less frequently from abdominal and pelvic organs. MLNs are generally characterized by a diffuse involvement and cytological features are usually significantly different from those of reactive LNs. The LN-FNC diagnosis of metastasis is generally straightforward, although exceptions may occur. Moreover, the FNC identification of MLN is generally immediate on direct smears when compared to lymphoproliferative processes, but the identification of unknown primary tumours may be difficult or impossible on routine smears. In fact, with the exclusion of specific cytological features, such as those of melanoma or PTC, and tumours with typical cytological patterns, like undifferentiated pharyngeal carcinoma or colonic adenocarcinoma (Fig. 4), many do not show specific characteristics or arise in different organs with the same cytological features, like squamous cell carcinoma. Therefore, the identification of a possible primary tumour is a challenging task and often requires the application of ancillary techniques. For this purpose, MLN FNC-ROSE may suggest the material management and require additional passes. Clinically, evident MLNs usually show a diffuse LN involvement, and as a consequence metastatic tumour cells outnumber lymphocytes in the background, if any are present. Conversely, in some cases, metastatic cells may be scanty and intermingled with or even hidden by lymphoid cells; lobular breast carcinoma is a typical example of this possibility (Fig. 5). In these cases, the differential diagnosis of metastatic cells with plasma cells, histiocytes, or large lymphocytes may be indicated. Cytological features of MLNs include the presence of cellular clusters, in comparison to the isolated lymphoid cells, and other cytological features such as "cell-in-cell," moulding, intranuclear inclusions, cytoplasmic vacuolization, an abundant, clear cytoplasm, the absence of lymphoglandular bodies, variably present necrosis and fibrosis. All these features may occur singularly or in combination, but none are pathognomonic and each feature should be evaluated within the whole cytological context. In some cases, metastatic carcinoma may simulate Hodgkin lymphoma (HL) and non-Hodgkin lymphoma (NHL). For example, nasopharyngeal "lymphoepithelial" carcinoma may simulate HL both clinically and cytologically because the 2 entities are common in young adults and show painless unilateral cervical LN enlargement (LNe). The corresponding FNC usually

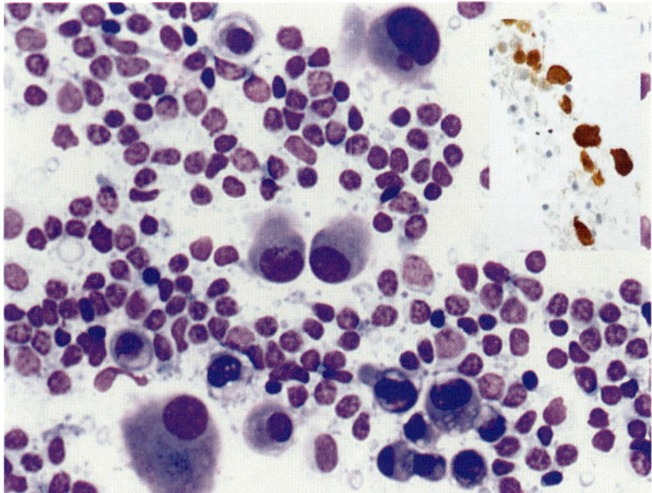

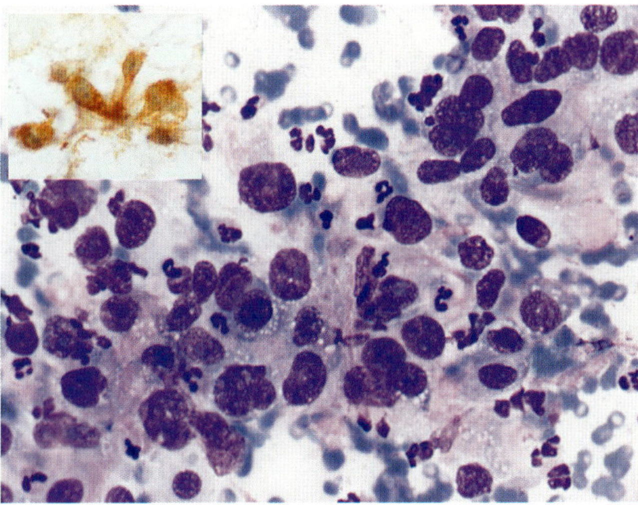

Fig. 2. LN metastasis from mesothelioma: scalene LN-FNC of a patient suffering from dyspnea showing lymphocytes and isolated cells with a wide dense cytoplasm and eccentric nuclei. Cells on the bottom show a kind of "window arrangement" and "barbed cytoplasm," suggesting a possible mesothelioma. Calretinin, which was added to a basic ICC panel, was positive (**inset**).

Fig. 3. LN metastasis from renal adenocarcinoma (CD10+; **inset**): a group of cells with a wide vacuolated cytoplasm, large irregular nuclei, and evident nucleoli.

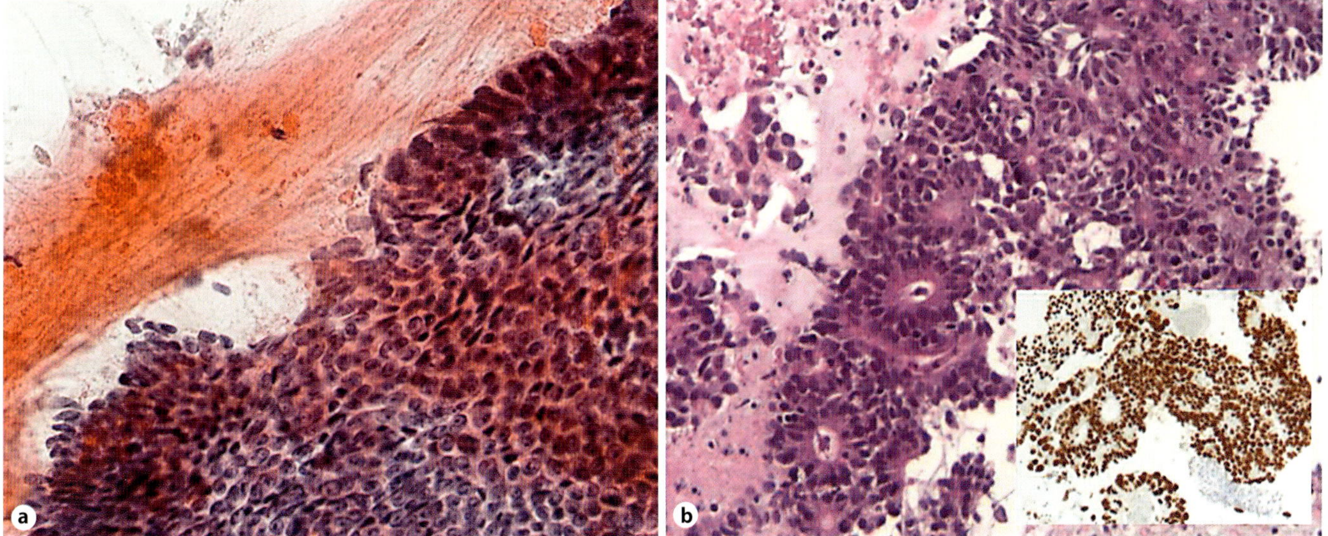

Fig. 4. a LN-FNC of metastasis from colonic adenocarcinoma; note the "picked-fence" arrangement of cells at the edge of the cell group and the mucoid background. **b** Cell block showing a glandular pattern of the cells that are CDX2+ (**inset**).

shows a polymorphous reactive cell population, including eosinophils, and a few malignant isolated cells that may simulate HL cells (Fig. 6). MLN from lobular carcinoma may also simulate NHL when the latter is composed of small, uniform, lymphocyte-like cells with occasional intracytoplasmic vacuoles that are a specific feature of lobular carcinoma. Metastatic neuroendocrine tumours may also simulate NHL; in these cases the key cytological features are a dense nuclear chromatin pattern, nucleoli absence, nuclear moulding, and focal necrosis, if present. Melanoma MLN

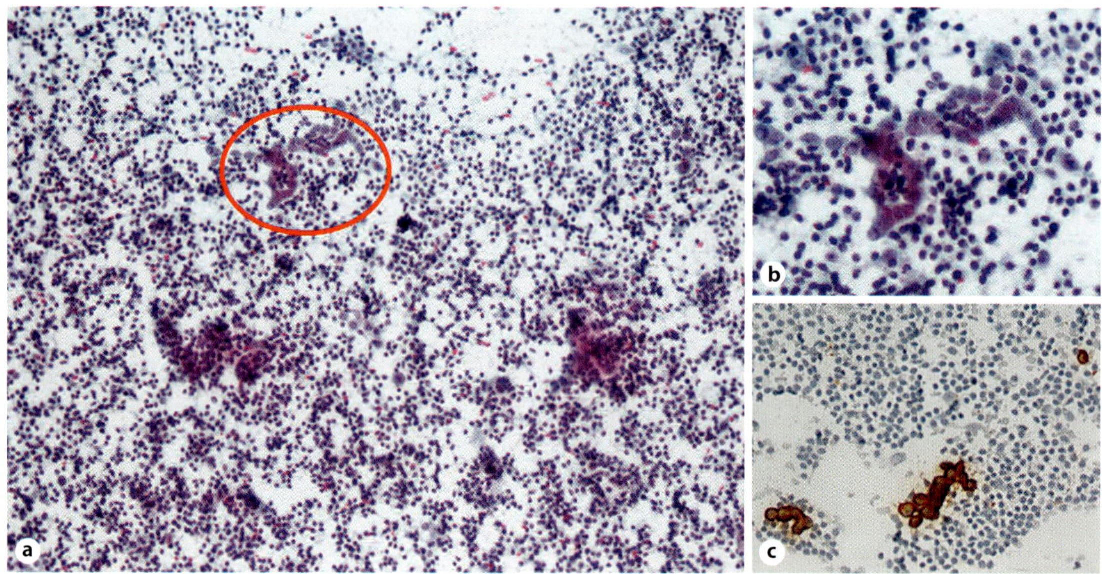

Fig. 5. LN-FNC of a breast carcinoma micrometastasis. **a** Few cohesive epithelial cells, organized into 2 small groups in a lymphoid background. **b** Epithelial cells are hardly larger than lymphoid. **c** CK19 positivity of the few epithelial cells on ICC.

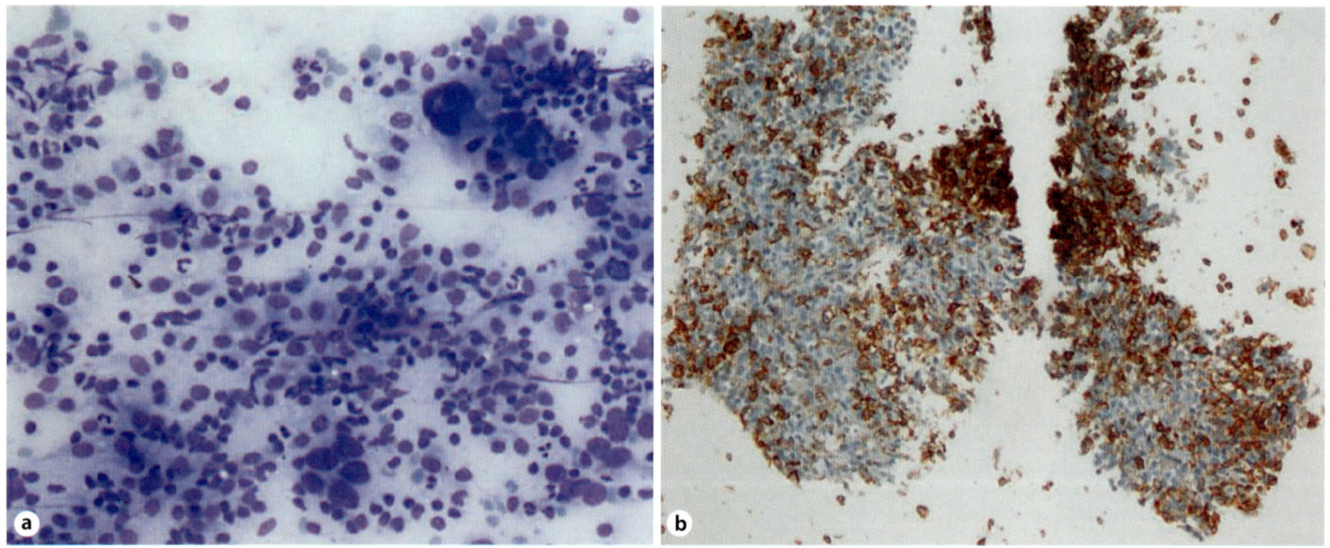

Fig. 6. LN-FNC metastasis from pharyngeal undifferentiated carcinoma. **a** A small group and isolated undifferentiated cells are scattered in a polymorphous background. Large atypical cells simulate Hodgkin or RS cells. **b** CK AE1-AE3 ICC on cell-block identifies the epithelial cells intermigled with lymphoid cells.

may also simulate large-cell NHL and plasmacytoma on FNC smears (Fig. 7). In all these cases, a definitive diagnosis requires the immunocytochemistry (ICC) identification of diagnostic cells. Conversely, some lymphoma, namely HL, DLBCL, anaplastic ALK+/– and some histiocytoses may simulate MLN. True or apparent cohesion, anaplasia of neoplastic cells, and the prevalence of a lymphoid background are possible causes of misinterpretation. ICC is mandatory,

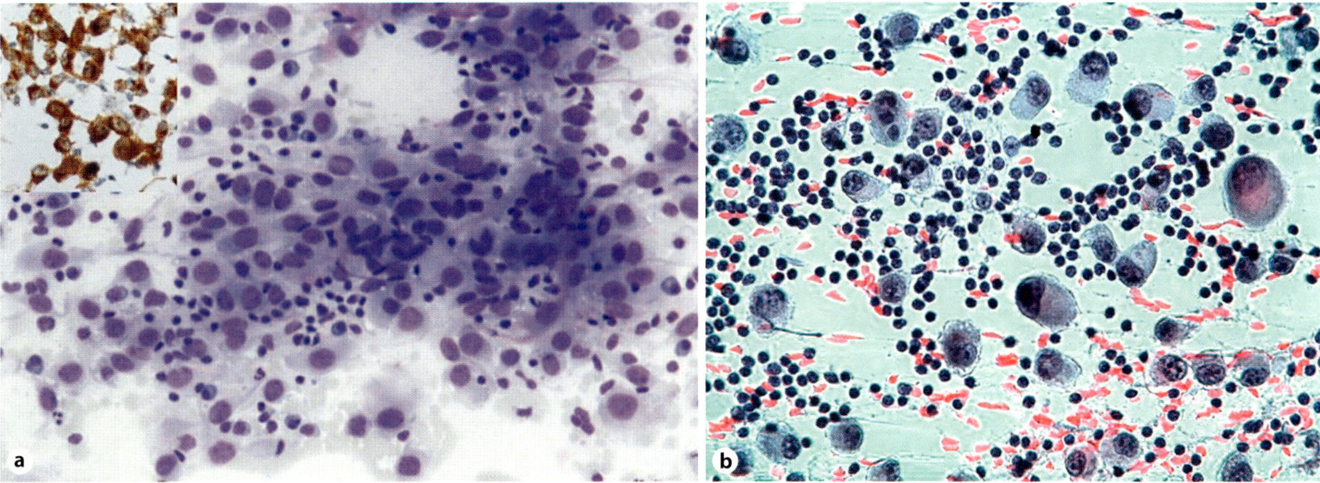

Fig. 7. Atypical (**a**) and typical (**b**) presentation of LN metastatic melanoma. **a** Cells are unusually aggregated with a dense cytoplasm and eccentric nuclei. Melanin and nuclear inclusions were absent, cells were HMB45 positive on the cell block (**inset**). **b** Isolated cells with a dense cytoplasm, eccentric nuclei, and nucleoli.

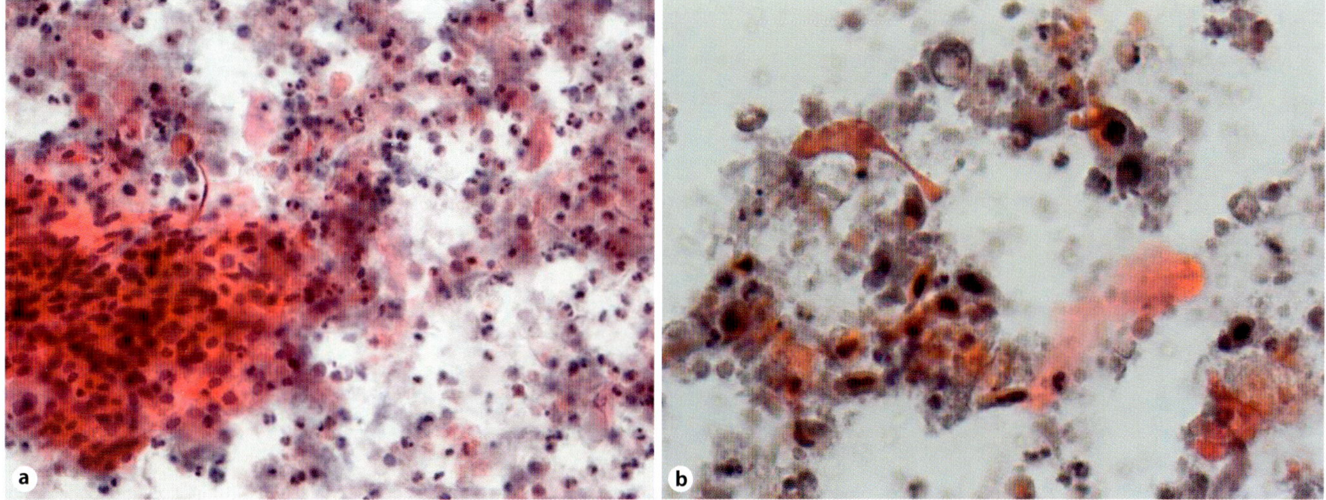

Fig. 8. Cystic modification in LN and LN-like nodules. **a** Group and isolated squamous cells with reactive atypical changes in a dysembriogenetic cyst. **b** Atypical keratinizing cells in a necrotic background in a "cystic" LN metastasis from epidermoid carcinoma.

though it is not always sufficient for an accurate FNC diagnosis. Other LN features, such as necrosis and cystic changes that frequently occur in metastatic squamous cell carcinoma, may hamper the FNC diagnosis of MLN. When necrotic and cystic changes are prominent, the collection of neoplastic cells by FNC may be scanty and limited to the most superficial and better-differentiated cell layers. As a

consequence, malignant cells may be missed or confused with benign squamous cells, especially when corresponding MLN are located in the neck and simulate dysembriogenetic cysts (Fig. 8). Cystic changes may also occur in the case of MLN from nasopharyngeal carcinoma and other tumours. In MLN from PTC, the thyroglobulin assay on FNC washout, combined with traditional smears, may be helpful [9].

Table 1. Basic and additional ICC panels for an "FNC discohesive pattern" or undifferentiated MLN

Basic panel	First diagnostic orientation	Additional panel
CKAE1AE3+	Undifferentiated carcinoma	CK7/CK20 and TTF1, Ca125, ER, CD56
LCA+	Lymphoma	CD20/CD3 and EMA, ALK, C30
S100+	Melanoma	HMB45, melan A
Vimentin+	Mesenchymal neoplasm	Desmin, S100, CD34

Table 2. Basic immunocytochemistry (ICC) for LN epithelial metastases

Cytological pattern or specific feature	ICC first diagnostic level	Diagnostic orientation	ICC second diagnostic level
Glandular, monolayered sheets	CK7+/CK20–	Lung, female genital tract	TTF1, CA125, WT1, Pax8
	CK7–/CK20+	Gastrointestinal tract	CDX2
	CK7+/CK20+	Biliopancreatic tract, urinary tract	CK19, CA19.9, GATA3
	CK7–/CK20–	Liver, prostate	HepPar1, PSA
Glandular, "picked fence"	CK7–/CK20+	Gastrointestinal tract	CDX2
Solid, multilayered	CK7–/CK20–	Breast, Lung	ER, P63, CK5-6
Papillary, monolayered, cytoplasmic nuclear inclusions	TTF1	Thyroid	TG
	CA125, WT1	Female genital tract	ER, Pax8
Clear cells	CD10, CD117	Kidney, female genital tract, soft tissue	RCC, PAX8, WT1, CA125, CA19.9, EMA
Signet ring cells	CK7+/CK20–	Pancreas, female genital tract	ER, CK19, WT1, PAX8
	CK7–/CK20+	Gastrointestinal tract	CDX2
Plasmacytoid cells, dispersed	ER, CD138, S100	Breast, melanoma, thyroid, myeloma	PR, HER2, HMB45, chromogranin, calcitonin, CD56, EMA
Small cells, no cytoplasm, nuclear crush	CD56, CK20	Neuroendocrine tumors, Merkel cell carcinoma	TTF1, chromogranin, synaptophysin
Indian rows, microvacuoles	ER	Breast	PR, GATA3

Micrometastases

LN micrometastases may hamper the detection of MLN by FNC. MLNs arise in the subcapsular sinus as little cellular aggregates or even as isolated cells that may easily be missed by FNC. However, with the exception of a few entities, the full LN involvement in the case of metastasis is a quite early event that generally characterizes clinically symptomatic LNs. At the same time, FNC is supported, nowadays, by ultrasound procedures that allow the sampling of specific areas of the LN, thus increasing diagnostic sensitivity in the case of partial LN involvement [10, 11] (Fig. 5, 7).

Immunocytochemistry and Diagnostic Algorithms

An FNC differential diagnosis of MLNs may concern the differentiation between high-grade NHL and MLN from a poorly differentiated carcinoma, as well as the identification of the primary tumour, when it is unknown. ICC is the most suitable ancillary technique for this purpose, but its application may be hampered by different factors. In fact, ICC may be applied on different FNC supports, including additional air-dried, fixed, or destained smears, cytospins, and cell blocks, each of them with specific characteristics in terms of fixation and treatment. This heterogeneity hampers the reproducibility evaluation of a single test and has determined

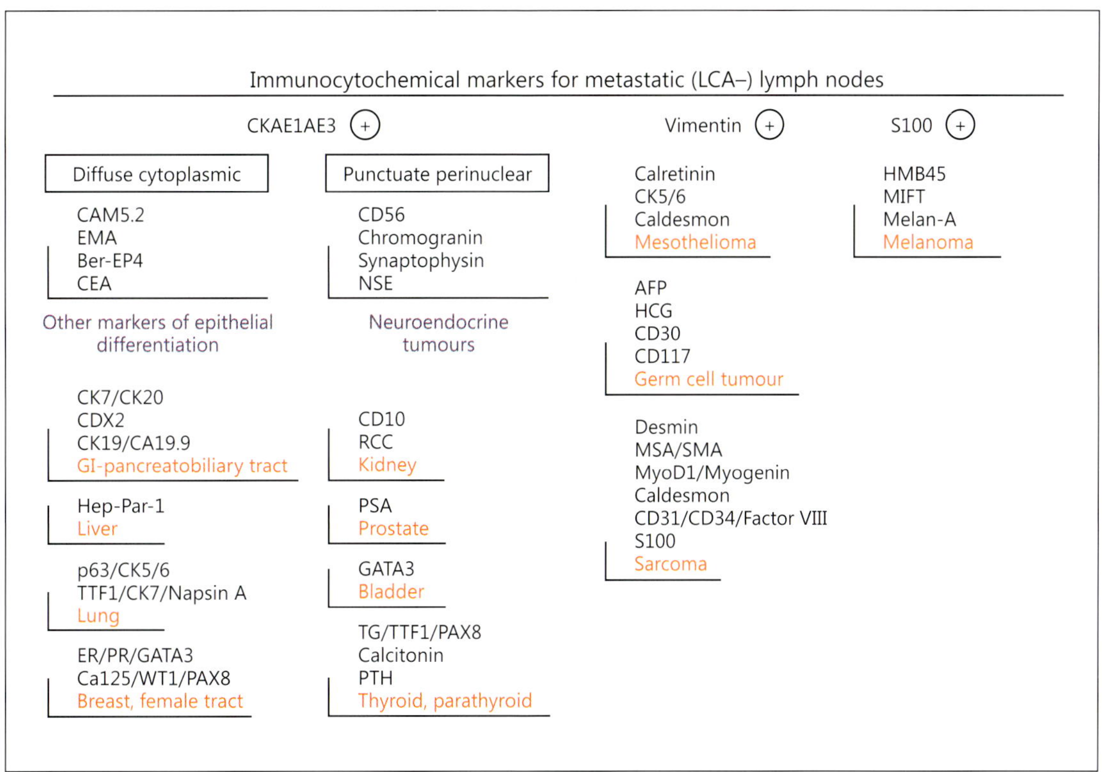

Fig. 9. Suggested immunocytochemical algorithm for LN metastases (LCA–), reporting basic antibodies and corresponding tumours.

the lack of specific guidelines and quality control procedures. The tumoral heterogeneity and the possible immunophenotypic differences between primary and metastatic tumours have to be taken into account when dealing with MLN, as well as the fact that FNC samples are quantitatively limited when compared to histological samples. These data should be considered in the choice of the antibodies for ICC together with clinical and cytological data. The choice of antibodies for MLN ICC should be based on their sensitivity and specificity, the possibility of internal and external controls, the rate of incidence of suspected primary tumours, and antigen specificity. A basic panel for poorly differentiated tumours may be CKAE1AE3, CD45 (LCA), vimentin, and S100 as markers for epithelial, lymphoid, mesenchymal, and melanocytic tumours, respectively (Table 1). A second panel of antibodies should be used in the case of better-differentiated tumours in which cytological features and clinical data suggest a possible primary tumour (Table 2). This wide group of reagents could include EMA, CAM5.2, Ber-EP4, CEA, CK20, CK7, CDX2, CK19, CA19.9, Hep-Par-1, p63, CK5/6, TTF1, napsin A, tireoglobulin,

PAX8, parathormone, calcitonin, mammaglobin, GCDFP-15, oestrogen, progesterone, HER2, Ca125, WT1, PSA, CD10, RCC, CD56, chromogranin, synaptophysin, NSE, HMB-45, MIFT, melan A, calretinin, caldesmon, AFP, HCG, CD30, and CD117 (Fig. 9). If properly applied and interpreted, the evaluation of these markers might solve most of the cases (Fig. 10). In a case of unknown primary squamous cell carcinoma MLN, FNC may rely on p16 protein evaluation (Fig. 11) and/or on tests to detect HPV (human papillomavirus) DNA. As with most head and neck MLNs from squamous cell carcinoma, mainly those originating from the palatine tonsil or the base of the tongue are HPV related [12–14].

Future Perspectives

"Occult" MLNs are the main weakness of FNC, but the application of new technologies is leading to interesting results. MicroRNA, namely MiR-203 and miR-205, determination by qRT-PCR for the detection of micrometastases in

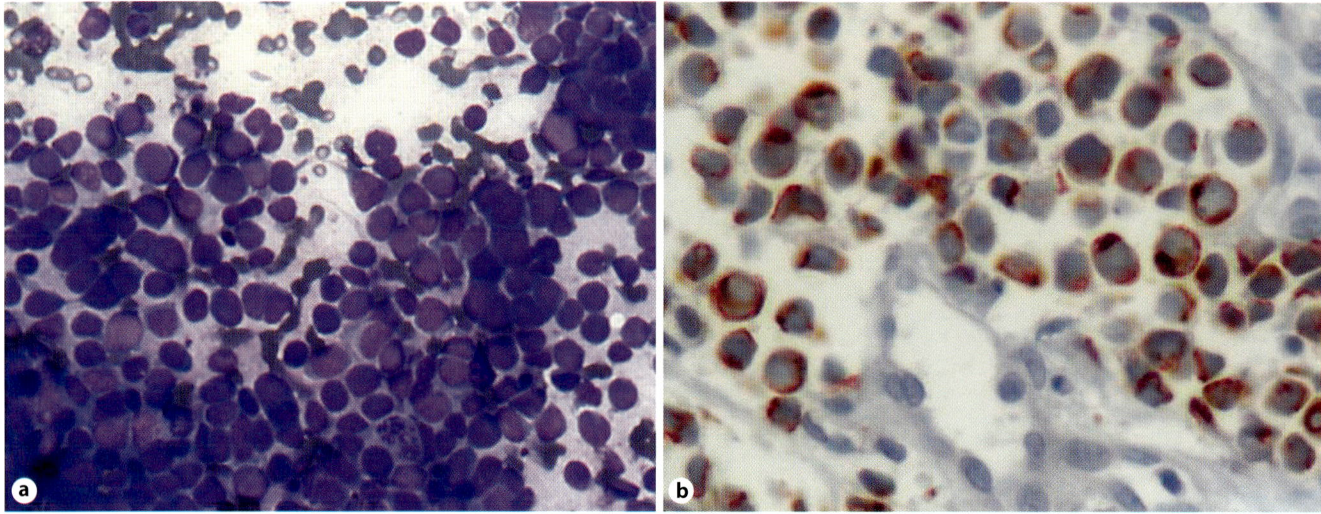

Fig. 10. LN metastasis from Merkel cell carcinoma. **a** Dispersed, monomorphous, medium-sized cells with round nuclei, dense chromatin, and inconspicuous or absent nucleoli. Cytoplasms are scanty or absent. **b** Cell bock: typical CK20, dot-like positivity.

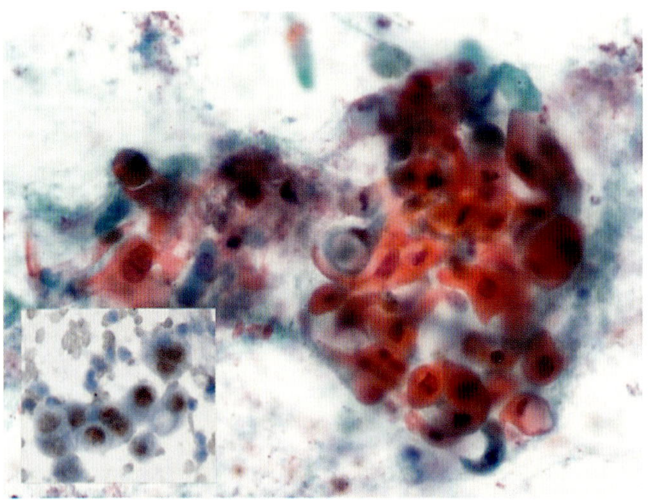

Fig. 11. Atypical keratinizing cells in an LN metastasis from a oropharyngeal carcinoma in a young patient. **Inset** ICC on an additional smear showed p16+.

cervical LNs has a role in the selection of treatment strategies and in the prognostic evaluation of patients with head and neck squamous cell carcinoma. MiR-203 and miR-205 determination has been successfully applied on FNC of sentinel LN (SLN) both at the time of treatment and during the follow-up [15]. OSNA (one-step nucleic acid amplification) is a rapid quantitative method to analyse cytokeratin 19

(CK19) mRNA expression, which may be used for SLN evaluation in breast cancer. The proteolytic cytokeratin fragment 21-1 (CYFRA 21-1) of CK19 is the most frequently used due to its high expression in body fluids and solid tumours of breast cancer patients. As a consequence, CYFRA 21-1 amplification by OSNA has also been successfully used on FNC [16, 17]. Occult MLN is a relevant problem in cases of melanoma; SLN may contain occult metastases that could easily be missed by FNC, as well as on histological sections, while a prompt and accurate diagnosis of MLN is important for staging, treatment, and prognosis. RT-PCR analysis of SLNs can detect MLN micrometastases from melanoma and has been successfully applied on FNC [18–20].

"Inclusions" and Other Conditions in Lymph Nodes

Benign squamous, glandular, or nevus cell inclusions may occur in LN due to developmental heterotopias [21, 22], with the upper lateral head and neck and axillary LNs being the most frequently involved sites. It is important to be aware of the possible occurrence of LN inclusions to avoid their misinterpretation on FNC. Salivary gland cell inclusions have been described in upper cervical LNs [22], thyroid follicular cells in lower cervical LNs, mammary gland cells in axillary LNs [23], and endosalpingiosis or endometriosis cells in pelvic LNs. Benign mesothelial cell inclusions in mediastinal LNs have also been reported [24], as well as the inclusion of nevus cells in LNs [25]. An FNC diagnosis of LN inclusions may be difficult or impossible due to the scant number of heterotopic cells and their lack of atypia. Sporadic reports have also documented the occurrence of intranodal leiomyoma, schwannoma, and myofibroblastoma; in these cases, the identification of LN cells on FNC is often impossible because they are present only on the edge of the nodule and are missed by FNC. Therefore, the definitive diagnosis is achieved by histological examination [26, 27].

References

1 Silvestri GA, Gonzalez AV, Jantz MA, Margolis ML, Gould MK, Tanoue LT, Harris LJ, Detterbeck FC: Methods for staging non-small cell lung cancer: diagnosis and management of lung cancer, 3rd ed: American College of Chest Physicians evidence-based clinical practice guidelines. Chest 2013;143(5 Suppl):e211S–e250S.

2 Gelberg J, Grondin S, Tremblay A: Mediastinal staging for lung cancer. Can Respir J 2014;21:159–161.

3 Park SH, Kim MJ, Park BW, et al: Impact of preoperative ultrasonography and fine-needle aspiration of axillary lymph nodes on surgical management of primary breast cancer. Ann Surg Oncol 2011;18:738–744.

4 Koelliker SL, Chung MA, Mainiero MB, et al: Axillary lymph nodes: US-guided fine-needle aspiration for initial staging of breast cancer – correlation with primary tumor size. Radiology 2008;246:81–89.

5 Jain A, Haisfield-Wolfe ME, Lange J, et al: The role of ultrasound guided fine-needle aspiration of axillary nodes in the staging of breast cancer. Ann Surg Oncol 2008;15:462–471.

6 Strojan P, Ferlito A, Langendijk JA, Corry J, Woolgar JA, Rinaldo A, Silver CE, Paleri V, Fagan JJ, Pellitteri PK, Haigentz M Jr, Suárez C, Robbins KT, Rodrigo JP, Olsen KD, Hinni ML, Werner JA, Mondin V, Kowalski P, Devaney KO, de Bree R, Takes RP, Wolf GT, Shaha AR, Genden EM, Barnes L: Contemporary management of lymph node metastases from an unknown primary to the neck. I. a review of therapeutic options. Head Neck 2013;35:123–132.

7 Strojan P, Ferlito A, Medina JE, Woolgar JA, Rinaldo A, Robbins KT, Fagan JJ, Mendenhall WM, Paleri V, Silver CE, Olsen KD, Corry J, Suárez C, Rodrigo JP, Langendijk JA, Devaney KO, Kowalski LP, Hartl DM, Haigentz M Jr, Werner JA, Pellitteri PK, de Bree R, Wolf GT, Takes RP, Genden EM, Hinni ML, Mondin V, Shaha AR, Barnes L: Contemporary management of lymph node metastases from an unknown primary to the neck. II. A review of diagnostic approaches. Head Neck 2013;35:286–293.

8 Ioachim HL, Medeiros LJ: Metastatic tumors in lymph nodes; in: Ioachim's Lymph Node Pathology, ed 4. Philadelphia, Lippincott, Williams & Wilkins, 2009, pp 590–598.

9 Jo K, Kim MH, Lim Y, Jung SL, Bae JS, Jung CK, Kang MI, Cha BY, Lim DJ: Lowered cutoff of lymph node fine-needle aspiration thyroglobulin in thyroid cancer patients with serum anti-thyroglobulin antibody. Eur J Endocrinol 2015;173:489–497.

10 Balu-Maestro C, Ianessi A, Chapellier C, Marcotte C, Stolear S: Ultrasound-guided lymph node sampling in the initial management of breast cancer. Diagn Interv Imaging 2013;94:389–394.

11 Ewing DE, Layfield LJ, Joshi CL, Travis MD: Determinants of false-negative fine-needle aspirates of axillary lymph nodes in women with breast cancer: lymph node size, cortical thickness and hilar fat retention. Acta Cytol 2015;59:311–314.

12 Boscolo-Rizzo P, Schroeder L, Romeo S, Pawlita M: The prevalence of human papillomavirus in squamous cell carcinoma of unknown primary site metastatic to neck lymph nodes: a systematic review. Clin Exp Metastasis 2015;32:835–845.

13 Pusztaszeri MP, Faquin WC: Cytologic evaluation of cervical lymph node metastases from cancers of unknown primary origin. Semin Diagn Pathol 2015;32:32–41.

14 Chernock RD, Lewis JS: Approach to metastatic carcinoma of unknown primary in the head and neck: squamous cell carcinoma and beyond. Head Neck Pathol 2015;9:6–15.

15 de Carvalho AC, Scapulatempo-Neto C, Maia DC, Evangelista AF, Morini MA, Carvalho AL, Vettore AL: Accuracy of microRNAs as markers for the detection of neck lymph node metastases in patients with head and neck squamous cell carcinoma. BMC Med 2015;13:108.

16 Yoon JH, Han KH, Kim E-K, et al: Fine-needle aspirates CYFRA 21-1 is a useful tumor marker for detecting axillary lymph node metastasis in breast cancer patients. PLoS One 2013;8:e57248.

17 Liscia DS, Detoma P, Zanchetta M, Anrò P, Molinar D, Favettini E, Paduos A: The use of CYFRA 21-1 for the detection of breast cancer axillary lymph node metastases in needle washouts of fine-needle aspiration biopsies. Appl Immunohistochem Mol Morphol 2017;25:190–195.

18 Voit C, Kron M, Rademaker J, Schwürzer-Voit M, Sterry W, Weber L, Ozdemir C, Proebstle T, Keilholz U: Molecular staging in stage II and III melanoma patients and its effect on long-term survival. J Clin Oncol 2005;23:1218–1227.

19 Scoggins CR, Ross MI, Reintgen DS, Noyes RD, Goydos JS, Beitsch PD, Urist MM, Ariyan S, Davidson BS, Sussman JJ, Edwards MJ, Martin RC, Lewis AM, Stromberg AJ, Conrad AJ, Hagendoorn L, Albrecht J, McMasters KM: Prospective multi-institutional study of reverse transcriptase polymerase chain reaction for molecular staging of melanoma. J Clin Oncol 2006;24:2849–2857.

20 Mocellin S, Hoon DS, Pilati P, Rossi CR, Nitti D: Sentinel lymph node molecular ultrastaging in patients with melanoma: a systematic review and meta-analysis of prognosis. J Clin Oncol 2007;25:1588–1595.

21 Lewis AL, Truong LD, Cagle P, Zhai QJ: Benign salivary gland tissue inclusion in a pulmonary hilar lymph node from a patient with invasive well-differentiated adenocarcinoma of the lung: a potential misinterpretation for the staging of carcinoma. Int J Surg Pathol 2011;19:382–385.

22 Daniel E, McGuirt WF Sr: Neck masses secondary to heterotopic salivary gland tissue: a 25-year experience. Am J Otolaryngol 2005;26:96–100.

23 Pantanowitz L, Upton MP: Benign axillary lymph node inclusions. Breast J 2003;9:56–57.

24 Paull G, Mosunjac M: Fine-needle aspiration biopsy and intraoperative cytologic smear findings in a case of benign mesothelial-cell inclusions involving a lymph node: case report and review of the literature. Diagn Cytopathol 2003;29:163–166.

25 Zaharopoulos P, Hudnall SD: Nevus-cell aggregates in lymph nodes: fine-needle aspiration cytologic findings and resulting diagnostic difficulties. Diagn Cytopathol 2004;31:180–184.

26 Martínez-Onsurbe P, Jiménez-Heffernan JA, Guadalix-Hidalgo G: Fine needle aspiration cytology of intranodal myofibroblastoma. a case report. Acta Cytol 2002;46:1143–1147.

27 Baldi C, Ieni A, Cozzolino I, Cerbone V, Memoli D, Zeppa P: Ultrasound-guided fine needle aspiration cytology of a primary lymph node leiomyoma: a flexible procedure for a complex case. Acta Cytol 2014;58:303–308.

Zeppa P, Cozzolino I: Lymph Node FNC. Cytopathology of Lymph Nodes and Extranodal Lymphoproliferative Processes.
Monogr Clin Cytol. Basel, Karger, 2018, vol 23, pp 102–112 (DOI: 10.1159/000478886)

Lymph Node Haematopoietic, Histiocytic, Dendritic Proliferations and Other Lymphoid Organs

Plasma cell, myeloid, histiocytic and dendritic neoplasms rarely arise in lymph nodes (LNs) as primary processes, although they may involve LNs in unusual presentations or in advanced stages of the same diseases. Fine-needle cytology (FNC) can be useful in their diagnosis but, as in other conditions, full knowledge of clinical and instrumental data available is essential for a correct diagnosis and management of the corresponding lesions.

Plasmacytoma

LN plasmacytomas (LNP) are rare [1, 2]. They may occur as primary LNP, representing one of the possible presentations of solitary extraosseous plasmacytoma, or as extramedullary localization of multiple myeloma. Primary LNP represents only 2% of all extramedullary plasmacytoma [1]. Some cases have been described arising in plasma cell-type Castleman disease [2] or associated with LN amyloidosis. LNP is frequently associated with serum monoclonal gammopathy (43%) of the IGG subtype [1]. LN-FNC shows plasmacytoid cells, either isolated or in clusters, with a variable degree of pleomorphism and bi- and multinucleation; mitoses may be observed [3, 4] (Fig. 1). Anaplasia, an increased number of plasmablasts, and numerous naked nuclei are frequently observed in extramedullary plasmacytoma, including LNP. The immunophenotype of LNP is CD138+ (Fig. 1), CD38+, VS38c+, and IRF4+. In contrast to medullary and extramedullary plasmacytoma or multiple myeloma, LNP may pre-

sent CD30 positivity and decreased MB2 (B-cell antigen) and CD45RO expression [1]. The diagnosis of LNP by FNC relies on its cytological features and on immunocytochemistry (ICC) or flow cytometry (FC) phenotype assessment. The differential diagnosis includes any reactive process with exuberant plasma cell proliferations and non-Hodgkin lymphoma (NHL) with relevant plasma cell differentiation, namely Castleman disease, lymphoplasmacytic, and marginal zone NHL. Plasma cell-rich reactive processes involving LNs, such as rheumatoid arthritis and syphilis, may be distinguished from LNP by FC or molecular polyclonality assessment. FNC of the plasmacellular variant of Castleman disease may have more polymorphous features, vascular structures, and polyclonal phenotypes. Regarding the diagnostic criteria for lymphoplasmacytic lymphoma and marginal zone lymphoma, plasma cells in NHL are more frequently CD19+, CD45+, and CD56– when compared to primary plasma cell neoplasms [for additional criteria, see Chapter 4, this vol., pp. 34–51].

Myeloid Leukaemia

Localized myeloid leukaemia, also termed granulocytic sarcoma or myeloid sarcoma, may occur as LN involvement in patients with known myeloid leukaemia, either acute or chronic, as well as in patients with the active disease. FNC of extramedullary localizations have been reported [5–10], including LN localization [11–13]. LN involvement may be

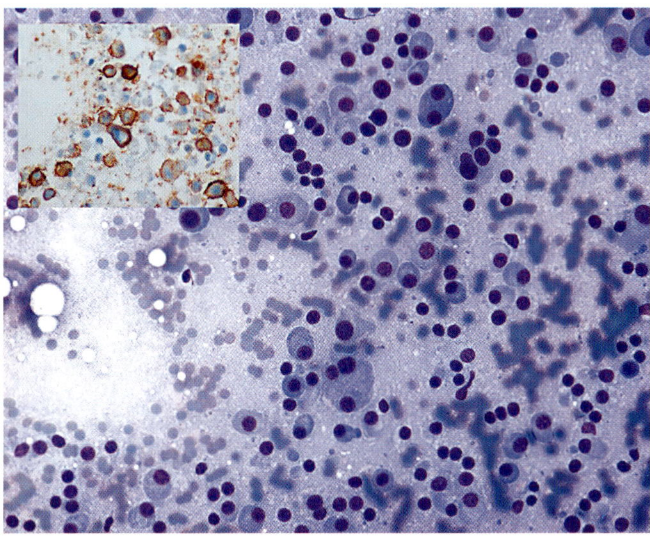

Fig. 1. Primary LNP showing differentiated, dispersed plasma cells with a wide, well-defined cytoplasm and 1 or more eccentrically located nuclei. **Inset** CD138 positivity on cell-block.

the first manifestation of myeloid leukaemia or the first sign of a relapse of the active disease, including its "blastic" transformation. Affected LNs may show partial involvement, either sinusoidal or interfollicular, a preserved structure, or diffuse effacement of the LN architecture. LN-FNC features depend on the differentiation grade of the corresponding process. High-grade myeloid leukaemia may show a uniform population of dispersed cells; the nuclei are generally medium-to-large with a scanty cytoplasm, if any (Fig. 2). Nuclear fragility is assessed by frequent nuclear crushes and strips. Auer rods and secondary granules are absent and numerous mitoses occur. A differential diagnosis with high-grade NHL or other undifferentiated neoplasms depends on the clinical data and specific myeloid phenotype. Better differentiated processes are more polymorphous, presenting medium-sized cells even with variable promyelocytic differentiation (Fig. 2); the nuclei show dispersed or vesicular chromatin and small nucleoli. The amount of cytoplasm may be scanty or moderate, and may contain granules [5–13]. The immunophenotype by ICC or FC may be positive for myeloperoxidase (Fig. 2), lysozyme, CD13, CD68, CD43, CD33, and CD117 [14, 15]. CD56, which is actually a prognostic marker, may further confirm the myeloid differentiation [16]. The main differential diagnosis concerns lymphoblastic lymphoma. Myeloid cells are often slightly larger than those in lymphoblastic lymphoma and usually contain

more prominent nucleoli. The identification of cytoplasmic granules should prompt the inclusion of specific myeloid markers to the ICC panel.

Mastocytosis

Mastocytosis is an abnormal mast cell proliferation with a heterogeneous clinical presentation. Mastocytosis commonly involves the skin (cutaneous mastocytosis), but may occur in haematopoietic, gastrointestinal, and hepatobiliary organs as localized or system mastocytosis (SM), with or without cutaneous lesions [17]. SM is further classified as indolent SM, SM with associated clonal, haematological non-mast cell lineage disease, aggressive SM, or mast cell leukaemia, based on their specific clinical-pathological features. The clinical presentation is extremely variable and depends on the organ system involved and the severity of the process, ranging from the paediatric, skin-limited disease, where a spontaneous regression generally occurs, to the more aggressive adult SM variants that may determine multiple organ dysfunction/failure and a fatal outcome [18]. SM patients generally do not present specific symptoms and rarely have LN involvement. LN enlargements (LNe) in SM may be caused by reactive hyperplasia, lymphadenopathic mastocytosis with eosinophilia, mast cell leukaemia, NHL, or even metastases. LNe occurs in patients with SM, mainly in deeply located stations, especially abdominal LN. Since the involvement of superficial LN stations in advanced SM is very rare [17, 18], LN-FNC features may present a partial involvement with the presence of both lymphoid and mast cells. Smears are generally scanty cellular. The mast cell shape may vary from round to fusiform, and the nuclei may be regular or atypical, with a roundish or oval shape, even with a monocytoid appearance (Fig. 3). The cytoplasm is variable, frequently elongated with long, polar processes and a variable amount of cytoplasmic granules, magenta stained with Diff-Quik (Fig. 4) [19–22]. These cells on LN-FNC smears may be scattered among polymorphous lymphoid cells, plasma cells, and eosinophils, or may represent the dominant cell population. An ICC expression of CD117 and CD25/CD2 co-expression by FC is helpful in the FNC diagnosis of mastocytosis (Fig. 3). In particular, CD117 differentiates mast cells from basophilic granulocytes, which may mimic mast cells for the fact that they are both positive with toluidine blue stain [20]. The aberrant CD25/CD2 co-expression may assess their clonality in adult mastocytosis [22]. Concerning the presence of eosinophils in LNs, other

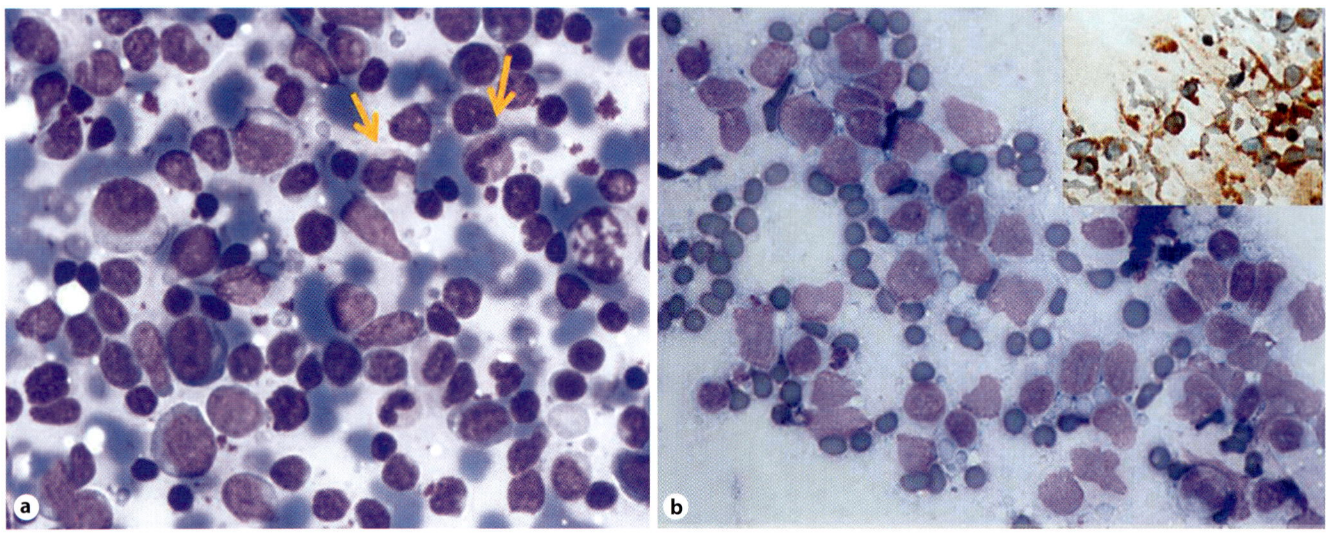

Fig. 2. a LN involvement from acute myeloid leukaemia showing large, immature blasts, a few scattered lymphocytes, and a few metamyelocytes (arrows). **b** Undifferentiated myeloblasts with immature chromatin and nuclear irregularities. **Inset** Myeloperoxidase positivity on an additional smear.

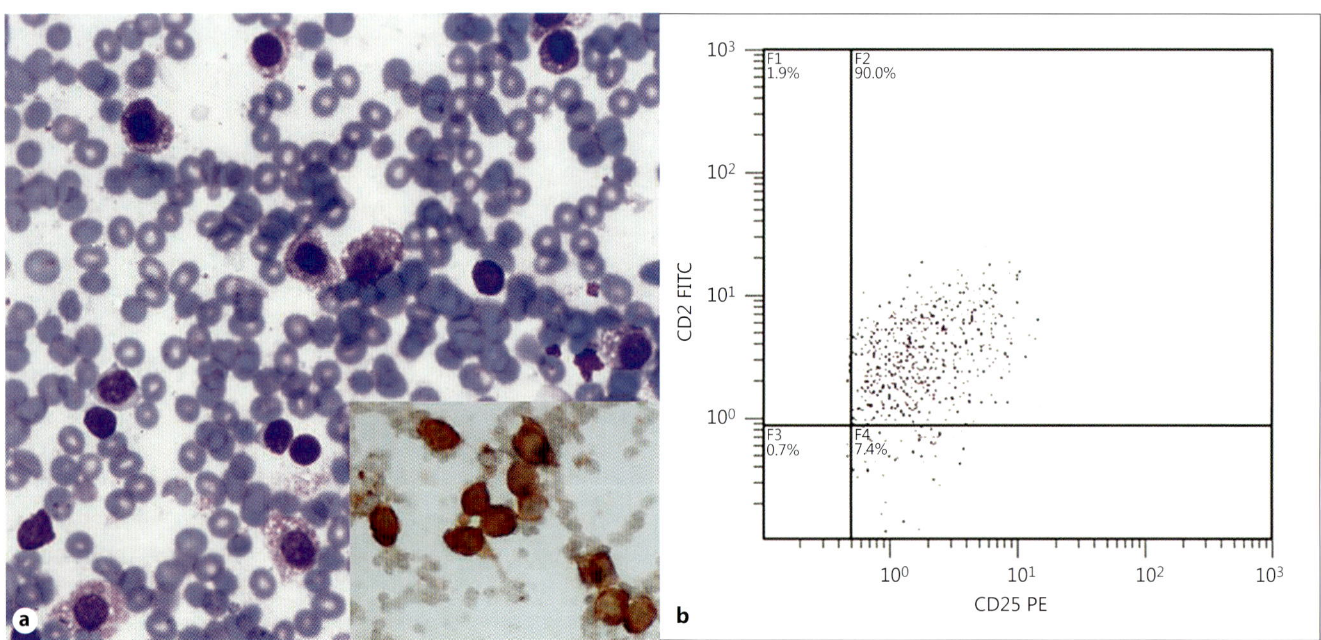

Fig. 3. a LN involvement by systemic mastocytosis showing dispersed mast cells with granular cytoplasm and centrally located nuclei; few lymphocytes are present in the background. **Inset** Cytoplasmic CD117 positivity on an additional smear. **b** Mast cell CD25/CD2 co-expression on FC.

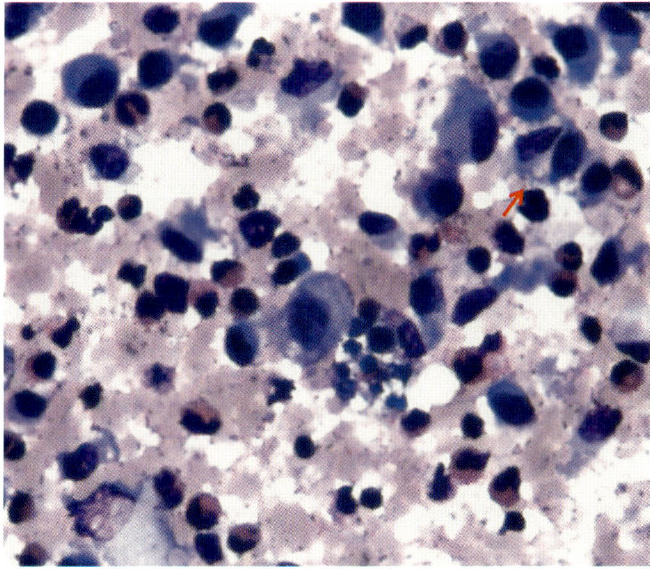

Fig. 4. LN involvement from LCHs showing large histiocyte-like isolated cells with cytoplasm and irregular nuclei with an occasional bilobed nucleus (arrow). The background is composed by lymphocytes, numerous eosinophils, and occasional plasma cells.

conditions, such as dermatopathic lymphadenopathy, Langerhans cell histiocytosis, or Hodgkin lymphoma, may show this feature, and a differential diagnosis with these entities should be considered [23].

Langerhans Cell Histiocytosis

Langerhans cell histiocytosis (LCH) is a rare clonal proliferation of Langerhans cells. LCH is also known as eosinophilic granuloma (single monostotic), Hand-Schüller-Christian disease (multiple polyostotic), and Abt-Letterer-Siwe disease (multisystemic), and the term histiocytosis X encompasses all the LCH clinical presentations [24]. LCH usually affects children between 1 and 15 years of age, with a peak incidence between 5 and 10 years. Adult forms are extremely rare and even more so in the elderly [24]. LCH is prevalent in Caucasians and affects males twice as often as females [25]. It is usually a sporadic and non-hereditary condition, although familial clustering has been reported in a limited number of cases [26]. LCH manifestations range from isolated bone lesions to a multifocal unisystem/multisystem disease. LN involvement in LCH commonly occurs as a systemic manifestation of LCH, with the involvement of other organs, mainly skin, lung, and bones.

Generally, a single LN is affected; indeed, LCH rarely presents as diffuse LN involvement. Isolated LN involvement with LCH, as with the single-site disease elsewhere, can be self-limiting or may fully respond to therapy. All LN stations may be affected by LCH and positron emission tomography may define the extension of the disease to bones and systemic localizations. Despite their clinical differences, all the LCH entities share the same pathological features, i.e., typical Langerhans cells in a polymorphous inflammatory background with a predominance of eosinophils. LN-FNC shows mononuclear cells with grooved and folded delicate nuclear membranes. Nucleoli are inconspicuous and mitoses are essentially absent (Fig. 4). "Birbeck granules" may be observed on electron microscopy. A varying number of eosinophils are present among Langerhans cells; when numerous, they may cause "eosinophilic abscesses" even with central necrosis. Multinucleated giant cells and hemosiderin in the background may occur in variable amounts. Langerhans cells are CD1a+, CD68+, langerin+, fascin+, and generally S100–. The differential diagnosis includes all the entities characterized by sinus histiocytic proliferation, like Rosai-Dorfman disease, and potentially eosinophilic-rich entities like Kimura disease in adults, Langerhans cell sarcoma, Hodgkin lymphoma (HL), ALCL, and PTL. Rarely, LCH may resemble poorly differentiated metastatic tumours and LCH should be considered when the first "run immunostaining" of a "metastasis" is cytokeratin negative.

Follicular Dendritic Cell Sarcoma and Interdigitating Dendritic Cell Sarcoma

Follicular dendritic cell sarcoma (FDCS) and interdigitating dendritic cell sarcoma (IDCS) are rare, spindle-ovoid cell neoplasms, arising from follicular dendritic cells and interdigitating dendritic cells located in the germinal centres and in T-zones, respectively, of LN and peripheral lymphoid tissues [27]. Both FDCS and IDCS usually arise in LNs, the cervical LNs being the most frequently involved; roughly one-third occurs in extranodal sites [28]. Most cases are asymptomatic but some patients, especially those with extra-nodal FDCS, may have systemic symptoms. Associations between FDCS and paraneoplastic pemphigus, HIV, myasthenia gravis and Castleman disease and between IDCS and NHL have been reported [28, 29]. The pathological features of both entities are those of sarcomas arising from LN or extranodal lymphoid tissue with diffuse, storiform or nodular patterns and variable cytological atypia. FDCS has a quite specific phenotype (CD21+, CD23+, CD35+, S100–, CD1a–, CD68–, CD31–, CD34–, ALK–, CD30–) that allows its diagnosis [29]. IDCS morphological features are similar to those of FDCS, but its phenotype is quite different (CD4+, CD11c+, CD14+, CD45+, lysozyme+, EMA+, S100+/–, CD68–/+, CD21–, CD23–, CD35–, CD1a–), supposedly having a more aggressive behaviour in comparison to FDCS [28]. FNC of FDCS has been described as a proliferation of large, spindle to ovoid epithelioid cells, isolated or arranged in small cohesive groups or in syncytial sheets, with moderate to abundant indistinct cytoplasm. Nuclei show irregular borders, fine granular or vesicular chromatin and one or more nucleoli; small lymphocytes are intermingled with the tumour cells [30–33]. Interconnecting long cytoplasmic processes giving FDCS cells a "medusa-head" or "starfish" appearance have been described and considered quite specific for FNC FDCS [34]. Differential diagnosis with other sarcomas, LCH, inflammatory myofibroblastic tumour, IDCS, sarcomatoid carcinoma, thymoma and schwannoma has to be pointed out. The rare incidence and the cytological features of FDCS do not allow a straightforward cytological diagnosis; nonetheless, the same cytological features if matched with its specific phenotype may suggest FDCS on FNC [30–33]. Few reports have described FNC features of IDCS, highlighting diagnostic mistakes more than the cytological features [35, 36]. FNC of IDCS has been described as isolated or clustered polygonal, atypical, large cells in a background of small lymphocytes. Nuclei are round to oval or irregular with fine chromatin and evident nucleoli; mitoses may be observed. Binucleated cells, cells with lobulated nuclei and high nuclear-cytoplasmic ratio, prominent nucleoli and clumping chromatin have also been reported [36, 37].

Histiocytic Sarcoma

Histiocytic sarcoma (HS) is an extremely rare neoplasm with histiocytic features and phenotype, and an aggressive clinical behaviour. In the past, several entities with neoplastic cells having histological similarities to the histiocytes were included in this entity; however, true HS should include only histiocytic tumours with histiocytic phenotype (CD45+, CD68+, CD163+, lysozyme+, MAC387+), in the absence of lymphoid, dendritic, epithelial, and melanocytic markers [27, 38]. Most HS arise in extranodal sites (skin, gastrointestinal tract, brain) and associations with different

NHL have been reported [27, 38, 39]. The differential diagnosis involves IDCS, DLBCL, anaplastic large cell lymphoma, metastatic melanoma and undifferentiated carcinoma. Few FNC reports of true LN HS are currently available [39, 40]. FNC of HS has been described as large pleomorphic cells with increased nuclear-cytoplasmic ratio and coarse chromatin seen in a background of mixed inflammatory infiltrate [40]. A case observed by the authors showed large histiocytes with abundant eosinophilic cytoplasm, large nuclei with mild atypia, coarse chromatin and nucleoli. Fibrous fragments were present and hampered the cell harvesting (Fig. 5).

Thymus and Thymoma

The thymus is a lymphoepithelial organ that promotes and controls T-cell differentiation. Thymoma are epithelial tumours of the thymus often associated with specific clinical and radiological features. Other than thymoma, germ-cell tumours, neuroendocrine tumours, and NHL may arise in the thymus with different incidences in children and adults. Thymic NHL occur mainly in children and young adults, with the T-lymphoblastic and the large B-cell NHL the most frequent subtypes. Cytological features of these entities have been previously described [see Chapters 5, 6, this vol., pp. 52–59, 60–76]. In B1 and B2, mixed, and lymphocyte-rich the tumoral epithelial cells are small, poorly differentiated, and often hidden by the reactive T cell. B1 and B2 thymoma may also occur as extramediastinal, often cervical nodules simulating LNe.

Ectopic Thymoma

Ectopic thymomas arise from thymic cells located in extramediastinal sites such as the pleura, pericardium, skin, or the cervical area [41, 42]. Ectopic cervical thymoma (ECT), albeit extremely rare, is the most frequently reported ectopic thymoma [41–48]. ECT may occur and develop as a palpable mass, reaching even remarkable sizes (50 mm or more), and may be clinically misdiagnosed as LNs or a thyroid nodule. FNC features of ECT have been described [45–47]. Smears are generally highly cellular, with a dispersed lymphoid cell population. Cells are medium or large in size, with a scanty or absent cytoplasm and nuclei, with finely dispersed chromatin (Fig. 6). Scanty large cells with evident nucleoli and occasional macrophages with a

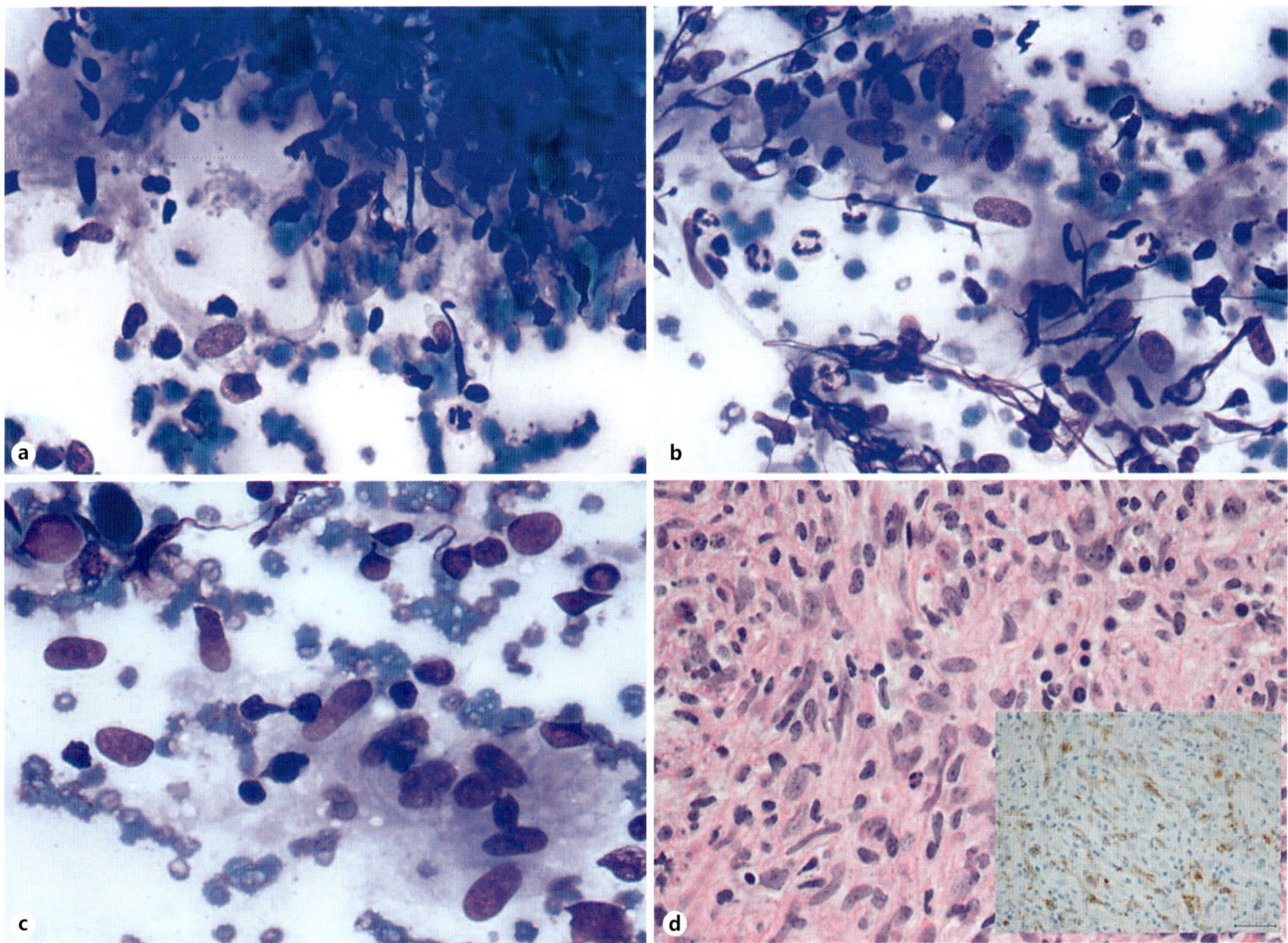

Fig. 5. LN-FNC of a histiocytic sarcoma (HS) showing fibrous fragments (**a**), loosely aggregated or isolated histiocyte-like cells with oval, eccentric, atypical nuclei and wide cytoplasm (**b**, **c**). This case was diagnosed as a "proliferation of atypical histiocytes." The histological control (**d**) revealed a HS with the same, atypical, CD68+ (**inset**) histiocytes.

wide debris-engulfed cytoplasm may be present. Cells are CD2+, CD3+, CD7+, CD5+, CD10+ (Fig. 6). CD4/CD8 may be co-expressed (Fig. 6), while B-cell antigens and light chains are not expressed. Epithelial cells, hallmark of thymoma, are hardly identified by Diff-Quik stain but may be revealed by cytokeratin ICC if ECT is suspected. In fact, thymomas may have variable amounts of epithelial and lymphoid cells, which determine their histological classification [48]. ECT are mainly B2-type with a prevalence of lymphoid cells, epithelial cells being represented by immature vesicular pale cells, with large nuclei and a scanty cytoplasm that easily escapes cytological and FC detection [45–47].

Spleen

FNC of the spleen was first used in 1916 for the diagnosis of leishmaniasis [49]. In 1970, Söderström [50] used FNC extensively to diagnose splenomegaly. Because of the general skepticism toward the cytological diagnosis of lymphoproliferative disorders and the fear of haemorrhage or rupture, splenic FNC has not become as widely used as in other organs. In addition, non-invasive diagnostic tools and imaging techniques have reduced the need for direct investigation of the spleen through biopsies or splenectomy. However, there are clinical situations, mainly concerning NHL and myeloproliferative disorders, in which direct diagnoses are needed, and FNC may represent an effective tool mainly if combined

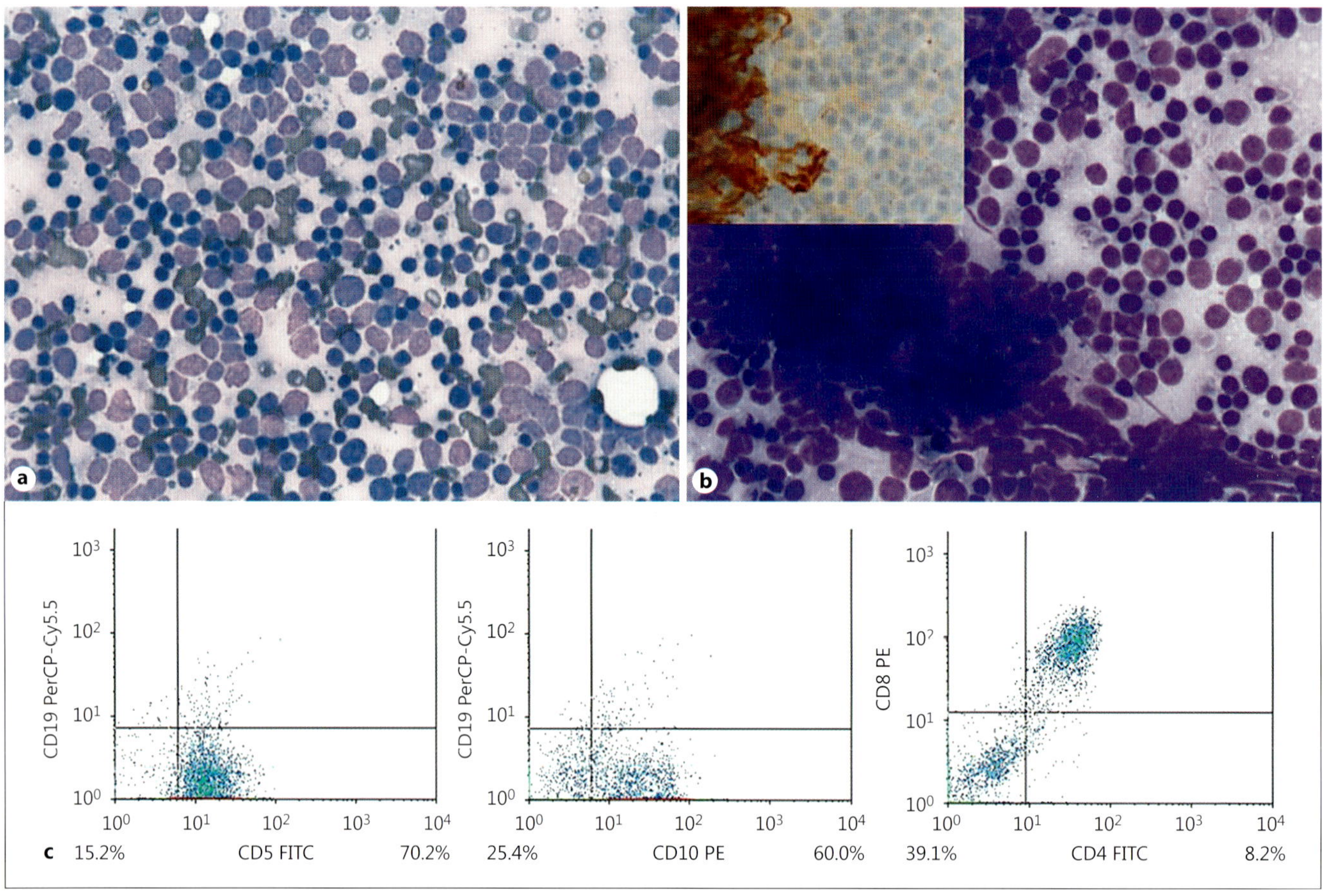

Fig. 6. FNC ectopic B2 thymoma. **a** Dispersed lymphoid cells and ill-preserved cells with large and air-dried nuclei. **b** Lymphoid cells and densely packed immature cells resulting CK positive on an additional smear with negative lymphocytes in the background (**inset**). **c** FC showing CD5+ and CD19–, CD10+ and CD4/CD8 co-expression as the typical phenotype of immature T lymphocytes.

Table 1. Focal and diffuse splenomegalies

Infections	Congestive	Autoimmune	Storage diseases	Lymphohematogenous	Miscellaneous
Abscess (f)	Banti disease (d)	Rheumatoid	Gaucher disease (d)	Castleman disease (f/d)	Amyloidosis (d)
Bacterial infections	Cardiac failure (d)	arthritis (d)	Mucopolysaccharidoses (d)	Haemolytic anaemia (d)	Cyst/hamartoma (f)
(endocarditis) (d)	Cirrhosis (d)	Sarcoidosis (d)	Niemann-Pick disease (d)	Histiocytoses (d)	Haemangioma/
Brucellosis (d)	Portal or splenic	Systemic lupus		LCH (f)	angiosarcoma (f)
Echinococcosis (f)	thrombosis (d)	erythematosus		HL (f)	Infarction (f)
Leishmaniosis (d)		(d)		High-grade NHL (f)	Metastases (f)
Histoplasmosis (d)				Low-grade NHL (d)	
Malaria (d)				Leukaemias (d)	
Mononucleosis (d)				Myeloproliferative syndromes (CML,	
Toxoplasmosis (d)				polycythemia vera, myelofibrosis,	
Tuberculosis (d)				myeloid metaplasia) (d)	

f, focal splenomegaly; d, diffuse splenomegaly; LCH, Langerhans cell histiocytosis; HL, Hodgkin lymphoma; NHL, non-Hodgkin lymphoma; CML, chronic myeloid leukaemia.

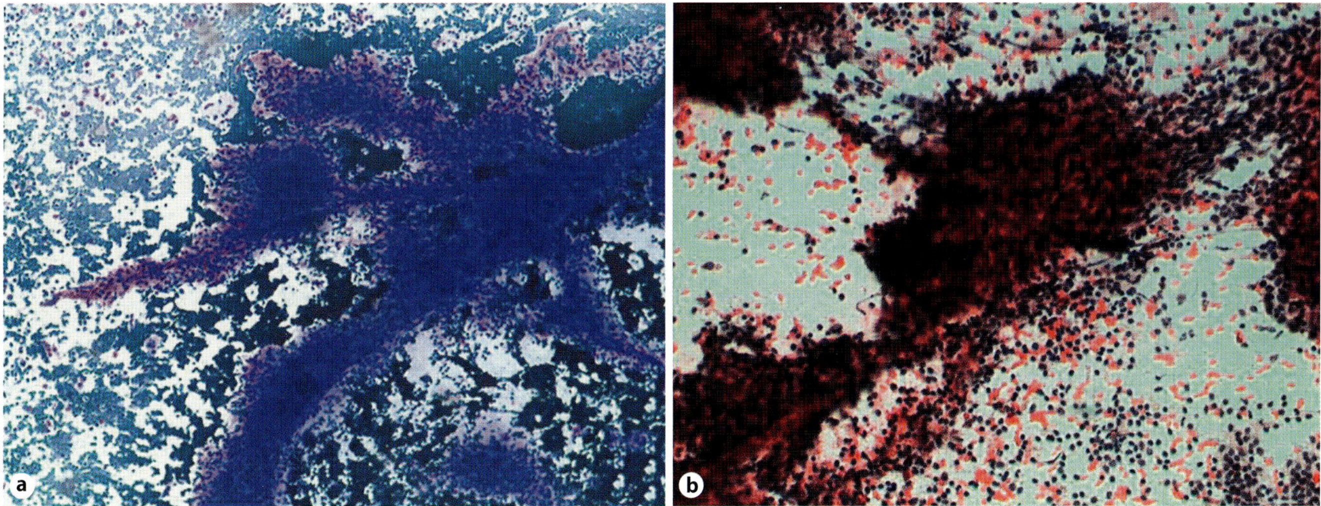

Fig. 7. a Splenic white pulp fragments on smears showing capillary structures with PALS. **b** Anastomosing capillaries and dispersed lymphocytes in the background.

with ancillary techniques (ICC or FC) [51–58]. The main disorders associated with splenomegaly are summarized in Table 1. Splenic FNC has to be performed under ultrasound (US) control and generally does not carry complications, provided that the procedure is properly performed, and being aware that mononucleosis and haemorrhagic diathesis are definitive contraindications. FNC has to be performed using a 23- to 25-G needle, the subcostal approach is preferable. The patient has to be prepared and invited to hold his breath upon insertion of the needle and during aspiration. A few quick movements back and forth may be made in aspiration. The smears, microscopic evaluation, and management of the material are described in Chapter 2 [this vol., pp. 14–18]. After splenic FNC, the patient should be prescribed bed rest, possibly with ice packs on the splenic area, for a few hours and US control should be performed.

Cytology of the Normal Components of the Spleen

The red pulp constituents are generally poorly represented on FNC. Platelets, macrophages, and scattered fibrous or endothelial cells may be observed. The white pulp is represented by dense fragments of lymphocytes tightly attached to each other, with nuclear details observable only at the edges of the fragments. Invariably, 1 or 2 vascular structures enter these groups, which represent the periarteriolar lymphoid sheaths (PALS; Fig. 7). In addition to PALS, scattered lymphoid cells at different stages of maturation may be present on the smear, representing the B cells component (Fig. 7). PALS and scattered lymphoid cells may vary at different ages and in different immunological stages, being numerous in childhood and in heightened immunological stages, and scanty in older patients.

Reactive and Neoplastic Processes

In white pulp hyperplasia, smears are highly cellular with numerous large PALS and dispersed lymphoid cells. White pulp hyperplasia may be observed in infectious diseases and immunological disorders. In children it is mainly related to a heightened immunological state. Abscesses may occur in blood-borne infections, sometimes associated with leukaemia or immunodeficiency syndromes. These processes may cause subacute inflammatory processes with histiocytes and multinucleated giant cells. Infarcts are common, mainly due to systemic or infective emboli determining coagulative or suppurative necrosis. Myeloid metaplasia may occur mainly in cases of myelofibrosis and myeloproliferative syndromes, but may be observed in different pathological conditions, such as NHL, previous infectious diseases, or after chemotherapy. The FNC hallmark of myeloid metaplasia are megakaryocytes, isolated

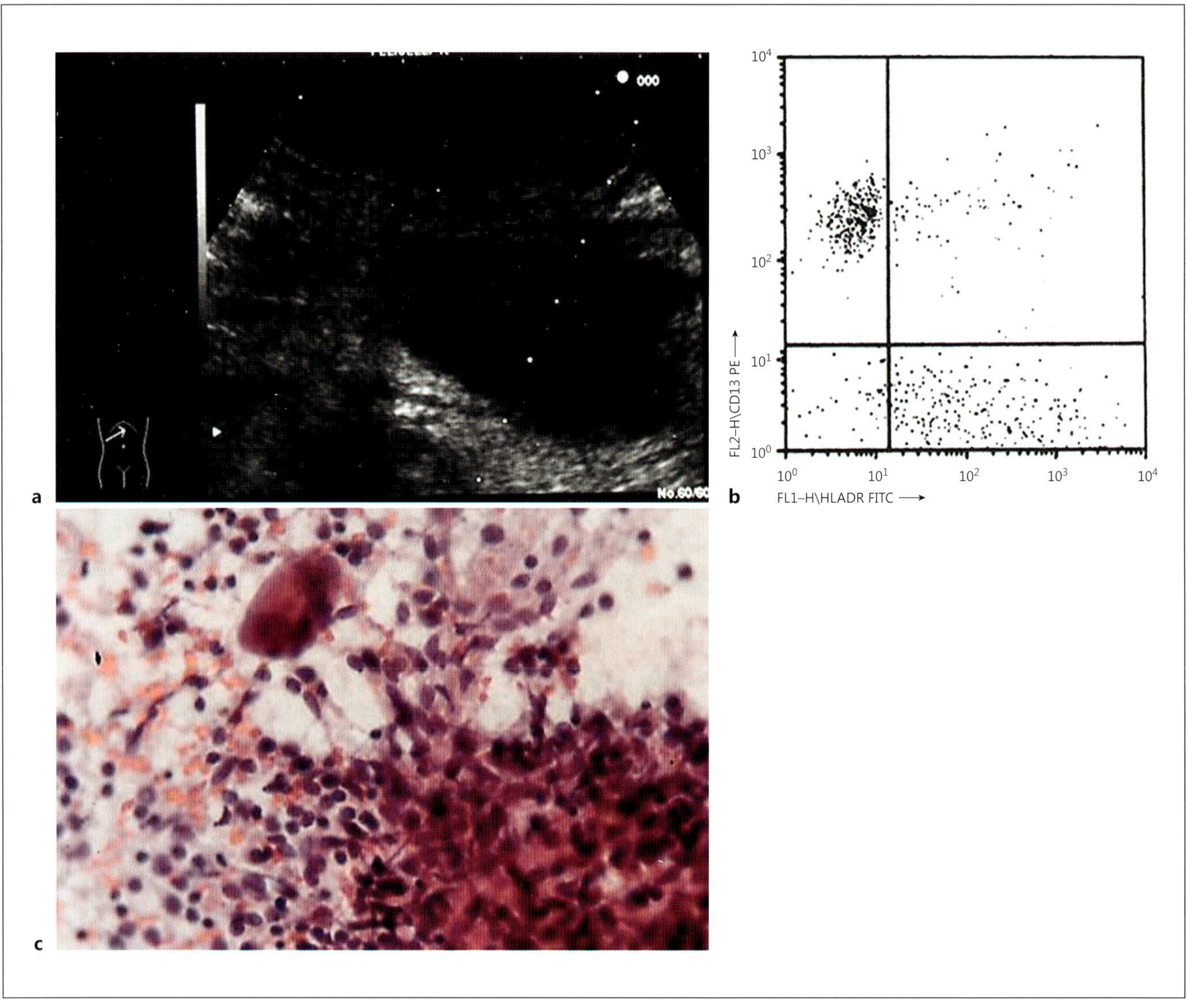

Fig. 8. a Myeloid metaplasia of the spleen: US shows large, diffuse splenomegaly. **b** FC showing CD13 positivity. **c** A dense fragment with mixed cellularity in the background and a megakaryocyte as a hallmark of splenic myeloid metaplasia.

or entrapped in PALS (Fig. 8), mature or immature, sometimes simulating Reed-Sternberg cells. Sarcoidosis and tuberculosis and other infective diseases may cause granulomatous lesions to the spleen. HL and NHL chemotherapy may cause granulomatous lesions showing equivocal clinical and imaging features. HL and systemic large-cell NHL may determine splenic nodular lesions, as well as primary splenic NHL, which is generally a B-cell, large NHL. Conversely, primary splenic small-cell NHL may show a diffuse or "miliaric" presentation. Cytological criteria (Fig. 9) and

ancillary techniques are almost the same as described for LNs, with the additional limitation of scanty diagnostic material, for which multiple passes are inadvisable. Splenic metastases are extremely rare [59]; lung, breast, melanoma, and colon tumours are the most frequently reported cases.

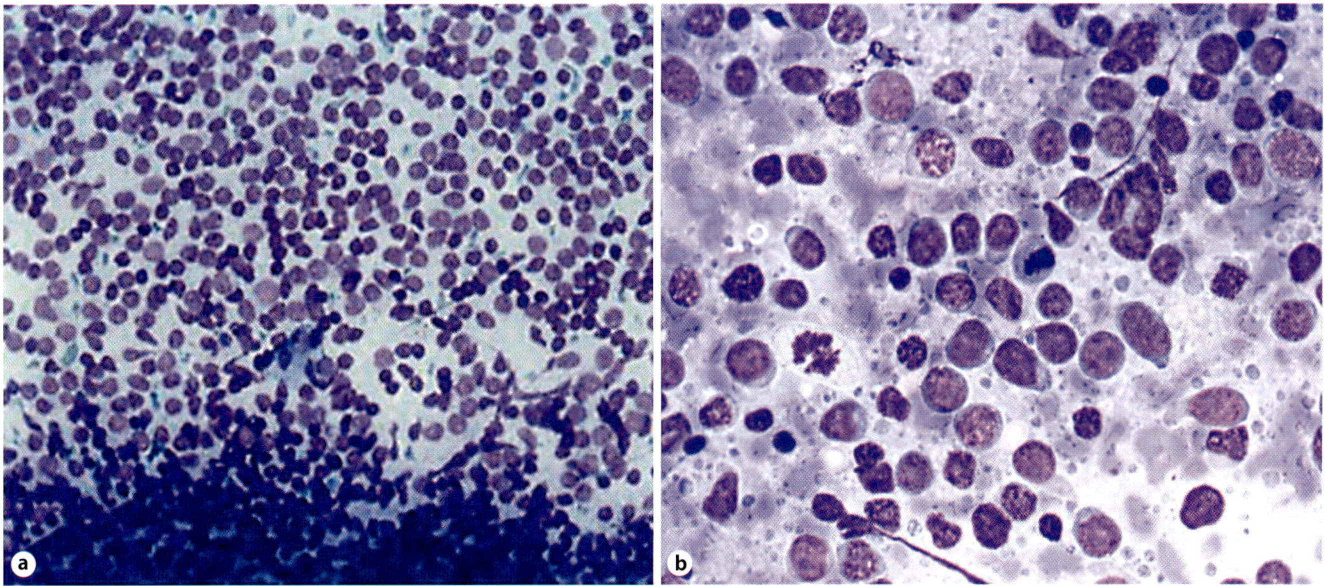

Fig. 9. a Small-cell splenic NHL FNC showing monomorphous small, immature lymphocytes and partial preservation of a PALS at the bottom. **b** Large-cell splenic NHL showing nuclear irregularities and mitoses. Cytological features for both small- and large-cell NHL are similar to the LN counterparts.

References

1　Menke DM, Horny HP, Griesser H, Tiemann M, Katzmann JA, Kaiserling E, et al: Primary lymph node plasmacytomas (plasmacytic lymphomas). Am J Clin Pathol 2001;115:119–126.

2　Lin BT, Weiss LM: Primary plasmacytoma of lymph nodes. Hum Pathol 1997;28:1083–1090.

3　Handa U, Chhabra S, Mohan H: Plasma cell tumours: cytomorphological features in a series of 12 cases diagnosed on fine needle aspiration cytology. Cytopathology 2010;21:186–190.

4　Sarin H, Manucha V, Verma K: Extramedullary plasmacytoma, a report of five cases diagnosed by FNAC. Cytopathology 2009;20:328–331.

5　Suh YK, Shin HJ: Fine-needle aspiration biopsy of granulocytic sarcoma: a clinicopathologic study of 27 cases. Cancer 2000;90:364–372.

6　Gaopande VL, Joshi SS, Joshi AR: Acute promyelocytic leukemia-associated Sweet's syndrome mimicking an axillary abscess: a case report with review of literature. Diagn Cytopathol 2015;43:1007–1010.

7　Fu J, Luo J: Granulocytic sarcoma of the breast in acute myeloid leukemia: two case reports. Oncol Lett 2014;7:145–147.

8　Thakur B, Varma K, Misra V, Chauhan S: Granulocytic sarcoma presenting as an orbital mass: report of two cases. J Clin Diagn Res 2013;7:1704–1706.

9　Gong X, Lu X, Fu Y, Wu X, Yan L, Zhang X, Wang L: Cytological features of chronic myelomonocytic leukaemia in pleural effusion and lymph node fine needle aspiration. Cytopathology 2010;21:411–413.

10　Cai G, Levine P, Sen F: Diagnosis of myeloid sarcoma involving salivary glands by fine-needle aspiration cytology and flow cytometry: report of four cases. Diagn Cytopathol 2008;36:124–127.

11　Elyamany G, Khan M, El Hag I, El-Zimaity M, Albalawi M, Al Abdulaaly A: Generalized lymphadenopathy as the first presentation of granulocytic sarcoma: a diagnostic challenge. Case Rep Med 2013;2013:483291.

12　Ojha SS, Kothari KS, Naik LP, Fernandes GC, Rangwala S, Agnihotri MA: Dysplastic megakaryocytes and eosinophilic precursors in the diagnosis of myeloid sarcoma on lymph node fine-needle aspiration cytology: a case series. Acta Cytol 2012;56:325–329.

13　Fulciniti F, Zeppa P, Marino G, Martinelli V, Ciancia R, Del Vecchio L, Rotoli B, Palombini L: Lymph node localization of extramedullary myeloid cell tumor in myelodysplastic syndrome: report of one case diagnosed by fine-needle cytology. Diagn Cytopathol 2003;28:136–139.

14　Liu K, Mann KP, Garst JL, Dodd LG, Olatidoye BA: Diagnosis of posttransplant granulocytic sarcoma by fine-needle aspiration cytology and flow cytometry. Diagn Cytopathol 1999;20:85–89.

15　Zeppa P, Marino G, Picardi M, Luciano L, Vetrani A, Palombini L: Expression of NK-associated antigens in extramedullary lymph nodal blast crisis of chronic myeloid leukemia on fine-needle cytology. Diagn Cytopathol 2002;27:158–160.

16　Coelho-Slva JL, Caralho LE, Oliveira MM, Franca-Neto PL, Andrade AT, Lima AS, Bezerra MF, Lima MM, Neves MA, Fonseca JM, Barros-Correia MC, Machado CG, Bezerra MA, Matos DM, Lucena-Araujo AR: Prognostic importance of CD56 expression in intermediate risk acute myeloid leukemia. Br J Haematol 2017;176:498–501.

17　Valent P, Akin C, Metcalfe DD: Mastocytosis 2016: updated WHO classification and novel emerging treatment concepts. Blood 2017;129:1420–1427.

18　Pardanani A: Systemic mastocytosis in adults: 2012 update on diagnosis, risk stratification, and management. Am J Hematol 2012;87:401–411.

19　Allpress SM, Silverman JF, Finley JL: Diagnosis of mastocytosis by fine-needle aspiration cytology. Diagn Cytopathol 1998;18:368–370.

20 Tongson-Ignacio JE, Gu M: Cytologic diagnosis of mastocytosis by fine needle aspiration biopsy: a case report. Acta Cytol 2007;51:814–819.

21 Steciuk M, Jhala D, Haber M, Jhala N: Endoscopic ultrasound-guided fine needle aspiration: a powerful modality in the diagnosis of aggressive systemic mastocytosis. Cytopathology 2011;22:130–132.

22 Cozzolino I, Picardi M, Lucci R, Petraroli A, Spadaro G, Marone G, Vetrani A, Zeppa P: Lymph node fine needle aspiration cytology in systemic mastocytosis: cytological features with ancillary tests and literature review. Cytopathology 2015;26:31–37.

23 Xu Z, Jamison B, Bence-Bruckler I: Smouldering systemic mastocytosis with lymph node involvement mimicking malignant lymphoma. Ann Hematol 2014;93:1603–1604.

24 The Writing Group of the Histiocyte Society: Histiocytosis syndromes in children. Lancet 1987;1:208–209.

25 Aricò M, Girschikofsky M, Généreau T, Klersy C, McClain K, Grois N, Emile J-F, Lukina E, De Juli E, Danesino C: Langerhans cell histiocytosis in adults: report from the International Registry of the Histiocyte Society. Eur J Cancer 2003;39:2341–2348.

26 Kapur P, Erickson C, Rakheja D, Carder KR, Hoang MP: Congenital self-healing reticulohistiocytosis (Hashimoto-Pritzker disease): Ten-year experience at Dallas Children's Medical Center. J Am Academy Dermatol 2007;56:290–294.

27 Swerdlow SH, Campo E, Harris NL, Jaffe ES, Pileri SA, Stein H, Thiele J: WHO Classification of Tumours of Haematopoietic and Lymphoid Tissues, ed 4. Lyon, IARC Press, 2017.

28 Ohtake H, Yamakawa M: Interdigitating dendritic cell sarcoma and follicular dendritic cell sarcoma: histopathological findings for differential diagnosis. J Clin Exp Hematop 2013;53:179–184.

29 Chen T, Gopal P: Follicular dendritic cell sarcoma. Arch Pathol Lab Med 2017;141:596–599.

30 Wang XI, Zhang S, Thomas JO, Adegboyega PA: Cytomorphology, ultrastructural, and cytogenetic findings in follicular dendritic cell sarcoma: a case report. Acta Cytol 2010;54(5 suppl):759–763.

31 Kure K, Khader SN, Suhrland MJ, Ratech H, Grossberg R, Oktay MH: Fine needle aspiration of follicular dendritic cell sarcoma in an HIV-positive man: a case report. Acta Cytol 2010;54:707–711.

32 Yang GC, Besanceney CE, Tam W: Histiocytic sarcoma with interdigitating dendritic cell differentiation: a case report with fine needle aspiration cytology and review of literature. Diagn Cytopathol 2010;38:351–356.

33 Fan YS, Ng WK, Chan A, Chan GS, Tsang J, Chim CS, Ip P: Fine needle aspiration cytology in follicular dendritic cell sarcoma: a report of two cases. Acta Cytol 2007;51:642–647.

34 Czapla A, Omman RA, Nam MW, Mehrotra S, Pambuccian SE: "Medusa-Head" cells, "Starfish" cells, and interconnecting long cytoplasmic processes as diagnostic cytologic clues for follicular dendritic cell sarcoma in fine needle aspiration samples. Diagn Cytopathol 2017;45:322–326.

35 Lupato V, Romeo S, Franchi A, Mantovani M, Dei Tos AP, Tirelli G, Da Mosto MC, Boscolo-Rizzo P: Head and neck extranodal interdigitating dendritic cell sarcoma: case report and review of the literature. Head Neck Pathol 2016;10:145–151.

36 Johnson RL, Boisot S, Ball ED, Wang HY: A case of interdigitating dendritic cell sarcoma/histiocytic sarcoma – a diagnostic pitfall. Int J Clin Exp Pathol 2014;7:378–385.

37 Jayaram G, Mun KS, Elsayed EM, Sangkar JV: Interdigitating dendritic reticulum cell sarcoma: cytologic, histologic and immunocytochemical features. Diagn Cytopathol 2005;33:43–48.

38 Vos JA, Abbondanzo SL, Barekman CL, Andriko JW, Miettinen M, Aguilera NS: Histiocytic sarcoma: a study of five cases including the histiocyte marker CD163. Mod Pathol 2005;18:693–704.

39 Mehrotra S, Pan Z: Fine needle aspiration cytology of histiocytic sarcoma with dendritic cell differentiation: a case of transdifferentiation from low-grade follicular lymphoma. Diagn Cytopathol 2015;43:659–663.

40 Mallya V, Bansal A, Kapoor S: Fine needle aspiration of histiocytic sarcoma. J Cytol 2014;31:205–206.

41 Weissferdt A, Moran CA: The spectrum of ectopic thymomas. Virchows Arch 2016;469:245–254.

42 Jing H, Wang J, Wei H, Liu M, Chen F, Meng Q, Tay Y: Ectopic hamartomatous thymoma: report of a case and review of literature. Int J Clin Exp Pathol 2015;8:11776–11784.

43 Lee YY, Wang WC, Li CF: Aspiration cytology of an ectopic cervical thymoma misinterpreted as a lymphoproliferative lesion of the thyroid: a case report. Oncol Lett 2015;10:1255–1258.

44 Tawaeevisit M, Sampatanukul P, Thorner PS: Ectopic thymoma can mimic benign and malignant thyroid lesions on fine needle aspiration cytology: a case report and literature review. Acta Cytol 2013;57:213–220.

45 Zeppa P, Varone V, Cozzolino I, Salvatore D, Vetrani A, Palombini L: Fine needle cytology and flow cytometry of ectopic cervical thymoma: a case report. Acta Cytol 2010;54(5 suppl):998–1002.

46 Gerhard R, Kanashiro EH, Kliemann CM, Juliano AG, Chammas MC: Fine needle aspiration biopsy of ectopic cervical spindle-cell thymoma: a case report. Diagn Cytopathol 2005;32:358–362.

47 Ponder TB, Collins BT, Bee CS, Silverberg AB, Grosso LE, Dunphy CH: Diagnosis of cervical thymoma by fine needle aspiration biopsy with flow cytometry: a case report. Acta Cytol 2002;46:1129–1132.

48 Fetsch JF, Laskin WB, Michal M, Remotti F, Heffner D, Ellis G, Furlong M, Miettinen M: Ectopic hamartomatous thymoma: a clinicopathologic and immunohistochemical analysis of 21 cases with data supporting reclassification as a branchial anlage mixed tumor. Am J Surg Pathol 2004;28:1360–1370.

49 Aravandinos A: Modification dans la technique de la ponction de la rate. Bull Soc Path Exot 1916;9:444–448.

50 Söderström N: Fine Needle Aspiration Biopsy. Stockholm, Almqvist and Wiksell/Gebers, 1966.

51 Gochhait D, Dey P, Rajwanshi A, Nijhawan R, Gupta N, Radhika S, Lal A: Role of fine needle aspiration cytology of spleen. APMIS 2015;123:190–193.

52 Handa U, Tiwari A, Singhal N, Mohan H, Kaur R: Utility of ultrasound-guided fine-needle aspiration in splenic lesions. Diagn Cytopathol 2013;41:1038–1042.

53 Kumar PV, Monabati A, Raseki AR, Arshadi C, Malek-Hosseini SA, Talei AR, Sadeghi E: Splenic lesions: FNA findings in 48 cases. Cytopathology 2007;18:151–156.

54 Sen R, Bhadani PP, Singh H, Sachdeva B, Sen J, Singh S, Gupta M, Mehta K: Myeloid metaplasia in aspirates from enlarged spleens: a clue in the absence of peripheral blood findings characteristic of myelofibrosis. Acta Cytol 2006;50:379–383.

55 Friedlander MA, Wei XJ, Iyengar P, Moreira AL: Diagnostic pitfalls in fine needle aspiration biopsy of the spleen. Diagn Cytopathol 2008;36:69–75.

56 Ramdall RB, Cai G, Alasio TM, Levine P: Fine-needle aspiration biopsy for the primary diagnosis of lymphoproliferative disorders involving the spleen: one institution's experience and review of the literature. Diagn Cytopathol 2006;34:812–817.

57 Zeppa P, Picardi M, Marino G, Troncone G, Fulciniti F, Vetrani A, Rotoli B, Palombini L: Fine-needle aspiration biopsy and flow cytometry immunophenotyping of lymphoid and myeloproliferative disorders of the spleen. Cancer 2003;99:118–127.

58 Zeppa P, Vetrani A, Luciano L, Fulciniti F, Troncone G, Rotoli B, Palombini L: Fine needle aspiration biopsy of the spleen: a useful procedure in the diagnosis of splenomegaly. Acta Cytol 1994;38:299–309.

59 Duggal R, Garg M, Kalra N, Srinivasan R, Chawla Y: Spleen metastasis from hepatocellular carcinoma: report of a case with diagnosis by fine needle aspiration cytology. Acta Cytol 2010;54(5 suppl):783–786.

Subject Index